BEHAVIORAL MEDICINE

International Perspectives

Volume 3

Development in Clinical Psychology

Glenn R. Caddy, series editor
Nova Southeastern University

MMPI-168 Codebook, by Ken R. Vincent, Iliana Castillo, Robert I. Hauser, H. James Stuart, Javier A. Zapata, Cal K. Cohn, and Gregory O'Shanick, 1984

Integrated Clinical and Fiscal Management in Mental Health: A Guidebook, by Fred Newman and James Sorensen, 1986

The Professional Practice of Psychology, edited by Georgiana Shick Tryon, 1986

Clinical Applications of Hypnosis, edited by Frank A. DePiano and Herman C. Salzberg, 1986

Full Battery Codebook, by Ken R. Vincent, 1987

Developments in the Assessment and Treatment of Addictive Behaviors, edited by Ted D. Nirenberg, 1987

Feminist Psychotherapies, edited by Mary Ann Douglas and Lenore E. Walker, 1988

Child Multimodal Therapy, by Donald B. Keat II, 1990

Psychophysiology for Clinical Psychologists, by Walter W. Surwillo, 1990

Strategic Health Planning: Methods and Techniques Applied to Marketing and Management, by Allen D. Spiegel and Herbert H. Hyman, 1991

Behavioral Medicine: International Perspectives (Vol. 1–3), edited by D.G. Byrne and Glenn R. Caddy, 1992

The MMPI: A Contemporary Normative Study of Adolescents, by Robert L. Colligan and Kenneth P. Offord, 1992

Reprogramming Pain, by Barry Bittman, 1995

BEHAVIORAL MEDICINE

International Perspectives

Volume 3

Edited by

Glenn R. Caddy, Ph.D., ABPP, AABM,
Academy of Medicine and Psychology
and Nova Southeastern University
Ft. Lauderdale, FL

D.G. Byrne, Ph.D., M.A.Ps.S., F.I.C.P.M
Department of Psychology
Australian National University
Canberra, A.C.T.

ABLEX PUBLISHING CORPORATION
NORWOOD, NEW JERSEY

Printed in the United States of America.

Library of Congress Cataloging-in-Publication Data

Behavioral medicine.
(Developments in clinical psychology)
Includes bibliographical references and index.
1. Medicine and psychology. 2. Medicine, Psychosomatic.
I. Byrne, D. G. (Donald Glenn). II. Caddy, Glenn R.
III. [DNLM; 1. Behavioral Medicine. 2. Psychology, Medical.
WM 90 B4194]
R726.5.B4256 1991 616'.001'9 91-26136
ISBN 0-89391-744-3

Ablex Publishing Corporation
355 Chestnut Street
Norwood, New Jersey 07648

To Janice Lynn and Gavin David,
with love, for permitting
me the time to work
so hard.

G.R.C.

To Annie

D.G.B.

Contents

Preface

There have been many landmarks in the history of clinical psychology. In the late 1950s and the 1960s, great progress in the theories and applications of behavior therapy signaled an inevitable but much welcomed shift in orientation from that of counselor and psychometrician to that of independent psychotherapist. The advent of behavior therapy gave the clinical psychologist, at last, a basis for the treatment of behavioral disorders and personal distress which was theoretically unique to the science of psychology. If there has been a professional landmark in the last decade, however, it must surely be seen in the arrival of behavioral medicine.

Behavorial medicine as a distinct discipline has existed for not much longer than 15 years, yet in that time it has made a considerable impact both on clinical psychology and on the practice of medicine. The course and magnitude of this impact are obvious in the amount of written material, both empirical and speculative, which has been generated in the past decade. In addition to a large array of texts documenting important areas of behavioral medicine, the area has given rise to its own specialized journal (the *Journal of Behavioral Medicine*) and several complete issues of other clinical and research journals (see, for example, *British Journal of Clinical Psychology*, No. 4, 1982, and *Journal of Psychosomatic Research*, No. 5, 1982). The sheer prominence of material emerging in the area provides adequate testimony to the seriousness and interest with which the formative years of behavioral medicine have been greeted.

In the early years of any field, definitions are often rather diverse, and those attached to behavioral medicine are no different. Schwartz and Weiss (1978) defined it as:

> The interdisciplinary field concerned with the development and integration of behavioral and biomedical science, knowledge and techniques relevant to health and illness and the application of this knowledge and these techniques to prevention, diagnosis, treatment and rehabilitation.

Somewhat more succinctly, Surwit et al. (1981) wrote:

> Behavioral medicine is broadly defined to encompass the application of principles from all behavioral sciences to medical problems.

Along more rigidly behavioral lines, Pomerleau and Brady (1979) claimed behavioral medicine to be:

> The clinical use of techniques derived from the experimental analysis of behavior—behavior therapy and behavior modification—for the evaluation, prevention, management or treatment of physical disease or physiological dysfunction.

Whichever position one takes, whether it be rigidly behavioral or more flexibily biopsychosocial, the essence of these definitions is clear. Behavioral medicine concerns the use of psychological evidence and techniques, typically but not exclusively those deriving from behavior therapy, in the diagnosis, prevention, and management of physically manifest illness.

Behavioral medicine is frequently confused with its close cousin, psychosomatic medicine, and the practitioner of the former is often asked to distinguish between the two. Surwit et al. (1981) argued that whereas psychosomatic medicine placed its emphasis on the pathogenic influence of personality traits leading, through neurotic conflicts, to physical illness, behavioral medicine was concerned with physiological responses arising initially through maladaptive environmental interactions, becoming established or learned by means of objectively testable chains of causal influence, and leading ultimately to physical pathology. In practice, behavioral medicine rejected psychodynamic labeling, emphasized the experimental principles of learning in treatment, and confirmed the importance of evaluation and replicability of treatment procedures.

If psychosomatic medicine takes its theoretical beginnings from the psychodynamic movement of Freud and his successors, behavioral medicine is firmly rooted in the stress theories of Selye and those who followed him, the learning theories of Skinner and those coming after, and the integrative work on biopsychosocial approaches to illness beginning with Levi and his colleagues.

Just as clinical psychology had developed scientifically to the point where it could legitimately give rise to a new area of practice, medicine too was demonstrating, by and large, a readiness to accept approaches more broadly based than those concerned with the strict application of technology. The recognition by both professions that the treatment of human disease required attention to the *environment* and the *psyche as well as the soma* created a fertile ground for the integration of knowledge and practice. This promise of growth, and the considerable body of evidence it had already produced, prompted the development of this series of books.

The intention of *Behavioral Medicine: International Perspectives* is not to supplant any of a number of excellent works in the field, but to provide, as far as possible, a very broad overview of contemporary thought and clinical wisdom. In doing so, it draws widely and diversely, mixing contributory chapters from North American, European, and Australian authors, with invitations to contribute being dependent only upon the judgment of the Editors that individual authors would produce the best possible overviews of the area. The deliberate diversity of sources is reflected in the title of the volumes. Any exercise involving such judgment is bound to attract disagreement; in recognizing this, the Editors are aware that many who are eminent in their own areas are not represented in these volumes. Nevertheless, we are confident that the breadth of authorship of each of the volumes in this series more than adequately compensates for individual omissions.

The organization of the three volumes of this series is traditional, and follows an "organ/system" approach. Importantly, however, we have attempted when appropriate to preface each section with a chapter outlining the anatomy, physiology, pathology, and epidemiology of the set of medical conditions under consideration. While the set of volumes will have a wide application across professional boundaries, the essentially interdisciplinary nature of behavioral medicine means that many readers will not have a background in the medical sciences. For them, it is important that concepts and terminologies in the substantive chapters are understood, and quick reference to an introductory summary seemed the best way of achieving this. Similarly, in the opening section of each volume, certain key issues in the clinical psychology of assessment and intervention have been discussed in summary chapters designed to acquaint the reader not trained in psychology with the unique contributions of this science to behavioral medicine. These additions, while somewhat increasing the length of the works, seek to establish the utility of these works across professional boundaries.

Volume One of this series begins with an overview of constructs in behavioral medicine and included topics on the vascular system, psychodermatology, and other issues including behavioral oncology, diabetes, and behavioral preparation for medical procedures.

Volume Two begins with various issues basic to the field such as health promotion and prevention, and international policy issues influencing behavioral medicine. Thereafter, the second volume presents perspectives on the musculoskeletal system, pain, behavioral neurology, and other issues, including exercise and health.

This third volume begins with Basic Treatment approaches in Behavioral Medicine and then includes material from the Gastrointestinal system, the Genitourinary system, Behavioral Pediatrics, Addictive Behavior, and finally, the Respiratory System.

It is our hope that this series of books will serve a wide audience. In guiding our large group of excellent contributors, we have attempted to encourage chapters encompassing the inextricably joined areas of empirical evidence and clinical skill and practice. It was our hope from the beginning that the series would be as useful to the clinical practitioner grappling with the problems of single patients as it would be to the researcher requiring contemporary and comprehensive reviews of the available evidence needed to guide further studies. In principle, we hold the view that the two areas cannot be separated; if this comes across in individual chapters, it is a tribute to the subject grasp and clear thinking of the many eminent scientists and practitioners who have contributed so ably to the series.

Enterprises such as these owe much to many people. In this respect, the contributing authors are most immediately deserving of our thanks. In spite of heavy teaching and research loads, and overwhelming clinical commitments, each contributor worked to the difficult deadlines imposed to produce chapters of both breadth and depth. To our contributors, then, we are inestimably grateful. The editing of a series of works, when editors themselves are separated by some thousands of kilometers of land and ocean, produces its own particular difficulties. One is inclined to thank the systems of international postage, but at times these have not proven the most reliable means of communication. Colleagues on both sides of the Pacific have, however, helped our task very considerably. Of course, families tolerate much from members who pursue such ephemeral activities as editing books, and for this tolerance, we are distinctly grateful.

The task of putting this work together has brought to each of us unique rewards. If we share one, however, it is the feeling that the series will have contributed palpably to the promotion of behavioral medicine as an area so new but with so much promise for the future.

Glenn R. Caddy
D. G. Byrne

I

BASIC TREATMENT STRATEGIES

1

Strategies of Treatment in Behavioral Medicine

Glenn R. Caddy
D. G. Byrne

TREATMENT OF PHYSICAL ILLNESS: MEDICAL VERSUS PSYCHOLOGICAL APPROACHES

By definition the symptoms of physical illness reflect an underlying state of organic disease. The outwardly observable symptom of fever points to underlying infection, the experience and reporting of pain to inflammation or perhaps ischemia, and the presence of blood in body fluids to a structural breakdown of tissue. The complex biological processes underlying human disease and the symptoms that give public or private manifestation to the disease process are, at face value, the rightful province of the pathologist, the physician, and—if all else fails—the surgeon. Generations of medical textbooks have proclaimed, confirmed, and reinforced the seemingly sacred view that exposure to pathogens precede the development of pathology and, once in train, this process gives rise to external indications of its existence in the form of objectively measurable signs and subjectively reported symptoms. All disease, therefore, has been seen traditionally in the context of biological processes, sometimes simple, other times patently complex, but always in principle understandable in terms of causal mechanisms anchored in the world of physical reality. Indeed, even when the physical basis of a disease process was unknown, biological bases for the process were presumed to be operating.

Adherence to this philosophical approach to the explanation of disease reduces uncertainty and choice in treatment to a very limited range of possibilities. The conviction that symptoms arise for no other reason than that there exists within the organism certain fundamental and knowable disturbances of physiological function or abnormalities in anatomical integrity lead inexorably to the view that the elimination or at least the alleviation of those symptoms involves no more than the physical correction of the physiological or anatomical dysfunction underlying the outward state. Indeed the very manifestation of symptoms as physical experiences underscores the view that their removal should also be a matter of physical correction to the presumed disequilibrium within the organism.

The selection of treatment strategies for the alleviation or remediation of physical symptomatology therefore reduces to the practitioner's view of the cause of the symptoms. If one adopts a "medical model" approach to symptomatology then the practitioner is likely to choose strictly medical (i.e., biological) strategies for treatment. Modern epidemiology theory does not, however, countenance the exclusively biological approach to disease formation and symptom onset for any but a very few diseases, these being typically of the infectious (both bacteriological and viral) kind. The overwhelming opinion in modern epidemiology is that disease formation and symptom onset follow from a manifestly complex and multivariate set of etiological factors only some of which are biological in their origins. The remainder of causal factors in contemporary epidemiological equations derive either from environmental, social, interpersonal, or individual sources. Thus they are to be seen as much in the behavior and emotions of the individual or in person-environment interactions as they are in the exposure to and response of the individual to "biological pathogens." Acceptance of this basic philosophic position broadens to a very substantial degree the therapeutic armory which the clinician may draw upon in the treatment of physical symptomatology since it opens up the possibility of a creatively interactionist approach to medical treatment whereby techniques from psychotherapy (in its broadest definition) as well as those from internal medicine may be used in conjunction with one another to the greatest benefit of the patient. Of course, this may also imply the need for interaction between clinicians where the psychologically or behaviorally trained practitioner works in close cooperation with the biologically trained physician to put together the most beneficial mix of treatments for the patients' unique set of symptoms and underlying pathologies.

THE PSYCHOLOGICAL TREATMENT OF PHYSICAL SYMPTOMS: PSYCHOSOMATIC OR BEHAVIORAL APPROACHES?

The use of psychological strategies in the treatment of physical symptoms is not at all new. The tradition of psychosomatic medicine has preached the use of a wide variety of psychological techniques for the alleviation or remediation of physical symptoms for more than 50 years (Lipowski, 1986). Traditional psychosomatic approaches were closely bound to psychoanalytic theory in which the genesis of the physical symptomatology was seen to arise in the form of intrapersonal conflicts, repressed into the unconscious and manifesting themselves as physical pathology and discomfort. Thus, traditional psychosomatic writings emphasized the use of classic psychoanalysis as a means of uncovering the nature and substance of repressed conflicts, working through these in a psychoanalytic sequence and (perhaps quite indirectly) eliminating the physical symptoms associated with these repressed conflicts. The use of psychoanalytic theory with its absence of an empirically testable theoretical basis bought the practice of psychosomatic treatment into some disrepute, particularly among clinical psychologists raised in the tradition of scientific psychology with its emphasis on experimental investigation. Indeed, the very advent of behavioral medicine as a distinct subdiscipline of clinical psychology arose out of a theoretical dissatisfaction with psychosomatic medicine and its reliance on psychoanalytic theory. Behavioral medicine sought to treat the same symptoms but conceptualized their origins not as repressed conflict but as learned patterns of maladaptive behavior producing, in turn, patterns of physiological responding to the environment which might produce immediate physical discomfort and, if prolonged, might result in long-term physical pathology. This is, of course, the basis of contemporary models of the stress/illness link with its beginnings in the works of James (1890), Selye (1976), and Mandler (1984). The emphasis that the early exponents of behavioral medicine placed on strictly behavioral treatments of physical symptomatology—that is, treatments based on the simple principles of reward and punishment, were, however, just as limiting to the creative clinician with a need to solve complex clinical problems as were the impositions arising out of a strictly psychoanalytic approach to physical symptomatology and its treatment. Contemporary behavioral medicine is, however, an area that in the broadest definition allows the use of a wide range of biopsychosocial strategies all directed towards the alleviation of physical symptoms.

Definitions of any broad field are frequently diverse and this is certainly true for behavioral medicine. Schwartz and Weiss (1978) defined behavioral medicine as:

> The interdisciplinary field concerned with the development and integration of behavioral and biomedical science, knowledge and techniques relevant to health and illness and the application of this knowledge and these techniques to prevention, diagnosis, treatment and rehabilitation.

More succinctly Surwit, Williams, and Shapiro (1982) wrote:

> Behavioral medicine is broadly defined to encompass the application of principles from all behavioral sciences to medical problems.

Adopting a somewhat more rigidly behavioral view, Pomerleau and Brady (1979) asserted that behavioral medicine was:

> The clinical use of techniques derived from the experimental analysis of behavior—behavior therapy and behavior modification—for the evaluation, prevention, management or treatment of physical disease or physiological dysfunction.

Whichever position one takes, whether it be rigidly behavioral or more flexibly socio-biomedical, the essence of these definitions is clear. Behavioral medicine concerns the use of psychological evidence and techniques, and principally those deriving from behavior therapy, in the diagnosis, prevention, and management of physically manifested illness.

The field of psychosomatic medicine has had a longer history and the practitioner of behavioral medicine is often asked to distinguish between the two. Surwit et al. (1982) argue that whereas the former focused on personality traits that were assumed to lead, through neurotic conflicts, to physical illness, the latter was concerned with physiological responses (ultimately pathology), arising initially through maladaptive environmental interactions and becoming established or learned by means of objectively testable paths of causal change deriving from mechanisms of psychobiological influence. In practice, behavioral medicine rejected psychodynamic labeling, emphasized the experimental principles of learning and treatment, and placed great value on the replicability of treatment procedures and the objective evaluation of therapeutic outcomes. The psychoanalytic underpinnings of psychosomatic medicine are obvious, and as we have previously stated, the tendency for experimentally-trained psychologists to reject the fundamental tenets of psychosomatic medicine has been strong, particularly in the last three decades.

Nonetheless, it is clear whether one speaks of psychosomatic medicine or behavioral medicine, and whatever definition of the latter one might take, a wide range of potential treatment strategies from a diverse set of theoretical backgrounds, relying on a copious assembly of practical procedures and based to a greater or lesser extent on empirically tested and testable evidence, is available to the practitioner who seeks to alleviate physical symptoms by psychological means. This imparts an essential polymorphism to any consideration of basic treatment strategies in behavioral medicine. The "purists" might continue to adopt the approach voiced by Pomerleau and Brady (1979), that behavioral medicine should strictly adhere to a behavioral set of strategies in its formulation of treatment. Others, and perhaps the majority nowadays, would hold that any treatment strategy from the broad armamentarium of psychology and psychiatry is a legitimate focus for practice in behavioral medicine, so long as that treatment strategy has scientific credibility and a degree of evidential support (the extent to which evidential support can be brought to bear for any particular therapeutic strategy will, of course, vary widely from one therapeutic approach to another).

With this conceptual background in mind, it is possible to divide basic treatment strategies in behavioral medicine between those relying on broad psychological or psychiatric concepts and those more specifically attuned to behavior therapy and behavior analysis. This does not mean that there is not or cannot be a constructive interaction between the two approaches, but simply that for the purposes of discussion the two approaches form relatively distinct conceptual entities.

STRATEGIES OF PSYCHOLOGICAL TREATMENT

What follows is a brief and inexhaustive overview of treatment strategies pertinent to the purview of behavioral medicine and based on psychotherapeutic intervention broadly defined. No attempt will be made to give any detailed theoretical account of the nature of these psychotherapeutic strategies nor an empirical justification of their merits or otherwise. They are merely mentioned in the sense that they represent broad categories of psychotherapy or of a psychotherapeutic approach and that they have pertinence to the broad concerns of behavioral medicine.

Individual Psychotherapy

The psychoanalytic beginnings of psychosomatic medicine dictated that individual (one-to-one or face-to-face) psychotherapy would be the only basis for treatment of the psychological causes of physical illness (Kimball, 1970). Indeed, the earliest forms of treatment involved lengthy individual psychotherapy based on traditional psychoanalytic method. More recently in the science of behavioral medicine, the psychoanalytic orientation has been replaced by a behavioral or cognitive orientation (or by a combination of these); however, much of the emphasis still involves individual psychotherapy (see, e.g., Meichenbaum, 1977). What this means in practice is that the psychological treatment of physical illness requires as intensive and extensive a set of interactions with the patient or client as does the treatment of psychological disorder.

The indications for individual psychotherapy in behavioral medicine are difficult to establish, since it is by an overwhelming degree the treatment of choice. As such, its sequence does not appreciably differ from that followed in many other areas of individual psychotherapy. Some early sessions are used to establish rapport with the patient and to assess the precise nature of the problem. These are followed by actual therapeutic sessions in which the problem is discussed and a more or less prescriptive attitude is taken towards the solution of the problem. Problem-solving sessions may or may not be interspersed with exercises involving home practice or other forms of self-directed activity, though the primary focus continues to be the individual interaction between therapist and patient on a regular basis (the frequency of contact will, of course, vary considerably from one therapist to another and from one problem to another). In some cases, evaluation or assessment sessions are arranged and may or may not be followed later in time by sessions aimed at consolidating the gains made during formal psychotherapy.

Once more, it is difficult to establish the range of problems for which individual psychotherapy is the treatment of choice. It may in many cases reduce, however, to matters of convenience or of personal preference by the therapist and/or the patient, such that there is a definite expression of preference by one or other parties at the outset of therapy. Individual psychotherapy is most certainly useful where work is required and in situations where the patient demands complete privacy, either for reasons of/or relating to the self-perception of the symptomatology (its sensitive or embarrassing nature) or where the patient feels unable to discuss symptomatology and disclose possible causes of that or responses to it to anyone but the therapist. Individual psychotherapy certainly allows the therapist to direct his or her entire attention towards a single patient during the therapy session, though it may carry with it the disadvantage that it is relatively open-ended and may give rise to less efficient forms of treatment.

Group Psychotherapy

Though the use of groups is less frequent than individual psychotherapy, the treatment of physical symptomatology using group methods is increasingly popular. One of the reasons underlying this is the development of structured packages focusing on the amelioration or removal of specific kinds of symptoms, whereby the somewhat rigidly defined structure of the program allows its convenient and efficacious use in a group setting. The primary advantage of the use of groups is that of time efficiency, so that a therapist may be able to treat a larger number of individual patients, all of whom suffer the same or similar symptomatologies, in one group. It carries with it, however, other advantages: groups allow discussion of symptomatology and therefore the essential normalization of perceptions of individual symptomatology. Thus, an individual who may have perceived his or her symptoms to be uniquely distressing may receive particular encouragement from the realization that others in similar circumstances suffer similar forms of symptomatology and distress. Groups also offer the possibility of practice and rehearsal using role-play techniques or other forms of psychological practice. This is particularly evident in such areas as stress management, where individuals may need to learn to control their stress reactions to particular situations by role-playing their responses to these situations within a confidential and supportive group.

Of course, there will continue to be a wide range of physical disorders for which group therapy is inappropriate, simply because they demand the intensive and extensive treatment which is provided by individual psychotherapy. Nonetheless, with the increasing availability of structured packages directed at very specific kinds of symptoms —for example, headache, eating disorders, and stress management for the reduction of blood pressure—the use of a group may add considerably to the therapist's overall collection of strategies and procedures, and may do so in a way that enhances the efficiency of the delivery of services to areas that do not require individual psychotherapy. With the expanding focus of managed (cost-constrained) health care delivery programs that have developed—in particular, in the United States—much more group-based therapeutic delivery may be anticipated in the future.

Treatment of Psychological Symptoms

Within the realm of behavioral medicine, physical symptoms frequently do not exist in isolation but are either preceded by or accompanied by psychological symptoms, typically those of emotional distress. The therapist, therefore, is often faced with the need not simply to address the physical symptom—whether it be pain, high blood pressure, or the like—but must also address the alleviation or removal of anxiety, depression, anger, or other emotional states (Byrne & Rosenman, 1990). The therapist in behavioral medicine must have at his or her disposal a range of techniques directed at more traditional psychotherapies in addition to those strategies and techniques directed more specifically to the physical symptomatology.

Often there is an essential complementarity within and between the treatment of psychological and physical symptoms so that the same kinds of treatment strategies may be employed to good effect with both kinds of symptoms. The therapist, however, is frequently faced with a problem of sequencing, in which the order of therapeutic intervention must be carefully planned and monitored so that psychological symptoms are accorded a degree of importance along with physical symptoms. This involves the process of ascertaining the interactive nature of psychological and physical symptoms and, in particular, of deciding when physical symptoms are exacerbated by the presence of emotional distress. It means, therefore, that the therapist must maintain a close monitoring function throughout the process of psychotherapy so that attention may be appropriately switched between the various demands of psychological treatment.

Education

Behavioral medicine involves the use of psychological techniques to treat physical symptoms that are in existence and that are of sufficient severity to distress those individuals who are experiencing them. One area of behavioral medicine that should not be forgotten, however, is that of education, since the range of symptoms that present to practitioners in behavioral medicine are frequently based at least in part on patterns of an unhealthy lifestyle. This raises the issue both of primary and secondary prevention, whereby the behavioral medicine practitioner may use simple educative procedures in order to persuade and direct the patient and, where appropriate, the family, towards the adoption of more healthy lifestyles, whatever these involve. Education, whether in the form of a verbal interaction between therapist and patient or in the form of the provision of written instructions or guidance, or a combination of these, presents a potentially powerful tool to the practitioner of behavioral medicine and one that should not be underrated as a therapeutic strategy.

STRATEGIES OF BEHAVIORAL TREATMENT

Behavior Therapy

The origins of behavioral medicine are most fundamentally to be found in the applications of the theory and skills of behavior analysis and behavior therapy to the treatment of physical symptoms. It is not surprising, therefore, that behavior therapy occupies a prominent position in the range of therapeutic strategies practiced by those involved in behavioral medicine. This is not the place to discuss the process and practice of behavior therapy in any detail. A wide variety of aspects of behavior therapy have been covered in individual chapters making up these volumes, and reference to any one of a number of excellent texts on behavior therapy will acquaint the nonpsychologically trained reader with the essential theoretical and practical underpinnings of this approach to therapy.

The focus of behavior therapy can be seen as taking two forms, the first of these relates to the process of symptom change or symptom removal, while the second has to do with risk factor management. Symptom change or symptom removal in behavioral medicine may be seen in many examples; however, the most clear cut are those involving single symptoms within a relatively simple etiological context. The behavioral treatment of pain or the use of behavioral techniques to reduce elevated blood pressure serve as good examples of situations in which direct behavioral management of a symptom for that symptom's change or removal acts as an end in itself. Within the context of preventive health or primary behavioral medical care, however, the issue of risk factor management is assuming a greater and greater level of importance. Risk factors for cardiovascular disease perhaps serve as the most clear cut examples in this area. If one considers the primary risk factors for cardiovascular disease to be those of elevated levels of some fraction of cholesterol in the blood, elevated blood pressure, cigarette smoking, or the presence of the Type A behavior pattern, then it is just a short step further to realize that there are a number of well-established, validated, and evaluated behavioral strategies which might be brought to bear on the control and removal of these risk factors. Once more, these strategies have been discussed in much greater detail both from a theoretical and practical perspective in individual chapters within these volumes and will not be considered to any greater extent here. Suffice to say that behavioral strategies have much to offer in the control of risk associated with a broad variety of disease conditions or states, and given the importance of prevention and of the psychological contribution to the public health field, the relative prominence of behavioral strategies for risk factor management is likely to increase over time.

Stress Management/Relaxation Therapy

While many would consider relaxation therapy and its involvement in composite packages of stress management to be part of behavior therapy, these strategies are often seen in behavioral medicine in relative isolation from the more exhaustive and systematic attempts at behavior modification based on thorough behavior analysis of presenting symptom problems. Practitioners of behavioral medicine frequently use relaxation therapy as a treatment strategy within more composite stress management programs as a means to reduce risk of illness. Both relaxation therapy and broadly based stress management programs are widely researched and evaluated, and they have been quite thoroughly documented in a number of chapters making up these present volumes. Specific examples may be gained from this material.

It is worth noting that relaxation in particular may offer too simple a form of therapy for a broad range of essentially complex problems; however the relative simplicity of relaxation will make it attractive for some, especially when initial change is sought with little expenditure of effort either by the therapist or the patient. It should be emphasized that relaxation therapy most probably serves no purpose other than might be achieved by the use of tranquilizing medication (except that it is unlikely to have side effects or to produce addiction and its use may facilitate the acknowledgment of an attribution of self-control). It is generally believed that its use alone, however, is unlikely to attack the real cause of many psychological disturbances underlying physical illness. Practitioners in behavioral medicine should be aware that relaxation therapy offers just one component to more broadly based treatment strategies and that any form of treatment must really be based on a thorough examination (whether by behavior analysis or more broadly based techniques) of the problem presented by the individual patient. Without this thorough analysis (as set out in the chapter on assessment strategies in behavioral medicine which may be seen in Volume I), treatment in behavioral medicine relying on relaxation alone will be at best incomplete, and at worst, seriously misguided.

Biofeedback

In a similar manner to behavior therapy, many will look to biofeedback as an "original science" in the field of behavioral medicine. Biofeedback is a set of strategies (based on a well-understood theoretical structure) that directs itself specifically to the behavioral control of single autonomic functions. Biofeedback is backed by a wealth of empirical evidence much of which is supportive, though this is not universally the case. However, it is one of the most widely and systematically researched of all areas in behavioral medicine and for this reason it continues to have a great attraction to the practitioner in behavioral medicine.

If biofeedback has one disadvantage in behavioral medicine it is that it requires sometimes complex and expensive equipment, and while this may frequently be available in the laboratory or consulting room it is less often practical to conduct biofeedback training in the natural environment. In recent times there have appeared on the market a number of light and inexpensive pieces of equipment that allow rudimentary biofeedback practice to be achieved either in the home or the field environments, and the use of such equipment is presently being evaluated. There is little doubt that this is an area of considerable growth potential and that with the increasing availability of portable technology, the use of biofeedback strategies will become increasingly important in behavioral medicine. Moreover, there is now much research into complex biofeedback training strategies—for example, those reliant on feedback of highly specific components of the electrocortical wave or equally highly specific components of the electrocardiographic impulse. These applications will continue for some time to require complex, bulky, and expensive equipment; however, they too will open new doors in the area of biofeedback, which in time are likely to offer very considerable treatment advantages of a noninvasive, nonpharmacological kind to patients with quite pronounced physical and pathophysiological dysfunction.

SPECIFIC CONCERNS IN BEHAVIORAL TREATMENT

A number of specific foci frequently present for attention in the practice of behavioral medicine. While these are often not central to the particular problem or illness, nonetheless they interact with it in such a way as to exacerbate its impact or impede the processes of recovery and rehabilitation. They should, therefore, be addressed as separate issues within the ambit of basic strategies of treatment.

Treatment of Illness Behavior

Illness behavior may be defined as the collective behavioral, emotional, and cognitive responses that an individual adopts in the face of the challenge of physical illness (Byrne & Whyte, 1978). Illness behavior is universal in this situation and is most frequently either adaptive or only mildly disruptive. It transforms to abnormal illness behavior when it either imposes additional stress on the individual already suffering from some kind of illness or when its components act to impair or interfere with the process of recovery and rehabilitation. In such cases, illness behavior must itself be seen as a focus for treatment, and appropriate therapeutic strategies applied. The nature of these therapeutic strategies is not unique to the field of illness behavior and will be drawn from the broad spectrum of therapeutic approaches available within the fields of clinical psychology and psychiatry. The issue that is unique to illness behavior is its assessment. While this cannot be covered in detail in this section, it should be noted that suspicion of the presence or the possibility of abnormal illness behavior should be carefully assessed by appropriate and available methods. This will allow the practitioner to more precisely and usefully direct the application of intervention strategies aimed at modifying behavior in directions that make it more adaptive to the illness it emerges in response to.

Enhancement of Compliance

A great deal of evidence is available in the area of compliance with treatment in behavioral medicine and much of this evidence has been discussed in other chapters within these volumes. Clearly, the success of much treatment in behavioral medicine depends on the capacity and willingness of the patient to comply with the therapeutic instructions and advice given by the practitioner. The evidence on compliance with such simple therapeutic strategies as medication indicate that compliance imposes a very substantial problem for the successful treatment of even simple and monosymptomatic illnesses. When one considers the complexity and the degree of patient involvement and responsibility required for the successful completion of many intervention strategies in behavioral medicine, one is struck with the potential difficulties that may arise through lack of compliance. Much of the success of behavioral and related strategies involves the close interaction of the patient with the therapist and the undertaking by the patient to transport the therapeutic advice and strategies suggested from the consulting room to practice in the real life setting. It is crucial to the success of many therapeutic strategies in behavioral medicine that compliance with complex and often time-consuming instructions is both understood and carried through by the patient.

There are specific techniques for the assessment of compliance and the detection of noncompliance in behavioral medicine, and these have been discussed in other chapters in the present volumes. Moreover, there are behavioral strategies aimed at enhancing compliance with therapeutic instructions within the setting of behavioral medicine, and once more the reader will find careful consideration of these in other areas of the present volumes. It is worth emphasizing however, that the practitioner in behavioral medicine must always be aware of the problems of compliance and should take steps to monitor that compliance with therapeutic instructions is indeed being carried out. Failure to do this may jeopardize the progress of primary treatment in behavioral medicine, since the clinician may frequently be unaware that the patient is failing to comply.

CONCLUSIONS

Behavioral medicine is both a science and an art which is fed by the contributions of many areas of the psychology, psychiatry, and internal medicine. It does not have a theoretical base that is unique, nor does it have a set of therapeutic strategies that it alone can claim proprietary rights over. Rather, behavioral medicine is essentially a derivative area drawing on the theories and therapies of many other areas for its advancement.

This does not mean that the applications of therapeutic strategies to the demands of behavioral medicine do not in themselves represent unique endeavours, or that the science underlying behavioral medicine is of secondary importance. It means simply that the practitioner in the area of behavioral medicine has the very substantial advantage of drawing widely on therapeutic strategies and on theoretical bases from a broad variety of disciplines within the health care professions.

Though the point has been made in previous chapters and particularly in the chapter on Strategies of Assessment in Volume I, it should always be borne in mind by the practitioner of behavioral medicine that monitoring and evaluation forms an essential component of any therapeutic exercise. The need to be continually aware of what one is doing and of the progress that is being made, both from the point of view of objective symptom or behavior change, and from the point of view of patient perception and satisfaction cannot be overemphasized.

REFERENCES

Byrne, D. G., & Whyte, H. M. (1978). Dimensions of illness behavior in survivors of myocardial infarction. *Journal of Psychosomatic Research, 22,* 485–491.

Byrne, D. G., & Rosenman, R. H. (1990). *Anxiety and the heart.* Washington: Hemisphere.

James, W. (1890). *The principles of psychology.* New York: Holt.

Kimball, C. P. (1970). Conceptual developments in psychosomatic medicine: 1939–1969. *Annals of Internal Medicine, 73,* 307–316.

Lipowski, Z. J. (1986). Psychosomatic medicine: Past and present. *Canadian Journal of Psychiatry, 31,* 8–13.

Mandler, G. (1984). *Mind and body: Psychology of emotion and stress.* New York: W. W. Norton.

Meichenbaum, D. (1977). *Cognitive behavior modification.* London: Plenum Press.

Pomerleau, O. F., & Brady, J. P. (1979). *Behavioral medicine: Theory and practice.* Baltimore: Williams & Wilkins.

Schwartz, G. E., & Weiss, S. M. (1978). Behavioral medicine revisited: An amended definition. *Journal of Behavioral Medicine, 1,* 249–251.

Selye, H. (1976). *Stress in health and disease.* Sydney: Butterworth.

Surwit, R. S., Williams, R. B., & Shapiro, D. (1982). *Behavioral approaches to cardiovascular disease.* New York: Academic Press.

II

THE GASTROINTESTINAL SYSTEM

2

Functional Bowel Disorders

Paul R. Latimer

Kelowna, B.C.
Canada

INTRODUCTION

The term *functional bowel disorder* covers an ill-defined group of conditions with clinically significant gastrointestinal symptoms but without demonstrable structural lesions or deficiencies of the gastrointestinal tract. The symptoms often suggest disordered function (hence, *functional*) although an actual demonstration of disordered function is not always included in diagnostic criteria for these disorders. In practice, the term *functional* indicates the absence of identifiable structural lesions more than it does the presence of well-defined disordered physiology; most of these conditions remain relatively poorly understood from a physiological viewpoint. This term includes (but is not limited to) disorders such as irritable bowel syndrome, painless diarrhea, simple constipation, nonspecific esophageal motor disorder, vomiting, proctalgia fugax, biliary dyskinesia, and globus hystericus. As a group, the functional bowel disorders have been estimated to account for between 13 and 70 percent of all new referrals to outpatient gastrointestinal clinics.

IRRITABLE BOWEL SYNDROME

Phenomenology

Irritable bowel syndrome (IBS) was first described in 1820 and since that time has been referred to by over two dozen names, reflecting changing fashions and ideas about etiology. The term IBS is devoid of etiological implications, is sufficiently general to encompass the various clinical manifestations, and has now gained wide acceptance.

There is no universal agreement on diagnostic criteria for IBS, but there is a growing consensus that the term should be restricted to patients with abdominal pain and change in bowel habit (constipation, diarrhea, or the one alternating with the other) occurring in the absence of structural abnormalities on the appropriate physical examination and laboratory investigations.

Patients with IBS are typically young adults whose symptoms began in late adolescence, although onset occurs before age 15 in a substantial proportion. Women are affected twice as often as men (Fielding, 1977a, 1977b).

Pain may vary widely in quality, site, and duration. Episodic left lower quadrant, colicky pain lasting from minutes to hours is most common. The pain is temporarily relieved following defecation and exacerbated following food in more than half the cases. In many, however, there are no specific relieving or aggravating factors (Chaudhary & Truelove, 1962; White & Jones, 1940).

Most commonly, the bowel habits are only imperfectly related to the pain; alternating periods of constipation, diarrhea, and relatively normal bowel movements are interspersed at irregular intervals. Abdominal distension, excessive flatus, rumbling and gurgling, mucus in the stool, urgency, bad taste in the mouth, loss of appetite, heartburn, regurgitation, nausea, and vomiting are among the other gastrointestinal complaints of IBS patients. Esophageal symptoms occur in over 50 percent of the cases (Keeling & Fielding, 1975; Watson, Sullivan, Corke, & Rush, 1978).

Less well appreciated are the prevalence and variety of nongastrointestinal symptoms such as weakness, fatigue, lack of energy, muscular pains, insomnia, palpitations, nervousness, dizziness, excessive perspiration, frequency of micturition, painful micturition, dysmenorrhea, dyspareunia, and headaches (Fielding, 1977a; Watson et al., 1978).

This latter group of symptoms suggests the possibility of anxiety and depressive disorders. Indeed, structured psychiatric interviews have shown that more than 70 percent of IBS patients have a psychiatric disorder and that a large proportion of these disorders go unrecognized by the attending physician (Young, Alpers, Norland, & Woodruff, 1976). From a psychiatric perspective the patients form a heterogeneous group (see Table 2.1). Although in some cases the identification of these psychiatric syndromes leads directly to an appropriate treatment strategy, it does not provide a sufficient basis for the understanding and treatment of all cases.

Studies using a wide variety of psychological assessment methods have shown that patients with IBS are psychologically disturbed when compared with the general population and with individuals suffering from other medical conditions. Assessment methods employed have included the Minnesota Multiphasic Personality Inventory (West, 1970), the Institute for Personality and Ability Testing Anxiety Scale (Esler & Goulston, 1973), the Eysenck Personality Inventory (Esler & Goulston, 1973; Latimer, Sarna, Campbell, Latimer, Waterfall, & Daniel, 1981; Palmer, Stonehill, Crisp, Waller, & Misiewicz, 1974), the Beck Depression Inventory, the Spielberger State-Trait Anxiety Inventory (Latimer et al., 1981), and the Edwards Personal Preference Schedule (Sjodin & Svedlund, 1985). These last authors found similar psychological characteristics in IBS and peptic ulcer patients.

Several of these studies have found that the psychological problems of the IBS patients are greater than those found in persons with much more severe and disabling gastrointestinal disease and therefore are unlikely to be solely a reaction to the digestive symptoms.

In interpreting these findings it is important to remember that there are equally neurotic, anxious, or depressed patients who have no bowel disturbances, and that not all patients with IBS, even in clinical populations, can be assigned a psychiatric diagnosis.

Prevalence and Social Impact

There are no satisfactory epidemiological data on the incidence and prevalence of IBS in the general population. There is, however, a consensus that IBS is the most common diagnosis among new referrals to outpatient gastrointestinal clinics with estimates varying from 13 to 52 percent (Ferguson, Sircus, & Eastwood, 1977; Fielding, 1977a; Harvey, Salih, & Read, 1983; Switz, 1976).

Even though only a small proportion of patients with IBS require hospitalization, in 1976 IBS was the primary diagnosis for 96,000 patients discharged from U.S. hospitals and the secondary diagnosis for 85,000 patients. "Psychogenic gastrointestinal disorder" appeared on about 37,000 discharge records and had been the primary reason for hospitalization for 19,000 patients. Together, patients with these two

Table 2.1.
Comparison of Psychiatric Studies of IBS

	Liss et al. (1973)	Young et al. (1976)	Latimer et al. (1981)	Wender and Kalm (1938)
Number	25	29	16	22
Source of Patients	G.I. Clinic	Private Practice	G.I. Clinic	G.I. Clinic
Females (%)	68	19	56	77
Psychiatric Illness (%)	92	72	100	73
(Feighner, Robins, Guze, Woodruff, Winokur, & Munoz Criteria)				
Undiagnosed Psychiatric Illness (%)	32	31	25	
Primary Affective Disorder Depressed (%)	8	17	31	
Hysteria (%)	28	17	13	
Anxiety Neurosis (%)	24	3.5	19	
Other (%)	0	3.5	13	
DSM-III				
Major Depressive Disorder (%)				23
Dysthmic Disorder (%)				27
Attention Deficit Disorder, Residual type (%)				27
Generalized Anxiety Disorder (%)				14
Other (%)				10

diagnoses accounted for over 450,000 hospital days, required heavy use of diagnostic facilities, and suffered no hospital mortality (Mendeloff, 1979). Unexplained abdominal pain is the tenth most common cause of hospital admission in men and the sixth most common in women (Lancet, 1972).

There have been two questionnaire studies of the prevalence of symptoms of functional bowel disorders in apparently healthy people. They found a symptom pattern consistent with a diagnosis of IBS is 13.6 and 17.1 percent respectively and symptoms characteristic of functional bowel disorders in general in almost one-third of the subjects studied; most had not consulted a physician (Thompson & Heaton, 1980; Drossman, Sandler, McKee, & Lovitz, 1982).

The symptoms are well known to run in families but there is insufficient data to distinguish genetic from environmental influences. There is evidence to suggest the importance of both (Latimer, 1983, pp. 34–35, 89–94).

Pathophysiology

There have been numerous attempts to identify a biologic marker for IBS. In support of a hypothesized gastrointestinal predisposition to abnormal motility have been studies reporting that IBS patients have an abnormal electrical rhythm in the smooth muscle of the rectum and rectosigmoid colon (Snape, Carlson, & Cohen, 1976; Taylor, Darby, & Hammond, 1978), as well as rectal and colonic motor hyperactivity during rest (Chaudhary & Truolove, 1961), and following food intake (Connel, Jones, & Rowlands, 1965), the injection of neostigmine (Chaudhary & Truelove, 1961; Wangel & Deller, 1965), and rectal distension (Whitehead, Engel, & Schuster, 1980). Primary colonic hyperalgesia has also been suggested as an underlying biologic determinant of the disorder (Ritchie, 1973).

The evidence in support of a unique abnormality of intestinal physiology is inconclusive. These findings have frequently not been replicated and differences between IBS patients and normal subjects have more often than not been absent. In most of these studies there has been inadequate attention to methodological issues such as scoring the data blindly and ensuring that the motility records can be scored reliably (Latimer et al., 1979, 1981; Latimer, 1983, pp. 61–82).

Since environmental events, stress, and psychological factors are known to be associated with changes in colonic physiology, any study intended to show definitively that there is a colonic abnormality peculiar to IBS patients must use a control group consisting of persons who are equally disturbed psychologically. In the only study to date in which this comparison has been made, patients with IBS could not be distinguished from neurotic patients without IBS on measures of colonic motor and myoelectrical activity or in their reports of pain in response to colonic distension. During rest, IBS patients did have a greater number and duration of colonic contractions than normal subjects (Latimer et al., 1979, 1981; Latimer, 1983, pp. 61–82).

Welgan, Meshkinpour, and Hoehler (1985) have recently replicated the Latimer et al. (1981) study without the neurotic control group and using different stressors. In all ways that the studies are directly comparable the results are identical.

These findings are equally problematic for all theories that attempt to account for IBS solely on the basis of distinctive intestinal physiologic characteristics, whether they be biologically determined or learned. If identical intestinal events occur in other individuals who do not exhibit IBS, the intestinal events themselves are not a sufficient explanation. For the same reason, treatment directed at eliminating or changing these intestinal characteristics, whether this be pharmacologic or behavioral (e.g., biofeedback) would be expected to be inadequate.

Another increasingly popular suggested etiology for IBS is food allergy. Although many IBS patients report food intolerances, these can often be demonstrated to be of psychological origin (Latimer, 1983, pp. 123–128). Bentley, Pearson, and Rix (1983) used exclusion diets and double-blind food provocation to investigate food hypersensitivity as a cause of abdominal symptoms in 27 IBS patients. There was consistent exacerbation of symptoms in 10 patients during open exclusion and dietary testing but food hypersensitivity as a cause of bowel symptoms was confirmed on double-blind provocation studies in only three. All three would be considered atopic by conventional criteria. As in other studies of IBS, most of the patients had significant psychiatric disorders.

It is well known that lactose intolerance may mimic IBS in those patients with lactose deficiency, but this is a relatively uncommon cause of IBS among non-Jewish whites of northern-western European background (Latimer, 1983, pp. 38–39; Newcomer & McGill, 1983).

An adequate model for IBS must account for all of the following characteristics:

1. Patients with IBS complain of a variety of symptoms including abdominal pain and alteration in bowel habits.
2. The symptoms are usually not confined to the gastrointestinal system alone.

3. On the average, these patients are more anxious, depressed, and neurotic than control subjects. A majority of persons with IBS meet strict criteria for a psychiatric diagnosis.
4. They are a heterogeneous group with respect to psychiatric diagnoses.
5. No distinctive biologic characteristics—physical, physiologic, biochemical—have been clearly demonstrated.
6. IBS patients closely resemble psychoneurotics in their psychological and physiologic characteristics, sex distribution, and nature of psychological problems.
7. They respond positively, albeit temporarily, to a variety of treatment procedures.
8. The symptoms run in families.

A behavioral model has been proposed to account for the above characteristics of IBS. As the name suggests, its emphasis is on observable behavior that can be reliably measured. As with any other disorder, the behavior observed may include what the patient says or does, and how that person responds physiologically. Thus the term behavior is used in an overall sense, which in the case of IBS may include the pattern of visits to the bathroom and the occurrence of colonic contractions. The behavioral approach is unique in emphasizing that each of these behaviors is capable of occurring independently. For example, when someone reports abdominal pain, a corresponding intestinal contraction may or may not occur. This model then allows for the possibility of disparity between symptom reports and intestinal events. Ample evidence shows that individuals can and do learn to report symptoms in the absence of disease, and that great individual variability is present in the tendency to report the symptoms.

Another important aspect of the behavioral model is the implication that IBS is a variation of the normal state rather than a categorically distinct disease. It is defined by changes in certain behaviors that are present to a greater or lesser degree in individuals among the general population. Exactly which behavioral variations are related to treatment-seeking cannot be assumed. The person seeking treatment is not necessarily the one with the most extreme changes in measures of intestinal physiology.

Finally, the evidence suggests that IBS patients are distinguishable from other psychoneurotic outpatients only in their emphasis on gastrointestinal complaints. Evidence exists of a genetic predisposition to neuroticism, and neuroticism may predispose to IBS. If IBS patients do come from the same stock as other neurotic individuals, then many features of IBS become less perplexing. Anxiety, depression, neuroticism, heterogeneous psychiatric disorders, multiple somatic and psychological symptoms, and positive response to various treatments are expected among such individuals. Likewise, it is generally accepted that neuroticism varies in the population in a dimensional way. The major question that remains is why some patients become identified as having IBS while others do not.

The answer to this question is not yet known, but several possibilities are worth exploring. From the parents or significant others with IBS, children may learn misconceptions about normal bowel habits. They may also learn that symptoms of IBS are a socially acceptable sign of distress, a way to avoid unpleasant responsibilities, and a way to elicit a show of concern and affection from family, friends, and health care providers.

Patients with IBS have been reported to respond to questions in a socially desirable way. It may be, as it often appears clinically, that many of these persons recognize that they have a psychological problem but find it more acceptable socially to be identified as having a medical problem. They therefore present themselves to the primary physician in a manner that contributes to nonrecognition of the psychological problem. This by no means exhausts the possibilities. Other factors that may contribute to a particular individual presenting with IBS include the way in which health care professionals approach the problem on initial contact, and other characteristics such as alexithymia and extraversion (Latimer, 1983, Chapter 6).

Assessment Procedures

The behavioral model suggests the appropriateness of a comprehensive approach to assessment that attends to the patient's behavior at several levels, from intestinal responses on the one hand to the psychosocial determinants of the symptomatic behavior on the other. A diagnosis of IBS and a behavioral treatment plan should be based not only on an adequate negative medical history and physical investigation but also on positive evidence for a behavioral formulation.

A comprehensive medical work-up would include:

1. Hemoglobin, hematocrit, white blood cell count, erythrocyte sedimentation rate
2. sigmoidoscopy
3. Air-contrast barium enema
4. Upper gastrointestinal tract radiography and/or endoscopy for upper abdominal pain
5. Stool cultures, parasite studies, and lactose tolerance tests where indicated.

Holmes and Salter (1982) followed up 77 of 84 patients in whom the IBS had been diagnosed at least six years previously using criteria very similar to these. Although 57 percent of the surviving patients still had their symptoms at follow-up, a different diagnosis was made in only four cases. This confirms other reports that IBS is often a chronic disorder, but one that can be relatively safely diagnosed using these criteria.

Behavioral analysis is the cornerstone of the behavioral approach to treatment. The term refers to the process of weaving the various threads of data collected, using the methods described below, into a coherent conceptual model of the client's problem. This model should lead logically to the answers of the following questions: Which treatment procedure should I employ with this particular individual, with this particular problem, at this point in time? Unless these questions are correctly answered, the technology of treatment is relatively impotent. The behavioral approach to treatment is not, as is often thought, the matching of treatment techniques to clinical disorders. Rather, the therapist, in collecting information, tries to understand why the patient's problem behavior began and why it has continued. In doing this, the therapist behaves like a detective, making hypotheses and systematically testing them. The nature of the hypotheses are obviously influenced by the therapist's knowledge base. In the case of IBS a wide base of knowledge about learning principles, gastrointestinal physiology, IBS, and behavioral assessment will increase efficiency. The goal is to develop a conceptual model or formulation which relates all of the patient's complaints to one another, explains why this person developed these problems at this time, and provides a basis for predicting the patient's behavior in various situations. The better the therapist can predict the patient's problem behavior, the more likely is the formulation to be correct. An individual treatment program is then based on this formulation.

An appropriate behavioral assessment for research or treatment must be comprehensive and trimodal, encompassing what the patient says (verbal behavior), what he or she does (overt nonverbal behavior), and how he or she responds physiologically (physiological behavior).

The concept of a trimodal assessment originated out of studies on anxiety (Lang, 1968; Rachman, 1978) in which it was observed that some subjects showing marked changes in overt behavior, like decreased avoidance, still continued to verbally label themselves as fearful. Others reported less fear while still exhibiting increased heart rate. Lang (1968) proposed that such results could stem from different behavioral systems (verbal, physiological, and motoric) being capable of at least some independent change through shaping by environmental demands. In the face of strong demands of performance and incentives for nonfearful behavior, fearful subjects can be induced to stop avoiding feared objects, whether or not they continue to react autonomically. Because of this, assessment methods sampling each of the three behavioral systems or modes have been widely advocated (see Table 2.2).

Interview. The clinical interview has been, and will continue to be, the predominant assessment method. No other method is capable of the flexibility, comprehensiveness, and the subtlety of the interview. Nor should the importance of the human relationship factor be underestimated. The quality of the information obtained is nowhere more sensitive to nuances of the therapeutic relationship than with IBS patients. This is especially true with those patients who have been referred for psychiatric/psychological therapy after first seeking medical treatment. Many patients view such a referral as a denial of the validity of their complaints. In all fairness, their perception that they have been labeled a "crock" is not always exaggerated.

The behavioral approach to this, or any other clinical problem, begins with a description of the symptomatic behavior. What exactly is the patient doing or experiencing that is problematic, under what circumstances, where and when do the symptoms occur, and what are their usual consequences? In behavioral jargon this is referred to as the ABCs (Antecedents, Behaviors, Consequences) of behavior analysis. Each of the antecedents, behaviors, and consequences may also be environmental. In many medical clinics the questions focus too narrowly on the physiological/gastrointestinal system, which results in a unimodal assessment. This not only limits the range of current behavior assessed but usually determines the other historical information

Table 2.2.
Assessment Procedures

Interview a) patient b) significant others
Self-Report Inventories
Self-Monitoring
Behavioral Observation
Physiological Recording

considered to be relevant. The opposite tendency is often present in psychiatric/psychological settings.

A comprehensive assessment should include descriptions of the following: the presenting complaint; the present problem including the ABCs of behavioral assessment; the development of each problem from its first occurrence to the present; the patient's present life circumstances including vocation, leisure activities, circle of friends, and financial situation and how these are affected by the presenting problems; previous medical and psychiatric/psychological investigation and treatment, including responses to and satisfaction with treatment; a general functional inquiry; family and personal history including descriptions of similar symptoms in other family members, responses of significant others to the patient's problems, and the usual survey of developmental and social milestones that reflect a person's level of functioning. At the conclusion it should be possible to provide the information necessary for a formal description of mental status.

It is generally the behavioral assessment of the presenting problem and its development that is most relevant to directing behavioral treatment. The comprehensive history may influence diagnosis and may help put the patient's current problems in perspective. Patients are frequently interested in knowing why they have their problems in addition to knowing how to solve them. The provision of a plausible explanation for the genesis of the problem behavior, in addition to an explanation for its maintenance, may enhance the therapist's credibility and hence facilitate therapy.

Once the patient has been interviewed, it is frequently helpful to interview a significant other. This may provide a corroboration of the patient's account, if it is done immediately so that there is no opportunity for discussion between the patient and the significant other. It is particularly important to get another, independent description of the problem behavior, its antecedents, and consequences. A patient's tendency to minimize problems or otherwise project a socially desirable impression may become transparent in the light of a spouse's answers to the same questions. Discrepancies that arise must be dealt with in a tactful and nonaccusatory manner. Such discrepancies may arise out of the fear of disapproval or genuine differences in perception. Deliberate deceptions are unusual but do occur. They sometimes involve patients with gastrointestinal symptoms as part of another syndrome such as anorexia nervosa or bulimia. The correct diagnosis is usually evident with the comprehensive assessment described above.

Self-report inventories. Self-report inventories are an extremely useful adjunct to the clinical interview. They are inexpensive and can be given to a patient to complete on his or her own time either in the office or at home. They may, like the Fear Survey Schedule (Wolpe & Lang, 1969), provide an efficient survey of a wide variety of potential problem areas or, like the Beck Depression Inventory (Beck, Ward, Mendelson, Mack, & Erbaugh, 1961), provide a quantitative measure of some behavior. These can serve as a check against clinical impressions, uncover overlooked, but potentially important problem areas, and provide a measure of the effectiveness of therapy. There are literally hundreds of available inventories from which to choose. Selection of appropriate instruments depends on the questions being asked, on the behavior being treated, and on the availability of adequate reliability and validity data for the inventory. To be clinically useful with IBS patients, an inventory must also be acceptable to general medical patients in the sense that it does not seem too psychiatric/psychological, and it must be practical. Some of the most widely used psychological inventories such as the MMPI (Minnesota Multiphasic Personality Inventory) are very lengthy. Both physicians and patients are reluctant to use these in many medical clinics.

There is a need for an inventory that provides a quantitative measure of severity of symptoms of the functional bowel disorders. This would allow better quantification of treatment results and would facilitate comparison of various clinical research studies on IBS (see Latimer, 1983, Appendix A).

Self-monitoring. It is frequently useful to ask patients to keep a daily log or diary of certain aspects of their behavior. This is a simple, practical, and very useful method which should be used with most cases.

The information collected in this way serves several functions. First, it may introduce a fresh and revealing perspective on the problem for both the patient and the therapist. We are not always attuned to the frequency of our behaviors or the circumstances in which they occur if we are not specifically monitoring these. Second, this increasing awareness may itself bring about behavior change in the desired direction. Third, at the very least, it provides a measure with which to gauge the effects of treatment on the behavior being monitored.

Direct behavioral observation. A picture is worth a thousand words and sometimes just observing a patient engage in a problem behavior is very illuminating. This is not a method that is practical in all cases, but where it is, it can be very useful. In certain situations a significant other may be able to directly observe and rate behavior under the direction of the therapist. This approach finds its widest application when the patient is a child and the parents are asked to collaborate in assessment and treatment procedures.

Physiological recording. The methods of recording gastrointestinal motor and myoelectrical activity are not yet widely used clinically, nor should they be until more standardized methods of recording and analyzing data are developed. Nevertheless, physiological recording methods can be useful in individual cases (Latimer, 1983, Chapter 4).

An indirect measure of physiological activity which may have more direct clinical application is observation of stool characteristics. Stool samples may be examined and rated for weight, volume, and consistency which have obvious clinical relevance. It must be remembered, however, that these characteristics are a function of both physiological activity and voluntary motor activity; diet and bowel habits, both with large voluntary components, make their contribution. Convenient stool collection systems are commercially available.

Target Symptoms for Treatment

As should now be obvious, the target symptoms are determined by the behavior analysis and may include a wide variety of symptoms in addition to those referrable to the gastrointestinal tract. To make matters even more complex, the symptoms targeted may be at any one of three levels; what the person says (verbal), what he/she does (overt nonverbal), and how he/she responds physiologically (physiological). Table 2.3 illustrates some common target symptoms and illustrates the importance of the three levels of behavior.

Table 2.3.
Target Symptoms

Verbal	Overt Nonverbal	Physiological
Anxiety	Phobic avoidance	Tachycardia
Abdominal pain	Medication use Lying down	Colonic contractions (frequency, duration, amplitude)
Constipation	Laxatives, enemas	Intestinal transit *Frequency and consistency of bowel movements.
Depression	Eating Weight Activity	Dexamethasone suppression test

Note: These symptoms are illustrative only. The list is not exhaustive.
*Frequency and consistency of bowel movements are a function of both overt nonverbal behavior (e.g., diet, trips to the bathroom) and physiological behaviors. The same may be true of the other physiological measures depending on the conditions of measurement.

In clinical practice, physiological measures are the least readily available. Nevertheless, it helps to be aware of the possibility that these various aspects of behavior may be changing independently.

Treatment

Dietary fiber. The use of dietary fiber in the treatment of IBS is based on the premise that these patients are distinguished from those without IBS by increased intraluminal pressure, which in turn is supposed to occur because less undigested fiber results in stools of smaller caliber.

Although the high fiber diet has become almost routine in the treatment of IBS, there is little rational basis for it. It has not been established that the diet, stool composition, or transit time of IBS patients differs from those of appropriate controls (Hillman, Stace, Fisher, & Pomare, 1982) or that the addition of dietary fiber is a useful treatment (Soltoff, Gudmand-Hoyer, Krag, Kristensen, & Wulff, 1976; Latimer, 1983, pp. 107–109; Cann, Read, & Holdsworth, 1984a).

It is reasonably well established that increasing fiber produces a larger stool and influences transit times; it speeds up slow transit and slows down fast transit (Eastwood, Kirkpatrick, Mitchell, Bone, & Hamilton, 1973; Harvey, Pomare, & Heaton, 1973; Connell, 1978; Cann et al., 1984a). Dietary fiber may, therefore, be useful in individual cases where these effects are desired. It is worth noting, however, that among healthy men, personality factors can account for about as much variance in stool output as dietary fiber (Tucker et al., 1981).

Antispasmodic pharmacotherapy. Next to the high-fiber diet, antispasmodic medications are probably the mainstay of physician-prescribed treatment for IBS. In a comprehensive review of the use of these medications for IBS, Goulston (1972) found that only five of the 29 drugs then in use had been evaluated by double-blind trial. Since over one-third of patients with IBS improved on placebo, double-blind placebo-controlled trials of drugs used for IBS are essential.

In another review, Ivey (1975) faulted the evidence concerning the efficacy of anticholinergics in IBS on two grounds. First, the evidence was unconvincing that the recommended oral doses of these drugs could produce the desired sustained reduction in colonic contractility. Second, like Goulston (1972), he found few double-blind placebo-controlled studies and concluded that the evidence for the clinical value of anticholinergics was at best dubious. The evidence has changed little since Ivey's (1975) review (Latimer, 1983, pp. 109–111). In a double-blind crossover design, Piai and Mazzacca (1979) demonstrated that three weeks of prifinium bromide (an anticholinergic) was significantly superior to three weeks of placebo in the treatment of patients with pain-predominant IBS. Although promising, these results should be accepted cautiously until they are replicated and the longer-term effects are assessed. In a chronic relapsing and remitting condition such as IBS, a really worthwhile treatment must be capable of producing positive effects at one and two years followup.

Miscellaneous. Several other drugs have been tried with little success in IBS (Latimer, 1983, pp. 109–113). Loperamide (Cann, Read, Holdsworth, & Barends, 1984b) is better than placebo in the treatment of diarrhea, urgency, and borborygmi in IBS patients and may therefore be a useful adjunct in patients who are particularly disabled with these symptoms.

Psychopharmacotherapy. Several published double-blind placebo-controlled studies have shown that benzodiazepines produce significantly greater improvement than placebos in both anxiety and somatic symptoms in patients with functional gastrointestinal symptoms (Baume, Tracey, & Dawson, 1975; Baume & Cuthbert, 1973; Samet, 1976). Unfortunately, these studies involved patients with a variety of functional gastrointestinal problems accompanied by anxiety and not just IBS patients. Similar results have been reported for the treatment of anxiety in several studies including both "functional" and "structural" gastrointestinal problems (Kasich, 1973; Furtado, 1976; Kasich, Richards, & Vanov, 1976; Chaplan & Vanov, 1977; Berkowitz, 1978).

Of the psychotropic medications, only antidepressants have been subjected to double-blind controlled investigation with IBS patients specifically. Heefner, Wilder, and Wilson (1978) conducted a double-blind comparison of desipramine hydrochloride with an inactive placebo in the treatment of IBS patients. Patients were assessed using self-rating scales for both depression and gastrointestinal symptoms over the course of the two-month treatment period. As with previous studies, a high proportion of IBS patients were found to be depressed (65 to 71 percent); both antidepressant and placebo produced a degree of improvement in a similar proportion of the depressed patients (60% and 64%, respectively). Both groups experienced considerable improvement in abdominal pain, bowel movements, and the degree of interference with daily life; the antidepressant group did somewhat better in each of those areas. The significance of those results is diminished by the fact that the study was almost certainly not double-blind since the side effects of the antidepressants caused three patients to drop out and there was no post-treatment follow-up.

Steinhart, Wong, and Zarr (1981) conducted a double-blind crossover trial of amitriptyline in IBS. During the active treatment phase, patients received 50 mg of amitriptyline at bedtime. Although the drug produced a significant improvement, it was not significantly superior to placebo. The authors pointed out that the doses used were subantidepressive doses.

Myren, Groth, Larssen, and Larsen (1982) compared 50 mg trimipramine at bedtime to placebo and found that both produced a significant improvement in most of the symptoms monitored. The antidepressant was significantly superior to placebo for sleeplessness, depression and mucous content of stools.

Lancester-Smith, Prout, Pinto, Anderson, and Schiff (1982) compared a combination preparation containing 1.5 mg. fluphenazine and 30 mg. nortriptyline (Motipress, Squibb) with a placebo in a double-blind study of IBS patients. At the end of the 12-week therapeutic trial the drug group were significantly better on only one of the four target symptoms—abdominal pain. There were no differences at 12 weeks with respect to diarrhea, constipation, or feeling of distension. At the start of the study 60 percent of the patients were classified as "probable psychiatric cases" and at the end 73 percent of these were classified as "probable normals." There was no difference between the drug and placebo groups in this respect.

In summary, benzodiazepines are better than placebo in providing relief for both anxiety and gastrointestinal symptoms in patients with functional gastrointestinal symptoms although there are little data for IBS specifically. Antidepressants appear to be only marginally better than placebo.

To demonstrate that benzodiazepines, the best anxiolytic medications available, relieve anxiety when administered to anxious patients (with gastrointestinal symptoms) over a brief period (typically two to four weeks) is a relatively trivial finding. In view of the fact that IBS is a chronic condition and that benzodiazepines are dependency-forming, these medications are unlikely to provide anything more than a temporary adjunct to therapy.

Psychotherapy. In view of the very high prevalence of psychiatric disorders among IBS patients, the well-known relationship between gastrointestinal symptoms and psychologically significant events and all of the other facts which form the basis for the behavioral model of IBS (see Pathophysiology and Assessment Procedures), it is surprising that there have not been more attempts to study the effects of psychotherapy on IBS. Among the few published reports, Jacobson (1927) reported the use of progressive muscular relaxation in the treatment of "spastic esoghagus" and "mucous colitis." Cohen and Reed (1968) also used progressive muscular relaxation but in the context of systematic desensitization to treat two cases of "nervous diarrhea." They regarded the diarrhea as a conditioned response and, once the conditioned stimuli were identified, systematic desensitization was used to overcome this learned maladaptive habit. Youell and McCullough (1975) reported the successful treatment of "mucous colitis" by helping the patient identify stressful antecedents to her symptoms and then teaching her coping skills to counter the stressful events. As interesting as these and other scattered reports of successful behavioral treatments are, all of this work is methodologically weak and can be considered only suggestive.

There have also been several reports of the use of biofeedback in the treatment of IBS. Furman (1973), using an electronic stethoscope to amplify bowel sounds, taught patients to both reduce and increase bowel sounds. He reported that all patients improved as a result of this training. The length of follow-up of these patients was not reported, nor were there adequate controls to indicate which aspect of treatment was effective. There has been at least one report (Weinstock, 1976) that this procedure was ineffective when tried on 12 patients with "functional colitis." Weinstock was subsequently able to produce clinical improvement in his patients when he switched to forehead EMG feedback plus twice-daily relaxation exercises.

Bueno-Miranda, Cerulli, and Schuster (1976) used feedback of pressure changes recorded from an intraluminal balloon in the sigmoid colons of 21 IBS patients. In a one-session pilot study, two-thirds of patients could decrease the frequency, amplitude, and duration of contractions and increase the volume of distension necessary to induce contractions. During repeat baseline studies eight weeks later, responders maintained the same levels of suppression of these responses. No clinical outcome data were reported.

Wise, Cooper, and Ahmed (1982) used a single group, pretest-posttest design to evaluate the effects of behaviorally oriented group therapy on twenty IBS patients. The group met for six 90-minute sessions which included didactic information about IBS, psychologically oriented group discussion, relaxation training, self-monitoring (of symptoms, emotional states, and stressors), and dietary advice. At posttest, patients reported improvement in both somatic and psychological symptoms which was maintained at a six-month follow-up. Obviously, given the single-group design it cannot be concluded that the treatment offered is any more effective than a placebo.

In what is probably the best study of psychotherapy for IBS to date, Svedlund, Sjodin, Ottosson, and Dotevall (1983) randomly assigned

101 outpatients with IBS to one of the two treatment groups. Both groups received similar medical treatment (bulk-forming agents, anticholinergic drugs, antacids, and minor tranquilizers as required) from gastroenterologists. Patients in one group also received 10 hour-long individual sessions of psychotherapy with a psychiatrist over a three-month period. Psychotherapy was aimed at modifying maladaptive behavior and problem solving. Sometimes a more educative strategy about relations between stressful life events and abdominal symptoms was used. Both the medical and psychotherapeutic treatments were tailored to the individual patient's needs. Patients were rated by the therapists and themselves on psychiatric and somatic symptoms before therapy, at three and fifteen months after the start of therapy. The psychotherapy group showed a significantly greater improvement in somatic symptoms after three months of therapy; one year after therapy they had improved further while the medical-only group showed some deterioration. Both groups improved to the same degree on psychological measures.

While this is the best study to date, it has a couple of serious methodological problems. The time spent with the patients in each group was not equal; hence, the advantage shown for psychotherapy plus medical treatment may be the result of nonspecific attention-placebo effects. Perhaps even more problematic is the fact that the raters were the therapists. One cannot, therefore rule out experimenter bias in accounting for the results.

Based on the behavioral model of IBS and on all of the treatment evidence reviewed above, Latimer (1983) has recommended a behavioral medicine approach to the treatment of IBS. In the context of the comprehensive assessment outlined above (Assessment procedures) and the behavior analysis, treatment has four major components, all or some of which may be required in any individual case:

1. Education
2. Symptom management
3. Stress management
4. Contingency management

1. *Education.* This takes place from the moment the initial interview begins. As the behavioral interviewer's approach to the problem gradually unfolds, the patient learns a new way of conceptualizing the disorder. The individual is viewed as having some learned maladaptive habits rather than a disease. The symptoms, whatever they are, are a variation of normal and are self-limited and benign. Contrary to what "common sense" frequently dictates, they are encouraged to cope

with rather than avoid situations precipitating the symptoms or in some cases the symptoms themselves. This is especially true in those cases where the physiological changes themselves are a phobic stimulus (Latimer, 1983, pp. 113–123).

Once a clear behavioral hypothesis has been formulated, the therapist explains this to the patient along with any other information necessary for its understanding. This may include basic information about the responsiveness of the gastrointestinal tract to stressful life events and emotional situations. It frequently also includes the correction of misconceptions about normal bowel habits and the significance of certain symptoms.

The behavior analysis and the process of self-monitoring frequently have the effect of increasing the patient's awareness of factors associated with the symptoms, and this in itself may produce some initial modest improvement.

2. *Symptom management.* The behavioral changes required of patients being treated for IBS may be substantial, and therefore symptomatic relief using behavioral methods alone is not always immediate. In those cases where a patient is significantly disabled, perhaps unable to work, or where the severity of symptoms makes it difficult for him or her to systematically cooperate in a behavioral treatment program, immediate symptom relief may be desirable and possible using nonbehavioral methods. This may involve the use of minor tranquillizers to relieve anxiety, antidepressants to relieve depression, or a bulk-forming agent and stool softener to relieve constipation. High-fiber diets and antispasmodic drugs are currently the main staples of symptomatic treatment by gastroenterologists; the evidence for their efficacy is reviewed above. In most cases, it is appropriate to present these measures as adjuncts to alleviate symptoms while the behavior analysis and treatment proceed.

3. *Stress management.* In few cases are patients simply told that their symptoms are due to stress. It is often not so simple, and such a facile explanation may lead to frustration and dissatisfaction when patients correctly observe an imperfect correlation between stressful life events and symptoms.

When it can be observed that symptoms result from an excessive autonomic reaction to certain stimuli, methods falling under the general category of stress management may be appropriate. The behavioral analysis may indicate the need for relaxation training, assertive training, marital therapy, or systematic desensitization of emotional reactions to certain situations (such as criticism or disapproval). Essentially, these and other stress management methods are aimed at helping the patient to either solve stressful problems or change emotional reactions to stressful circumstances that cannot be changed.

Since stress management is so often equated with relaxation training, it needs to be said that relaxation training alone, whether it includes Frontalis EMG biofeedback or not, is very seldom sufficient.

4. *Contingency management.* As discussed above (Pathophysiology), symptom reports do not necessarily correlate with excessive autonomic reactions. A child may report abdominal pain to avoid school or an adult to avoid sex, where these activities have become anxiety-producing for some reason. Others may simply complain to get attention from otherwise undemonstrative family members. When such factors are playing a part, stress management will be inadequate and misdirected. Appropriate treatment in these cases involves helping the patient to deal with fears or to get attention in more adaptive ways. The most crucial step, however, is to recognize the nature of the problem and the fact that certain reinforcing events (avoidance of anxiety, attention) are contingent on symptom complaints. In behavioral terms, treatment then involves making the reinforcing events contingent on more adaptive behavior—thus contingency management.

PAINLESS DIARRHEA

The diagnostic criteria for IBS (see above) specifically require both abdominal pain and change in bowel habit, thus excluding painless diarrhea. There is evidence that among patients with IBS, those characterized predominantly by pain have a greater number and duration of colonic segmental contractions than those in whom diarrhea predominates (Chaudhary & Truelove, 1961; Wangel & Deller, 1965). Segmental contractions in the colon are believed to mix the colonic contents and to retard transit thus facilitating absorption of fluids in the colon. An increased number and duration of segmental contractions would thus be consistent with constipation and a decrease with diarrhea (Latimer, 1983, Chapter 4).

Diarrhea-predominant IBS patients have also been distinguished from pain-predominant IBS patients by higher anxiety indices including scores on self-report anxiety inventories and urinary epinephrine excretion (Esler & Goulston, 1973). Increased excretion of the catecholamine metabolite vanillylmandelic acid in patients with "nervous diarrhea" has also been reported (Wright & Das, 1969).

Although diarrhea-predominant IBS and painless diarrhea are not symptomatically identical it seems unlikely that they are fundamentally distinct disorders. There is relatively little research on painless diarrhea which is less common than diarrhea-predominant IBS.

Among apparently healthy people, 3.7 percent report painless diarrhea (Thompson & Heaton, 1980).

PAINLESS CONSTIPATION

Painless constipation has been reported to occur in six percent of apparently healthy people (Thompson & Heaton, 1980). The diagnosis of constipation must be approached with caution since the term is often applied incorrectly. Connell, Hilton, Irvine, Lennard-Jones, and Misiewicz (1965) conducted population surveys of bowel habit and found that, for 99 percent of the population, the frequency of bowel movements fell within the range of three actions a week to three a day, inclusive. In spite of this, 19.7 percent took laxatives and 16 percent of those surveyed in a general practitioner's office regarded themselves as "constipated." The use of this term often bore no relation to frequency or consistency of bowel movements. For many people, anything less than one bowel movement per day is constipation. Although there is no universal agreement on the diagnostic criteria for constipation, most would agree that the consistency of stools is more relevant than their frequency; stools should be of small caliber and/or pellet-like.

Unlike IBS (pain and constipation), painless constipation is associated with a hypotonic, lax, and often distended rectum and colon. Factors which may contribute to its development include: inadequate dietary fiber, depression, chronic laxative use, and suppression of regular bowel movements due to pain or embarrassment.

It is well established that increasing dietary fiber produces a larger, looser stool and speeds up slow transit (Connell, 1978; Eastwood et al., 1973; Harvey, Pomare, & Heaton, 1973). It is necessary to ensure adequate fluid intake to complement the hydrophilic action of the fiber.

Depression is well known to be accompanied by constipation which usually improves along with the depression. Many antidepressants contribute to constipation as a side effect and it is difficult to predict the net effect of antidepressant drug therapy on bowel habit.

There may be both psychological and physiological contributions to the constipation resulting from chronic laxative abuse. Damaged myenteric neurons can result from chronic administration of anthracene cathartics (Smith, 1968). More important, however, is the psychological dependence on laxatives which leads to a disruption of the many learned aspects of a regular bowel habit (see Chapter 3, this volume).

If the urge to defecate is ignored, the rectum accommodates, and the urge passes. When this occurs repeatedly the rectum and colon can

Table 2.4.
Organic Contributions to Constipation

1.	Obstruction, e.g., carcinoma
2.	Metabolic, e.g., myxedema
3.	Defective innervation, e.g., spinal cord injury
4.	Pharmacologic, e.g., opiates
5.	Painful anorectal lesions, e.g., fissure-in-ano

become distended, the urge to defecate ceases to occur, and, at the extreme, fecal soiling occurs. Such suppression may occur because defecation is painful due to an anal fissure or following an operation, because it is socially inconvenient to go to the bathroom or because of anxiety about defecating in a strange environment.

The hypotonic colon may produce infrequent, large stools. Paradoxically, diarrhea may occur in impacted patients because only fluid finds its way around the solid fecal mass in the rectum. This may go unrecognized unless digital rectal examination is performed. In addition, fecal incontinence may occur if anal sphincter function is impaired by a large rectal mass; this is a frequent cause of encopresis in children (see Chapter 3, this volume).

Appropriate treatment of painless constipation depends on accurate diagnosis and behavior analysis. It must be remembered that not all constipation is functional; structural problems must be considered before making a diagnosis of functional constipation (see Table 2.4).

ESOPHAGEAL DISORDERS

Esophageal disorders have, to date, received relatively little attention from behavioral scientists. Several appear to be good candidates for research in the future; of these, nonspecific motor disorder is the prime example. Only a small percentage of patients with esophageal symptoms such as difficulty swallowing and/or chest pain, are eventually given a specific diagnosis such as diffuse esophageal spasm, achalasia, or scleroderma. Many more have a nonspecific motor disorder or perhaps no demonstrable manometric abnormality at all. Several facts suggest the possibility that these patients are analogous to and perhaps simply an upper gastrointestinal variation of IBS: (a) The motility tracings of these patients are frequently either normal or exhibit nonspecific abnormalities of a kind that may also be found in asymptomatic individuals (Pope, 1977); (b) a high percentage of these patients may be given a psychiatric diagnosis on psychiatric examination (Clouse & Lustman, 1983); (c) over 50 percent of IBS patients also have esophageal symptoms (Watson et al., 1978); (d) similar motility patterns have been reported to result from emotional stress (Wolf & Almy, 1949; Rubin, Nagler, Spiro, & Pilot, 1962) and acoustic stimulation (Stacher, Schmierer, & Landgrat, 1979).

Clouse and Lustman (1983) studied 50 consecutive patients who were referred for clinical esophageal manometry. Patients had both manometry and a structured psychiatric interview. Twenty-five (50%) had some form of contraction abnormality and a nonspecific motor disorder accounted for 18 of these. Thirteen had normal manometry. Fifty-eight percent had one or more lifetime psychiatric diagnoses and 84 percent of those with contraction abnormalities had a psychiatric condition. Depression, anxiety, and somatization disorder were the most frequent diagnoses.

Much of what has been written about applying the behavioral approach to IBS may therefore also apply to this disorder. Apart from the symptomatic use of progressive muscular relaxation in the treatment of "spastic esophagus" (Jacobson, 1927), I am unaware of any other published results of behavioral intervention for this disorder.

Intriguing possibilities for behavioral intervention are suggested by the report of the successful behavioral treatment of a woman with dysphagia, weight loss, and chest pain due to diffuse esophageal spasm (Latimer, 1981). In this case, failure of conventional medical treatment in the face of continued weight loss led to consideration for surgery. The need for surgery was obviated by the successful application of relaxation training which resulted in a significant reduction in painful esophageal spasms, weight gain, and an improvement in psychological state; there was, however, no change in the underlying esophageal motor disorder. After an initial unsuccessful attempt to eliminate the disordered motility using biofeedback of esophageal motility, it was discovered that by swallowing twice the patient could effectively normalize her motility. The optimal interval between swallows (about 7s) was arrived at by trial and error. It was hypothesized that the distal inhibition associated with the second swallow effectively inhibited the continuing maladaptive spasms initiated by the first swallow; the effect was demonstrated manometrically. The use of this "double swallowing" coping strategy had a beneficial effect in addition to that of the relaxation training and clinical improvements were maintained and increased at six-month follow-up. It must be emphasized, however, that this treatment allowed more effective coping and did not permanently alter the basic motility disorder which was still present at follow-up manometry.

More common in the behavioral literature are reports of the successful treatment of patients with a fear of swallowing, but who do not have any demonstrable disorder of motility. These patients are phobic and where there is no objective obstruction to ingestion, the treatment, as with other phobias, involves exposing the patient to the feared stimuli. This may be accomplished in a variety of ways, including the use of graded exposure in vivo, systematic desensitization, paradoxical intention, or aversion relief (Solyom & Sookman, 1980). Since many of these patients are rather obsessional in character graded exposure in vivo is, in my experience, usually the most straightforward and rapid method of treatment. In the therapist's presence the patient, whose fear of choking increases with the consistency of food, is asked to eat food of progressively firmer consistency. A food hierarchy might begin with liquids, purees, and minced foods and end with steak. The major guidelines for this therapeutic approach are that fear not be the reason to stop eating at any given session, and that the patient continue eating until there has been some decrement in anxiety level. They are encouraged to practice similar exposures at home between sessions. As with behavior therapy for other problems, the most appropriate treatment depends on the behavior analysis and frequently involves multiple interventions.

Finally, mention should be made of the use of biofeedback for the treatment of reflux esoghagitis. Schuster (1979) has reported that patients undergoing esophageal manometry can be taught to increase their lower esophageal sphincter pressure when given appropriate feedback; the magnitude of the increases achieved appear to be clinically significant to the extent that esophageal reflux is a function of lower esophageal sphincter pressure. This would appear to be a potentially useful treatment. Unfortunately, in all the years since the first report there have been no controlled trials to clearly demonstrate the clinical efficacy of this procedure.

VOMITING

Several distinct syndromes fall under this heading. Nausea and vomiting associated with cancer chemotherapy and bulimia (see Chapter 14, this volume) have received considerable attention. Infant rumination and adult psychogenic vomiting will be discussed here.

Rumination refers to the voluntary regurgitation of food from the stomach to the mouth where it may be chewed and reswallowed or spit out; it occurs primarily in infants and retarded individuals but may also occur in adults of normal intelligence. Rumination and chronic vomiting in infants and the mentally retarded can be life-threatening and therefore often require rapid suppression. For this reason, response-contingent punishment has frequently been used. Aversive electrical shock has been used contingent upon either the onset of vomiting or the occurrence of some consistent prevomiting behavior in infant ruminators (Lang & Melamed 1969; Toister, Colin, Worley, & Arthur, 1975; Cunningham & Linscheid, 1976; Linscheid & Cunningham, 1977) and mentally retarded patients (White & Taylor, 1976; Luckey, Watson, & Musick, 1968; Galbraith, Byrick, & Rutledge, 1970; Kohlenberg, 1970; Watkins, 1972; Wright & Thalassinos, 1973). Others have reported that the injection of lemon juice into the mouth can be substituted for electric shock in the treatment of the infant ruminator (Sajwaj, Libet, & Agras, 1974; Becker, Turner, & Sajwaj, 1978). In cases requiring less immediate results, the mentally retarded have also been treated using extinction procedures (Wolf, Brinbrauer, Williams, & Lawler, 1965), positive practice and restitution (Azrin & Wesolowski, 1975), forced vomiting (Spergel, 1975), and overcorrection (Duker & Seys, 1977).

An entirely different approach to this disorder is based on the theory that rumination is a self-stimulatory behavior that is a symptom of maternal social deprivation. An increase in noncontingent mothering or holding has been an effective treatment procedure in a number of published cases (Whitehead & Schuster, 1985).

In adult patients of normal intelligence, the methods described above are generally less applicable; fortunately, there has been no shortage of alternatives suggested. Since all of the reports to date are single cases, it is difficult to make many generalizations. Nevertheless, there appear to be two major subgroups of vomiters and intervention strategies. In the first group, vomiting appears to be an operant reinforced by attention from family, friends, physicians, or by the avoidance of difficult or anxiety producing special situations; these patients are often labeled hysterical. Treatment involves rearranging social contingencies so that reinforcement of the vomiting is eliminated and replaced by reinforcement of more adaptive, incompatible behavior (Alford, Blanchard, & Buckley, 1972; Ingersoll & Curry, 1977; Munford & Pally, 1979).

The second group appears to vomit in response to unpleasant internal sensations such as nausea, feeling full, pain and anxiety usually associated with eating; the vomiting itself is an avoidance response. These cases are akin to phobias; the unpleasant subjective state, which may be associated with a characteristic physiological response, occurs in response to specific identifiable stimuli and their identification leads to avoidance of these stimuli. These patients are frequently labeled obsessional or anorexic and treatment involves gradually exposing them to the feared stimuli (Peck, 1978; Welch, 1979; Mogan & O'Brien, 1972; Lang, 1965; Burgess, 1969; Stoffelmayer, 1970).

Our understanding of these problems could benefit from a tripartite (verbal, motoric, physiological) behavioral assessment as demonstrated by Latimer, Malmud, and Fisher (1982). They successfully treated a woman with a 30-year history of vomiting after eating. In this case, eating was followed by duodenal spasm demonstrated radiologically and by markedly delayed gastric emptying demonstrated by gastric scintiscan. Ingestion was consistently followed in 15 min by epigastric discomfort, belching, and regurgitation. Vomiting usually occurred after 15–30 min and was followed by a sense of relief and well-being. Failure to vomit led to increasing discomfort, a heavy, full feeling, and anxiety. The fact that in 30 years the patient had never had an "accident" in public but always made it to the washroom suggested that she had some control despite her perception of the vomiting being involuntary. Treatment by graded exposure in vivo and response prevention involved having the patient eat foods of progressively greater difficulty in the therapist's presence and without recourse to the washroom. Frequency of vomiting was dramatically reduced after one outpatient session and more slowly thereafter until it was completely eliminated. Following the initial large changes in overt behavior, the topography of her responses to eating began to change more slowly, the latency to epigastric discomfort increased, and the intensity of discomfort gradually decreased. When vomiting had entirely ceased, gastric emptying time had returned to normal and eating was unassociated with discomfort or belching.

SUMMARY

Although this review is by no means complete, it is apparent that the integration of behavioral and biomedical methods of assessment and treatment holds promise for the several functional gastrointestinal disorders discussed. It is my contention that the conceptual framework provided in the behavioral model of IBS is equally applicable to all functional gastrointestinal disorders and indeed to functional disorders in other systems as well; it could form the basis for a progressive research program. Nevertheless, it should be recognized that this way of thinking about these disorders is quite foreign to most of the professionals involved in both their treatment and research. This presents real obstacles in communicating that may have to be overcome before substantial progress occurs.

REFERENCES

Alford, G. S., Blanchard, E. G., & Buckley, T. M. (1972). Treatment of hysterical vomiting by modification of social contingencies: A case study. *Journal of Behavior Therapy and Experimental Psychiatry, 3,* 209–212.

Azrin, N. H., & Wesolowski, M. D. (1975). Eliminating habitual vomiting in a retarded adult by positive practice and self-correction. *Journal of Behavior Therapy and Experimental Psychiatry, 6,* 145–148.

Baume, P., & Cuthbert, J. (1973). The effect of medazepam in relieving symptoms of functional gastrointestinal distress. *Australian and New Zealand Journal of Medicine, 3,* 457–460.

Baume, P., Tracey, M., & Dawson, L. (1975). Efficacy of two minor tranquillizers in relieving symptoms of functional gastrointestinal distress. *Australian and New Zealand Journal of Medicine, 5,* 503–506.

Beck, A. T., Ward, G. H., Mendelson, M., Mack, J., & Erbaugh, J. (1961). An inventory for measuring depression. *Archives of General Psychiatry, 4,* 53–61.

Becker, J. F., Turner, S. M., & Sajwaj, T. E. (1978). Multiple behavioral effects of the use of lemon juice with a ruminating toddler-age child. *Behavior Modification, 2,* 267–268.

Bentley, S. J., Pearson, D. J., & Rix, K. J. B. (1983, August). Food hypersensitivity in irritable bowel syndrome. *Lancet, 6,* 295–297.

Berkowitz, J. M. (1978). A clinical assessment of lorazepam in the treatment of anxiety associated with gastrointestinal symptomatology. *Journal of Clinical Psychiatry, 39,* 46–52.

Bueno-Miranda, F., Cerulli, M., & Schuster, M. M. (1976). Operant conditioning of colonic motility in IBS. *Gastroenterology, 70,* 867.

Burgess, E. P. (1969). Elimination of vomiting behavior. *Behavior Research and Therapy, 7,* 173–176.

Cann, P. A., Read, N. W., & Holdsworth, C. D. (1984a). What is the benefit of coarse wheat bran in patients with irritable bowel syndrome? *Gut, 25,* 168–173.

Cann, P. A., Read, N. W., Holdsworth, C. D., & Barends, D. (1984b). Role of loperamide and placebo in management of irritable bowel syndrome. *Digestive Diseases And Sciences, 29,* 239–247.

Chaplan, A., & Vanov, S. K. (1977). G.I. illness: Treatment of the anxiety component. *Psychosomatics, 18,* 49–54.

Chaudhary, N. A., & Truelove, S. C. (1961). Human colonic motility: A comparative study of normal subjects, patients with ulcerative colitis and patients with irritable colon syndrome. *Gastroenterology, 40,* 1–36.

Chaudhary, N. A., & Truelove, S. C. (1962). The irritable colon syndrome. A study of the clinical features, predisposing causes and prognosis in 130 cases. *Quarterly Journal of Medicine, 31,* 307–322.

Clouse, R. E., & Lustman, P. J. (1983). Psychiatric illness and contraction abnormalities of the esophagus. *The New England Journal of Medicine, 309,* 1337–1342.

Cohen, S. I., & Reed, J. L. (1968). The treatment of "nervous diarrhea" and other conditioned autonomic disorders by desensitization. *British Journal of Psychiatry, 114,* 1275–1280.

Connell, A. M. (1978). The effects of dietary fiber on gastrointestinal motor function. *American Journal of Clinical Nutrition, 31,* S152–S156.

Connell, A. M., Hilton, C., Irvine, G., Lennard-Jones, J. E., & Misiewicz, J. J. (1965). Variation of bowel habit in two population samples. *British Medical Journal, 2,* 1095–1099.

Connell, A. M., Jones, F. A., & Rowlands, E. N. (1965). Motility of the pelvic colon. Part IV. Abdominal pain associated with colonic hyperactivity after meals. *Gut, 6,* 105–112.

Cunningham, C. E., & Linscheid, T. R. (1976). Elimination of chronic ruminating by electric shock. *Behavior Therapy, 7,* 231–234.

Drossman, D. A., Sandler, R. S., McKee, D. C., & Lovitz, A. J. (1982). Bowel patterns among subjects not seeking health care. *Gastroenterology, 83,* 529–534.

Duker, P., & Seys, D. (1977). Elimination of vomiting in a retarded female using restitutional overcorrection. *Behavior Therapy, 8,* 255–257.

Eastwood, M. A., Kirkpatrick, J. R., Mitchell, W. D., Bone, A. & Hamilton, T. (1973). Effects of dietary supplements of wheat bran and cellulose on faeces and bowel function. *British Medical Journal, 4,* 392–394.

Esler, M. D., & Goulston, K. J. (1973). Levels of anxiety in colonic disorders. *New England Journal of Medicine, 288,* 16–20.

Feighner, J. P., Robins, E., Guze, S. B., Woodruff, R. A., Winokur, G., & Munoz, R. (1972). Diagnostic criteria for use in psychiatric research. *Archives of General Psychiatry, 26,* 57–63.

Ferguson, A., Sircus, W., & Eastwood, M. A. (1977). Frequency of 'functional' gastrointestinal disorders. *Lancet, 2,* 613–614.

Fielding, J. F. (1977a). A year in out-patients with irritable bowel syndrome. *Irish Journal of Medical Science, 146,* 162–166.

Fielding, J. F. (1977b). The irritable bowel syndrome. *Clinical Gastroenterology, 6,* 607–622.

Furman, S. (1973). Intestinal biofeedback in functional diarrhea: A preliminary report. *Journal of Behavior Therapy & Experimental Psychiatry, 4,* 317–321.

Furtado, J. D. (1976). Lorazepam in gastrointestinal disorders with anxiety overlay. *Psychosomatics, 17,* 32–34.

Galbraith, D. A., Byrick, R. J., & Rutledge, J. T. (1970). An aversive conditioning approach to the inhibition of chronic vomiting. *Canadian Psychiatric Association Journal, 15,* 311–313.

Goulston, K. (1972). Drug usage in the irritable colon syndrome. *Medical Journal of Australia, 1,* 1126–1131.

Harvey, R. F., Pomare, E. W., & Heaton, K. W. (1973). Effect of bran on bowel function. *British Medical Journal, 4,* 614.

Harvey, R. F., Salih, S. Y., & Read, A. E. (1983, March). Organic and functional disorders in 2000 gastroenterology outpatients. *Lancet, 19,* 632–634.

Heefner, J. D., Wilder, R. M., & Wilson, I. D. (1978). Irritable colon and depression. *Psychosomatics, 19,* 540–547.

Hillman, L. C., Stace, N. H., Fisher, A., & Pomare, E. W. (1982). Dietary intakes and stool characteristics of patients with irritable bowel syndrome. *American Journal of Clinical Nutrition, 36,* 626–629.

Holmes, K. M., & Salter, R. H. (1982). Irritable bowel syndrome—a safe diagnosis? *British Medical Journal, 285,* 1533–1534.

Ingersoll, B. & Curry, F. (1977). Rapid treatment of persistent vomiting in a 14-year-old female by shaping and time-out. *Journal of Behavior Therapy and Experimental Psychiatry, 8,* 305–307.

Ivey, K. J. (1975). Are anticholinergics of use in the irritable colon syndrome? *Gastroenterology, 68,* 1300–1307.

Jacobson, E. (1927). Spastic esophagus and mucus colitis. *Archives of Internal Medicine, 39,* 433–445.

Kasich, A. M. (1973). Chlorazepate dipotassium in the treatment of anxiety associated with chronic gastrointestinal disease. *Current Therapeutic Research, 15,* 83–91.

Kasich, A. M., Richards, D. J., & Vanov, S. K. (1976). Lorazepam in the management of anxiety associated with chronic gastrointestinal disease: A double blind study. *Current Therapeutic Research, 19,* 292–307.

Keeling, P. W. M., & Fielding, J. F. (1975). The irritable bowel syndrome: A review of 50 consecutive cases. *Journal of the Irish College of Physicians, 4,* 91–94.

Kohlenberg, R. J. (1970). The punishment of persistent vomiting: A case study. *Journal of Applied Behavior Analysis, 3,* 241–245.

Lancaster-Smith, M. J., Prout, B. J., Pinto, T., Anderson, J. A., & Schiff, A. A. (1982). Influence of drug treatment on the irritable bowel syndrome and its interaction with psychoneurotic morbidity. *Acta Psychiatrica Scandinavica, 66,* 33–41.

Lancet. (1972). Unruly guts [Editorial]. *Lancet, 4,* 960–961.

Lang, P. J. (1965). Behavior therapy with a case of nervous anorexia. In L. P. Ullmann & L. Krasner (Eds.), *Case studies in behavior modification* (pp. 217–221). New York: Holt, Rinehart & Winston.

Lang, P. J. (1968). Fear reduction and fear behavior: Problems in treating a construct. In T. M. Shlien (Ed.), *Research in psychotherapy* (Vol. III). Washington, DC: American Psychological Association.

Lang, P. J., & Melamed, B. G. (1969). Case report: Avoidance conditioning therapy of an infant with chronic ruminative vomiting. *Journal of Abnormal Psychology, 74,* 1–8.

Latimer, P. R. (1981). Biofeedback and self-regulation in the treatment of diffuse esophageal spasm: A single-case study. *Biofeedback and Self-Regulation, 6,* 181–189.

Latimer, P. R. (1983). *Functional gastrointestinal disorders. A behavioral medicine approach.* New York: Springer.

Latimer, P. R., Campbell, D., Latimer, M. R., Sarna, S. K., Daniel, E. E., & Waterfall, W. E. (1979). Irritable bowel syndrome: A test of the colonic hyperalgesia hypothesis. *Journal of Behavioral Medicine, 2,* 285–295.

Latimer, P. R., Malmud, L. S., & Fisher, R. S. (1982). Gastric stasis and vomiting: Behavioral treatment. *Gastroenterology, 83,* 684–688.

Latimer, P. R., Sarna, S. K., Campbell, D., Latimer, M. R., Waterfall, W. E., & Daniel, E. E. (1981). Colonic motor and myoelectrical activity: A comparative study of normal subjects, psychoneurotic patients and patients with irritable bowel syndrome (IBS). *Gastroenterology, 80,* 893–901.

Linscheid, T. R., & Cunningham, C. E. (1977). A controlled demonstration of the effectiveness of electric shock in the elimination of chronic infant rumination. *Journal of Applied Behavior Analysis, 10,* 500.

Liss, J. L., Alpers, D., & Woodruff, R. A. (1973). The irritable colon syndrome and psychiatric illness. *Diseases of the Nervous System, 34,* 151–157.

Luckey, R. E., Watson, C. M., & Musick, J. K. (1968). Aversive conditioning as a means of inhibiting vomiting and rumination. *American Journal of Mental Deficiency, 73,* 139–142.

Mendeloff, A. I. (1979). Epidemiology of the irritable bowel syndrome. *Practical Gastroenterology, 3,* 12–18.

Mogan, J., & O'Brien, J. S. (1972). The counterconditioning of a vomiting habit by sips of ginger ale. *Journal of Behavior Therapy and Experimental Psychiatry, 3,* 135–137.

Munford, P. R., & Pally, R. (1979). Outpatient contingency management of operant vomiting. *Journal of Behavior Therapy and Experimental Psychiatry, 10,* 135–137.

Myren, J., Groth, H., Larssen, S. E., & Larsen, S. (1982). The effect of trimipramine in patients with the irritable bowel syndrome. *Scandinavian Journal of Gastroenterology, 17,* 872–875.

Newcomer, A. D., & McGill, D. B. (1983). Irritable bowel syndrome. Role of lactose deficiency. *Mayo Clinic Proceedings, 58,* 339–341.

Palmer, R. L., Stonehill, E., Crisp, A. H., Waller, S. L., & Misiewicz, J. J. (1974). Psychological characteristics of patients with the irritable bowel syndrome. *Postgraduate Medical Journal, 50,* 416–419.

Peck, C. L. (1978). Modification of a learned vomiting ritual by change in stimulus conditions and self-controlled response prevention. *Journal of Behavior Therapy and Experimental Psychiatry, 9,* 359–363.

Piai, G., & Mazzacca, G. (1979). Prifinium bromide in the treatment of the irritable colon syndrome. *Gastroenterology, 77,* 500–502.

Pope, C. E. (1977). Motor disorders of the esophagus. *Postgraduate Medicine, 61,* 118–125.

Rachman, S. J. (1978). *Fear and courage.* San Francisco: W. H. Freeman.

Ritchie, J. (1973). Pain from distension of the pelvic colon by inflating a balloon in the irritable colon syndrome. *Gut, 14,* 125–132.

Rubin, J., Nagler, R., Spiro, H. M., & Pilot, M. L. (1962). Measuring the effect of emotions on esophageal motility. *Psychosomatic Medicine, 24,* 170–176.

Sajwaj, T., Libet, J., & Agras, S. (1974). Lemon-juice therapy: The control of life-threatening rumination in a six-month-old infant. *Journal of Applied Behavior Analysis, 7,* 557–563.

Samet, C. M. (1976). The evaluation of Bellergal tablets compared to Librium and placebo in the treatment of symptoms of anxiety tension states associated with functional gastrointestinal disorders. *Psychosomatics, 17,* 202–209.

Schuster, M. M. (1979). Biofeedback control of gastrointestinal motility. In J. V. Basmajian (Ed.), *Biofeedback-principles and practice for clinicians.* Baltimore: Williams & Wilkins.

Sjodin, I., & Svedlund, J. (1985). Psychological aspects of non-ulcer dyspepsia: A psychosomatic view focusing on a comparison between the irritable bowel syndrome and peptic ulcer disease. *Scandinavian Journal of Gastroenterology, Supplement No. 109,* 51–58.

Smith, B. (1968). Effect of irritant purgatives on the myenteric plexus in man and the mouse. *Gut, 9,* 139–143.

Snape, W. J., Carlson, A. M., & Cohen, S. (1976). Colonic myoelectric activity in the irritable bowel syndrome. *Gastroenterology, 70,* 326–330.

Soltoft, J., Gudmand-Hoyer, E., Krag, B., Kristensen, E., & Wulff, H. R. (1976). A double-blind trial of the effect of wheat bran on symptoms of irritable bowel syndrome. *Lancet, 1,* 270–272.

Solyom, L., & Sookman, D. (1980). Fear of choking and its treatment: A behavioral approach. *Canadian Journal of Psychiatry, 25,* 30–34.

Spergel, S. M. (1975). Induced vomiting treatment of acute compulsive vomiting. *Journal of Behavior Therapy and Experimental Psychiatry, 6,* 79–82.

Stacher, G., Schmierer, G., & Landgrat, M. (1979). Tertiary esophageal contractions evoked by acoustical stimuli. *Gastroenterology, 77,* 49–54.

Steinhart, M. J., Wong, P. Y., & Zarr, M. L. (1981). Therapeutic usefulness of amitriptyline in spastic colon syndrome. *International Journal of Psychiatry in Medicine, 11,* 45–57.

Stoffelmeyer, B. E. (1970). The treatment of a retching response to dentures by counteractive reading aloud. *Journal of Behavior Therapy and Experimental Psychiatry, 1,* 163–168.

Svedlund, J., Sjodin, I., Ottosson, J., & Dotevall, G. (1983). Controlled study of psychotherapy in irritable bowel syndrome. *Lancet, 2*(8350), 589–591.

Switz, D. M. (1976). What the gastroenterologist does all day. *Gastroenterology, 70,* 1048–1050.

Taylor, I., Darby, C., & Hammond, P. (1978). Comparison of rectosigmoid myoelectrical activity in the irritable colon syndrome during relapses and remissions. *Gut, 19,* 923–929.

Thompson, W. G., & Heaton, K. W. (1980). Functional bowel disorders in apparently healthy people. *Gastroenterology, 79,* 283–288.

Toister, R. P., Colin, J., Worley, L. M., & Arthur, D. (1975). Faradic therapy of chronic vomiting in infancy: A case study. *Journal of Behavior Therapy and Experimental Psychiatry, 6,* 55–59.

Tucker, D. M., Sandstead, H. H., Logan, G. M., Klevay, L. M., Mahalko, J., Johnson, L. K., Inman, L., & Inglett, G. E. (1981). Dietary fiber and

personality factors as determinants of stool output. *Gastroenterology, 81,* 879–883.
Wangel, A. G., & Deller, D. J. (1965). Intestinal motility in man: III Mechanisms of constipation and diarrhea with particular reference to the irritable colon syndrome. *Gastroenterology, 48,* 69–84.
Watkins, J. T. (1972). Treatment of chronic vomiting and extreme emaciation by an aversive stimulus: Case study. *Psychological Reports, 31,* 803–805.
Watson, W. C., Sullivan, S. N., Corke, M. & Rush, D. (1978). Globus and headache: Common symptoms of the irritable bowel syndrome. *Canadian Medical Association Journal, 118,* 387–388.
Weinstock, S. A. (1976). The re-establishment of intestinal control in functional colitis. *Biofeedback and Self-Regulation, 1,* 324.
Welch, G. J. (1979). The treatment of compulsive vomiting and obsessive thoughts through graduated response delay, response prevention, and cognitive correction. *Journal of Behavior Therapy and Experimental Psychiatry, 10,* 77–82.
Welgan, P., Meshkinpour, H., & Hoehler, F. (1985). The effect of stress on colon motor and electrical activity in irritable bowel syndrome. *Psychosomatic Medicine, 47,* 139–149.
Wender, P. H., & Kalm, M. (1983). Prevalence of attention deficit disorder, residual type, and other psychiatric disorders in patients with irritable colon syndrome. *American Journal of Psychiatry, 140,* 1579–1582.
West, K. L. (1970). MMPI correlates of ulcerative colitis. *Journal of Clinical Psychology, 26,* 214–219.
White, B. U., & Jones, C. M. (1940). Mucous colitis: A delineation of the syndrome with certain observations on its mechanism and on the role of emotional tension as a precipitating factor. *Annals of Internal Medicine, 14,* 854–872.
White, J. D., & Taylor, D. (1976). Noxious conditioning as a treatment for rumination. *Mental Retardation, 5,* 30–33.
Whitehead, W. E., Engel, B. T., & Schuster, M. M. (1980). Irritable bowel syndrome: Physiological and psychological differences between diarrhea-predominant and constipation-predominant patients. *Digestive Diseases and Sciences, 25,* 404–413.
Whitehead, W. E., & Schuster, M. M. (1985). *Gastrointestinal disorders. Behavioral and physiological basis for treatment.* Toronto: Academic Press.
Wise, T. N., Cooper, J. N., & Ahmed, S. (1982). The efficacy of group therapy for patients with irritable bowel syndrome. *Psychosomatics, 23,* 465–469.
Wolf, M., Brinbrauer, J., Williams, T., & Lawler, J. (1965). A note on apparent extinction of the vomiting behavior of a retarded child. In L. P. Ullmann & L. Krasner (Eds.), *Case studies in behavior modification* (pp. 364–366). New York: Holt, Rinehart & Winston.
Wolf, S., & Almy, T. P. (1949). Experimental observations on cardiospasm in man. *Gastroenterology, 13,* 401–421.
Wolpe, J., & Lang, P. J. (1969). *Fear survey schedule.* San Diego: Educational and Industrial Testing Service.

Wright, J. T., & Das, A. K. (1969). Excretion of 4-hydroxy-3-methoxy mandelic acid in cases of ulcerative colitis and diarrhea of nervous origin. *Gut, 10,* 628–630.

Wright, L., & Thalassinos, P. A. (1973). Success with electroshock in habitual vomiting: Report of two cases in young children. *Clinical Pediatrics, 12,* 594–597.

Youell, K. J., & McCullough, J. P. (1975). Behavioral treatment of mucous colitis. *Journal of Consulting and Clinical Psychology, 43,* 740–745.

Young, S. J., Alpers, D. H., Norland, C. C., & Woodruff, R. A. (1976). Psychiatric illness and the irritable bowel syndrome. *Gastroenterology, 70,* 162–166.

3

The Behavioral Medicine Approach to Fecal Incontinence

Paul R. Latimer

Kelowna, B.C.
Canada

Fecal incontinence among adults is a relatively uncommon and much neglected clinical problem. It is for most patients a serious social embarrassment which confines many to their homes. Although there are idiopathic cases, most arise as sequelae to a variety of medical and surgical disorders (see Table 3.1). Recent advances in the assessment and treatment of this disorder provide an excellent model of the behavioral medicine approach. They reflect a true integration of concepts and methods from the biomedical and behavioral sciences (Latimer, 1980).

PATHOPHYSIOLOGY

Incontinence occurs predominantly at the two ends of the age spectrum. Defecation is initially an unlearned reflexive response usually

Table 3.1.
Causes of Fecal Incontinence

SPHINCTER INJURY	
	— childbirth
	— surgical
	— hemorrhoids
	— anal fissures
	— imperforate anus
	— Hirschsprung's disease
	— tumors
	— inflammatory bowel disease
NEUROLOGICAL	
	— myelomeningocele
	— multiple sclerosis
	— cerebrovascular accident
	— spinal cord injuries or tumors
	— diabetic neuropathy
OTHER MEDICAL	
	— rectal prolapse
	— inflammatory bowel disease
	— scleroderma
IDIOPATHIC	

initiated by meals which stimulate the gastroileocolic reflex. The learning of continence is one of the earliest socialization experiences and as such is a function of the child's biological capability and the interaction between the child and his parents. Defecation in socially inappropriate situations by children over the age of five is usually referred to as encopresis. Although encopresis can result from some of the same disorders as incontinence among adults, it usually results from either constipation (with overflow incontinence) or psychological disturbances.

At the other end of the age spectrum are the demented, whose incontinence, along with that of psychotic and severely retarded individuals, often results from social indifference much as it does in children prior to toilet training. The demented may require diapers and/or other toileting assistance just as infants do, the psychotics require treatment of their psychosis and the retarded may respond to intensive behavioral training programs which have been developed for them (Foxx & Azrin, 1973).

This chapter is concerned predominantly with fecal incontinence among adults which results neither from inadequate childhood toilet training nor from social indifference. Although there are a variety of physical structures and physiological mechanisms involved in the maintenance of continence, it is the anal sphincters and rectosphincteric reflexes which are most accessible to study, best understood, and which have so far been most relevant to behavioral medicine approaches to treatment.

According to current understanding there are two components to the anal sphincter: an internal and external sphincter. The internal sphincter is an extension of the smooth muscle of the wall of the rectum and is involuntary. The external sphincter consists of three bundles of striated muscle and is under voluntary control. When the rectum is distended, as it is when stool descends from the proximal colon prior to a bowel movement, there is a reflex relaxation of the internal anal sphincter which is tonically contracted at rest. Continence depends on the rectal distension being sensed, the external sphincter being contracted, and that contraction being of sufficient magnitude and duration to oppose the forces of elimination (Schuster, 1975). Unlike most other skeletal muscles the external anal sphincter is tonically contracted at rest. In continent adults distension of the rectum is associated with a further brief contraction of the external sphincter.

The relaxation of the internal sphincter allows rectal contents to come into contact with the sensory epithelium which lines the proximal anal canal. These sensors are capable of discriminating solids, liquids, and gas. When the urge to defecate has been felt, a conscious sampling may be done by increasing abdominal tension and voluntarily increasing the activity of the external sphincter. In a continent individual the solids can be retained and gas expelled to relieve intrarectal pressure. Fluid contents can be detected and retained by voluntary contraction of the external sphincter.

Until recently the external sphincter response was thought to be an unlearned reflex but it now appears to be learned, probably during toilet training. That the external sphincter response to rectal distension is a voluntary response cued by the perception of rectal distension is suggested by the following observations:

1. Many constipated patients do not show this response, presumably because they have little need for it
2. Normal subjects can omit the response with little or no practice when requested to do so
3. In spinal cord transected humans, the reflex response to rectal distension is an inhibition of resting tone in the external sphincter rather than a contraction
4. The response is significantly less likely to occur in normal subjects during sleep (Whitehead, Orr, Engel, & Schuster, 1982).

This distinction has obvious clinical significance. The absence of an unlearned reflex response would strongly suggest interruption of the reflex arc, that is, a neurological disorder. The absence of an operant response to a discriminative stimulus could occur because of lack of motivation, failure to perceive the stimulus, inability to emit the response, or because of the association between stimulus and response was never learned.

Other factors which are undoubtedly relevant to continence include stool consistency, anal, rectal, and colonic motility, rectal compliance, and angulation of the anorectal junction. Liquid stool may compromise continence particularly in the presence of a marginally competent sphincter. The combination of liquid stool with strong propulsive colonic contractions as with certain types of diarrhea or following certain enemas or laxatives make continence particularly difficult.

Within certain biological limits the rectum is compliant or accommodating. An initial urge to defecate and relaxation of the internal sphincter precipitated by a fecal mass in the rectum gradually subsides if defecation is socially inhibited. Receptive relaxation occurs, and the rectum expands to accommodate the stool and intraluminal pressure returns to normal. As the fecal mass increases, the limits of compliance are reached and there is a gradual increase in rectal pressure accompanied by a persistent urge to defecate. In certain conditions such as inflammatory bowel disease and scleroderma there is fibrosis and loss of elasticity of the rectum. This results in urgency and, potentially, incontinence if there is no toilet immediately available.

The angulation of the anorectal junction is due to the continuous activity of the puborectalis muscle (which also forms the deep bundle of the external anal sphincter) which encircles this region like a sling (see Figure 3.2). This angulation is extremely important for continence. Defecation is associated with straightening of this angulation due to relaxation of the puborectalis muscle. Any fecal mass in the lower rectum acts gravitationally on the internal aperture of the anal canal. When the anal canal is vertically oriented, the whole weight of the mass must be opposed by the sphincter. When the anal canal is obliquely directed, as it is when the puborectalis muscle is tonically contracted, only a component of the force of the fecal mass must be opposed by the strength of the sphincter. The greater the angulation the less the squeeze force necessary for continence. Compromise of this puborectalis sling, as sometimes occurs due to surgery or due to congenital malformations, usually results in incontinence (Kerremans, 1969).

ASSESSMENT

Assessment naturally includes the usual history, physical examination, and self-monitoring of episodes of incontinence. Particular attention is paid to identifying the various causes of incontinence that are outlined in Table 3.1, and to ensuring that adequate assessment and treatment of underlying medical conditions has occurred. Self-monitoring focuses not only on episodes of frank fecal incontinence but also on stained underwear, changes of underwear, and use of laxatives or enemas. It is also important to distinguish actual incontinence from fear of incontinence. The latter is not uncommon and may lead to an agoraphobia-like syndrome. There is often, in such cases, a history of a single episode of incontinence which may have occurred for obvious medical reasons, that is, during an episode of gastroenteritis with severe diarrhea and urgency. Irrational fear of incontinence may be treated by graduated exposure in-vivo (as may other phobias) without recourse to the methods to be described later which are directed at actual fecal incontinence.

The assessment of the anal sphincters is quite specific and owes its origin to biomedical science. Although there are various methods available, the most commonly used is a system of tandem balloons (Schuster, Hookman, Hendrix, & Mendeloff, 1965). This method is safe, requires no bowel preparation, and is about as uncomfortable as a digital rectal examination. The device consists of a hollow steel cylinder around which is tied a double latex balloon, creating two separate compartments. A third rectal balloon is affixed to polyethylene tubing and inserted through the hollow core of the steel cylinder.

With the patient in the left lateral position and following a digital rectal examination to ensure the absence of obstructions, the rectal balloon (fully deflated and lubricated) is inserted first and advanced into the rectum. The metal cylinder with tandem balloons is next advanced along the tubing of the rectal balloon which was previously inserted through the hollow core of the metal cylinder. With both balloons deflated and lubricated the cylinder is inserted into the anal canal until the second balloon is almost out of sight. The internal sphincter balloon is now inflated with 10 cc of air, and during this process it should slip farther into the rectum. Gentle traction is now applied to the external cross member of the metal cylinder while the external sphincter balloon is inflated with 10 cc of air. The device should assume the position shown in Figure 3.1. When the sphincters are normal the device will usually remain in place without assistance; in other cases adhesive tape from the cross member of the metal cylinder to the buttocks may be required to maintain this position. Polyethylene tubing joins each balloon to a pressure transducer; the electrical output from these devices is amplified and recorded by a direct-writing polygraph.

The rectal balloon is primarily for distending the rectum and thereby simulating the usual stimulus to defecation; pressure can also be measured from it but this is not usually necessary. The other two balloons are specifically designed by their configuration to reflect the activity of the internal and external sphincter separately. The separation of the activity of the two sphincters is complicated by the fact that they overlap as can be seen in Figure 3.1.

A typical manometric assessment might include determination of the resting tone of the sphincters, the patient's maximal voluntary sphincteric contraction, sphincteric responses to brief distension of the rectal balloon at a series of standard volumes and for various durations of distension and minimum volume of distension necessary to evoke sensation, external sphincter contraction, and internal sphincter relaxation. Incontinence is associated with an elevated threshold for detecting distension, a lowered threshold for urgency to distension, reduced external sphincter strength (Latimer, Campbell, & Kasperski, 1984), and elevated threshold for phasic external sphincter contraction (Wald & Tunuguntla, 1984). Incontinence can result from impairment of either sensation or external sphincter strength.

This method does have certain limitations. The pressures recorded are a function of the balloon's elasticity, shape, and volume and cannot be taken as absolutes. Open-ended perfused catheters provide a more accurate measure of intraluminal pressure (Latimer, 1983, p. 51).

Even an accurate measure of intraluminal pressure, however, does not necessarily accurately reflect sphincter function. Intraluminal pressure can be influenced by the gluteal muscles and by anatomical variables such as the amount of adipose tissue in the buttocks. These problems can be overcome where necessary by measuring sphincter EMG activity directly, using needle or flexible fine wire electrodes. These have the disadvantage of causing pain and thus causing reactive changes in sphincter activity. Surface electrodes can also be used for measuring EMG activity but they cannot discriminate sphincter EMG activity from that of the surrounding muscles (Latimer, 1983, Chapter 4; Schuster, 1975; Whitehead & Schuster, 1983). Thus, each of these methods has potential specific application and each has limitations. Recently, there have been attempts to develop simpler, less expensive devices for use at home. MacLeod (1983) has developed a particularly compact unit suitable for home use. It involves a dumbbell-shaped intra-anal plug containing two ring electrodes connected to an electromyometer so that electrical impulses generated by sphincter contractions can be presented to the patient both as a meter reading and as an audible sound. This device does not allow differentiation of internal and external sphincter activity nor does it provide for assessment of sensory deficits.

Constantinides and Cywes (1983) have described a simple pneumatic device for home biofeedback training in patients who have failed to develop social fecal continence following sacroabdominoperineal pull-through operations for anorectal anomalies. This device is intended to measure contractions of the puborectalis muscle. It provides no information about the response of the internal sphincter. It is simple and inexpensive but no data are provided with respect to its effectiveness.

TREATMENT

Before the application of behavioral principals to the problem of fecal incontinence, there were low-residue diets, carefully timed enemas, and various techniques of sphincteroplasty, but their efficacy was poorly documented.

The development of biofeedback for fecal incontinence illustrates the essential nature of behavioral medicine. Methods that had already been developed in the service of understanding the physiology of continence were simply combined with behavioral principles. What had been a physiological assessment procedure became treatment. It was truly a marriage of behavioral and biomedical methods.

The first attempt at biofeedback for anal incontinence was made by Haskell and Rovner (1967). This early report has not been widely recognized and was not even referenced by Engel, Nikoomanesh, and Schuster (1974) who are frequently credited with the first published report of the use of biofeedback for fecal incontinence. Haskell and Rovner used needle electrodes, auditory and visual feedback, and combined low-voltage electrostimulation with encouragement to maximize voluntary contractions. Treatments were given three times a week for two weeks and then once a week. The mean number of treatments necessary is not reported. They reported success in 71 percent of patients with a normally innervated sphincter and partial anal incontinence. Only 36 percent of patients with an abnormally innervated sphincter improved. The criterion for classifying a patient as improved and the duration of follow-up were not reported. The authors did not believe that improvement resulted from the passive muscle response to the surging electric current.

The method that has been most widely applied was first described by Engel, Nikoomanesh, and Schuster (1974) and utilized the three-balloon manometric system shown in Figure 3.1. Patients were shown their rectosphincteric responses to inflation of a balloon in the rectum and were shown how their responses differed from those of continent subjects. In these patients the external sphincter response was either diminished or absent. The patients were then encouraged to attempt to approximate the normal response each time the rectal balloon was inflated. Patients were praised for approximations to the normal response. Using praise and visual feedback the patients were also taught to synchronize sphincteric responses so that the external-sphincter contraction occurred simultaneously with internal sphincter relaxation. Finally, patients were gradually weaned from the need for the apparatus by periodically withholding visual feedback.

Using this method they initially reported on seven patients whose incontinence arose from a variety of medical and surgical causes. Four became completely continent after treatment, two were much improved and one dropped out (Table 3.2). In a subsequent progress report, Cerulli, Nikoomanesh, and Schuster (1979) followed 50 consecutive patients with severe daily fecal incontinence from a variety of medical and surgical causes, who received this treatment (see Table 3.2). Thirty-six of 50 patients achieved a decrease in frequency of incontinence of at least 90 percent. Seventy-five percent of these required only one training session!

Using an entirely different approach, Schiller, Santa Ana, Davis, and Fordtran (1979) treated a patient with incontinence secondary to chronic diarrhea of unknown etiology (see Table 3.2). In this case the patient was urged to retain as much of a 25-min rectal infusion of 1500 ml of saline as possible. After 10 training sessions, the patient increased her ability to retain the fluid sevenfold. In spite of continued diarrhea she became continent. Anal sphincter pressure and her ability to retain a solid sphere against traction did not change during or after training. She had a hypotensive sphincter mechanism and normal sensitivity both before and after treatment. The mechanism of improvement is therefore obscure. The authors speculated that rectal compliance may have been enhanced. A reduction in urgency was consistent with this but there was no change in stool frequency as one might have expected.

This example is interesting because it involved feedback of a complex function, that is, continence, rather than of a single specific physiological variable. Any or all of the physiological mechanisms involved in continence may have been trained.

Goldenberg, Hodges, Hersh, and Jinich (1980), utilizing the three-balloon manometric method, treated 12 patients whose incontinence resulted from a variety of medical and surgical conditions (see Table 3.2). Ten patients had good responses with complete continence in six patients. Nine of ten responders required only one treatment session.

Olness, McParland, and Piper (1980), utilizing a three-balloon manometric system (not the Schuster apparatus), treated 50 children, 10 of whom had had surgical repair, in infancy, of imperforate anus and 40 of whom had chronic constipation and overflow incontinence (see Table 3.2). All had had extensive investigations and previous treatment methods before being referred for biofeedback. Of the 10 patients with surgical repair of imperforate anus six achieved complete continence while one had minor soiling. Among the functional constipation group, 24 developed normal bowel habits with no incontinence, 14 developed normal bowel movements with minor soiling, while the remaining two continued to have major problems.

Wald (1981a), using the three-balloon manometric system, treated 17 incontinent patients with mixed medical and surgical problems (see Table 3.2). Ten were completely continent while an additional two achieved at least a 75 percent decrease in the frequency of incontinence. Biofeedback led to a decrease in the volume of rectal distension required to elicit an external sphincter contraction in both good and poor responders, and there were no significant differences between these two groups. Several poor responders were incontinent in spite of

Table 3.2.
Outcome Studies of Biofeedback for Fecal Incontinence

Authors	Method	Patient Population	Number of Patients	Age of Patients (years)	Duration of Follow-Up	Results
Haskell and Rovner (1967)	Needle electromyography	Patients undergoing assessment for surgery for incontinence	54	6–73	?	27 of 38 (71%) with normally innervated sphincter became completely continent 6 of 16 (36%) with abnormally innervated sphincter became completely continent
Engel, Nikoomanesh, and Schuster (1974)	Three-balloon manometric system	Mixed medical-surgical	7	6–54	6 months–5 years	4 completely continent 2 much improved 1 drop-out due to pain
Cerulli, Nikoomanesh, and Schuster (1979)	Three-balloon manometric system	Mixed medical-surgical	50	5–97	4–108 months	20 completely continent 16 at least 90% decrease in frequency of incontinence
Schiller, Santa Ana, Davis, and Fordtran (1979)	Rectally infused saline	Chronic diarrhea—etiology unknown	1	31	10 weeks	complete continence

MacLeod (1979)	Intra-anal plug electromyography	Mixed medical-surgical incontinence of gas and liquid only	17	25–79	1–2 years	6 complete continence 4 almost complete 3 moderately improved 2 slight improvement 2 no improvement
Goldenberg, Hodges, Hersh, and Jinich (1980)	Three-balloon manometric system	Mixed medical-surgical	12	12–78	10–96 weeks	6 complete continence 3 < 1 minor episode/month 1 < 1 minor episode/week 2 no improvement
Olness, McParland, and Piper (1980)	Three-balloon manometric system (not the Schuster system)	10 surgical repair of imperforate anus 40 chronic functional constipation	50	4–18	6 months–3 years	*Imperforate Anus* 6 complete continence 1 minor soiling 1 major soiling 2 no improvement *Functional Constipation* 24 complete continence 14 minor soiling 1 major soiling 1 no improvement
Wald (1981)	Three-balloon manometric system	Mixed medical-surgical	17	10–79	2–38 months	10 completely continent 2 at least a 75% decrease in frequency of incontinence

Table 3.2. (cont'd.)
Outcome Studies of Biofeedback for Fecal Incontinence

Authors	Method	Patient Population	Number of Patients	Age of Patients (years)	Duration of Follow-Up	Results
Wald (1981) (1983)	Three-balloon manometric system	**Meningomyelocele**	15	5–33	8–30 months	3 complete continence 4 90% decrease in frequency of incontinence 8 no improvement
Whitehead, Parker, Masek, Cataldo, and Freeman (1981)	Three-balloon manometric system	**Myelomeningocele**	8	5–15	13–24 months	4 ≤ 1 episode/mo. 2 1 episode/day 2 no change
MacLeod (1983)	Intra-anal plug electromyography	**Mixed medical-surgical** **Partial anal incontinence**	50	25–76	1 year	36 at least 90% decrease in frequency of incontinence
Latimer, Campbell, and Kasperski (1984)	Three-balloon manometric system	Mixed medical-surgical 3 with surgical repair of imperforate anus	8	8–72	6 months	3 complete continence 4 minor soiling 1 incontinent but improved
Wald and Tunuguntla (1984)	Three-balloon manometric system	Diabetes mellitus	11	25–72	4–30 months	5 complete continence 3 incontinent but improved 3 no change

normal rectosphincteric responses. The authors hypothesized that psychological problems contributed to the poor outcome in these cases.

Wald (1981b, 1983), using the same methods, treated 15 incontinent children with meningomyelocele. Children with inability to sense rectal distension were excluded. Three became completely continent, four achieved a 90 percent decrease in incontinence while eight had no improvement (see Table 3.2). Although these results are quite impressive, when compared to other available treatments, they are not as good as those achieved in studies of adults with incontinence due to mixed medical and surgical conditions. Wald (1983) found that responders to biofeedback had a significantly lower threshold for rectal sensation than did nonresponders. No responder had a threshold of rectal sensation which exceeded 20 ml of distension, whereas five of eight nonresponders did.

Whitehead et al. (1981) also studied the effects of rectosphincteric biofeedback on eight incontinent children with myelomeningocele (see Table 3.2). Like Wald they only achieved moderate improvement. Four children were incontinent once per month or less, two improved but were still incontinent once per day and two were no better.

More impressive results can be obtained with this difficult group using a comprehensive bowel training program. Shepherd, Hickstein, and Shepherd (1983) used a combination of timed regular evacuations, stool consistency modification by diet, and biofeedback in 22 patients (aged 3–11 years) with spina bifida. Eighteen of these patients had perianal anaesthesia, flail anus, and absent anorectal reflex but some degree of rectal sensation. Twenty-one of the 22 achieved satisfactory continence following the comprehensive program. The design of the study did not allow evaluation of the effectiveness of the separate treatment components. Timed, regular, complete evacuations 2–3 times a day were accomplished, if necessary using enemas and/or digital stimulation.

In spite of the substantial clinical improvement, there were no changes in perianal sensation or internal sphincter relaxation. However, the ability to voluntarily contract the "external sphincter" and the ability to evacuate the rectal balloon were improved in all but one patient. Rectal sensation was improved in many patients.

MacLeod (1979), using an intra-anal plug, reported preliminary results on 17 patients with partial anal incontinence due to mixed medical and surgical disorders (see Table 3.2). These patients were incontinent to gas and liquid feces but not to formed stool. Six patients were completely continent with a 50 percent or greater increase in strength of sphincter contraction, while four more were almost completely continent with a 25–49 percent increase in strength of sphincter contraction. All patients had failed to improve as a result of sphincter exercises prior to biofeedback.

Of interest in this report is the substantial discrepancy between the patients' reported improvement in symptoms and the improvement in sphincter strength as measured by electromyography. Of the six patients who achieved complete continence, only two showed electromyographic improvement. In no case was electromyographic improvement greater than reported symptomatic improvement. The author attributed this discrepancy to insensitivity of the electromyography recording method.

Using the same method on a similar patient population, MacLeod (1983) demonstrated that 36 of 50 patients could achieve at least a 90 percent decrease in frequency of incontinence. The number of sessions (20 minutes) required ranged from two to six; 23 needed only two sessions.

Latimer, Campbell, and Kasperski (1984) used the three-balloon manometric system on eight patients with mixed medical-surgical causes of incontinence (see Table 3.2). All eight patients were substantially improved and only one continued to be incontinent of formed stool. Three were completely continent, while four continued to have minor soiling.

Latimer et al. (1984) also attempted to differentiate the effects of three separate components of the usual biofeedback procedure: (a) exercise of the external sphincter muscle, (b) training in discrimination of rectal sensation, and (c) training in synchrony of the internal and external sphincter responses. Three distinct treatment procedures were devised which isolated these potentially effective components while utilizing the same instrumentation.

The exercise treatment consisted of inflating the rectal balloon for two to three second durations with volumes above the established threshold for sensation. The patients were instructed to contract the anal sphincter in response to each inflation, just as they would if they were trying not to have a bowel movement. They were given verbal feedback and encouragement to produce stronger contractions. They were given no other feedback and were not allowed to view their sphincter responses being recorded.

The sensory discrimination training consisted of inflating the rectal balloon, beginning with volumes just greater than the threshold of sensation. Patients were asked to report each inflation and to estimate the volume of inflation. They were given verbal feedback concerning their estimate and praised when correct. When accurate discriminations for supra-threshold inflations had been made for three consecutive trials the inflation was decreased in 5–10 cc steps.

The training in synchronchy was essentially the procedure described by Engel et al. (1974). Because this procedure included all three components it was always done last; the only novel component was synchrony training. All three procedures employed the same instrumentation and the same number and duration of rectal distensions during the same time period.

These three treatments were employed in a series of single-case experiments which demonstrated that each of the three potentially effective components of the usual biofeedback procedure was effective in some cases.

One patient responded to exercise training alone, and he had normal sensation to rectal distension at initial assessment. Three patients responded to the sensory discrimination training procedure, and all three of these individuals had an elevated threshold to first sensation at their initial manometric assessment. One patient required training in synchrony of the internal and external sphincter responses. One patient got better with no treatment indicating that this condition, like all others, is susceptible to expectancy effects and must be evaluated accordingly. One patient responded to and relapsed following each treatment and did not finally maintain treatment gains until contingency management procedures were also employed. In this case the fecal soiling was maintained in part by the effects it had on significant others; it was a way of getting attention. Finally, one patient responded partially to sensory discrimination training but was clearly much better at six months follow-up than immediately following any of the treatments. This patient's incontinence was the result of an intradural cyst excision at L-2 and was associated with paraparesis and urinary incontinence. The improved incontinence at six months follow-up may have been partly due to gradual recovery of neurological function over time. At six months follow-up she was no longer incontinent of urine and her gait was much improved.

The group manometric data, when compared to that of continent control subjects, demonstrated that incontinence was associated with an elevated threshold for detecting rectal distension, a lowered threshold for urgency on rectal distension, and reduced sphincter strength. Treatment improved the first and last of these, which is consistent with current understanding of the mechanism of continence. In contrast, the configuration of rectosphincteric responses to rectal distension did not appear to be a reliable predictor of treatment outcome; none of these patients had normal rectosphincteric reflexes after treatment.

The findings of this study suggest the possibility that the treatment component necessary could be identified at initial assessment and that effective treatments could be developed that are even simpler and less invasive than the three-balloon manometric system.

Wald and Tunuguntla (1984) compared the anorectal sensorimotor functioning in four groups of patients: continent and incontinent diabetics and nondiabetics. They then studied the effects of biofeedback in 11 incontinent diabetics (see Table 3.2). The incontinent diabetics were distinguished from the other three groups by their higher mean sensory threshold to rectal distension. There was no relation between thresholds of conscious rectal sensation and internal-sphincter relaxation, suggesting that these two phenomena are mediated by different neural mechanisms. A rectal sensory conditioning procedure similar to the sensory discrimination training described by Latimer et al. (1984) (see above) was used prior to external sphincter biofeedback. Unfortunately, the effects of these two procedures are not reported separately.

Eight of the 11 diabetic biofeedback patients decreased fecal soiling; five were completely continent. Sensory thresholds decreased in six of seven patients with threshold levels above 20 ml of distension; bowel control improved in five of these. Biofeedback also lowered substantially the threshold for external-sphincter contraction in all nine patients with thresholds of 30 ml or higher; in eight of these soiling decreased.

Three responders had repeat anorectal manometry at various intervals posttreatment. All maintained their improvement in both rectal sensory threshold and the threshold for external sphincter contraction. Interestingly, none contracted the external sphincter in response to rectal distension as they had been taught to do during biofeedback. A similar finding was reported by Latimer et al. (1984).

CONCLUSION

This series of studies demonstrates that the integration of the behavioral and biomedical sciences in the treatment of fecal incontinence has merit. Not surprisingly, there are limitations; this approach is not successful with every patient. The criteria for selecting appropriate patients have not yet been rigorously defined but the following guidelines are suggested by the studies reviewed:

1. Ability to understand the instructions
2. Motivation to be continent
3. Some ability to sense rectal distension although the threshold may be elevated

4. Adequate anorectal angulation
5. Some external sphincter function although it may be weak.

Complete absence of any one of these characteristics is probably incompatible with achieving continence using the methods described. The greater the deviation from normal on any of them the more difficult the task of achieving continence.

Although the results to date are impressive, many questions remain unanswered. Several authors (Schiller et al., 1979; Wald, 1981, 1983; Wald & Tunuguntta, 1984; MacLeod, 1979; Latimer et al., 1984) have reported an apparent lack of concordance between clinical outcome and physiological variables which were assumed to underlie continence. It now seems likely that biofeedback can be effective through a variety of mechanisms which include: expectancy, improved sensory discrimination, strengthening the external sphincter muscles, training synchrony of internal and external sphincter responses, increased rectal compliance and increasing angulation of the anorectal junction.

It is clear that not all of these mechanisms are equally relevant to each incontinent patient. The thrust of future research will likely be to refine assessment procedures and attempt to tailor treatment to specific deficits in anorectal sensorimotor functioning.

REFERENCES

Cerulli, M. A., Nikoomanesh, P., & Schuster, M. M. (1979). Progress in biofeedback conditioning for fecal incontinence. *Gastroenterology, 76,* 742–746.

Constantinides, C. G., & Cywes, S. (1983). Fecal incontinence: A simple pneumatic device for home biofeedback training. *Journal of Pediatric Surgery, 18,* 276–277.

Engel, B. T. (1978). The treatment of fecal incontinence by operant conditioning. *Automedica, 2,* 101–108.

Engel, B. T., Nikoomanesh, P., & Schuster, M. M. (1974). Operant conditioning of rectosphincteric responses in the treatment of fecal incontinence. *New England Journal of Medicine, 290,* 646–649.

Foxx, R. M., & Azrin, N. H. (1973). *Toilet training the retarded.* Champaign, IL: Research Press.

Goldenberg, D. A., Hodges, K., Hersh, T., & Jinich, H. (1980). Biofeedback therapy for fecal incontinence. *American Journal of Gastroenterology, 74,* 342–345.

Haskell, B., & Rovner, H. (1967). Electromyography in the management of the incompetent anal sphincter. *Diseases of the Colon and Rectum, 10,* 81–84.

Kerremans, R. (1969). *Morphological and physiological aspects of anal continence and defecation.* Bruxelles: Editions Arscia S. A.

Latimer, P. R. (1980). Behavioural medicine: Scope and definition. *International Journal of Mental Health, 9,* 3–8.

Latimer, P. R. (1983). *Functional gastrointestinal disorders. A behavioral medicine approach.* New York: Springer.

Latimer, P. R., Campbell, D., & Kasperski, J. (1984). A components analysis of biofeedback in the treatment of fecal incontinence. *Biofeedback and Self-Regulation, 9,* 311–324.

McLeod, J. H. (1979). Biofeedback in the management of partial anal incontinence: A preliminary report. *Diseases of the Colon and Rectum, 22,* 169–171.

McLeod, J. H. (1983). Biofeedback in the management of partial anal incontinence. *Diseases of the Colon and Rectum, 26,* 244–246.

Olness, K., McParland, F. A., & Piper, J. (1980). Biofeedback: A new modality in the management of children with fecal soiling. *The Journal of Pediatrics, 96,* 505–509.

Schiller, L. R., Santa Ana, C., Davis, G. R., & Fordtran, J. S. (1979). Fecal incontinence in chronic diarrhea. Report of a case with improvement after training with rectally infused saline. *Gastroenterology, 77,* 751–753.

Schuster, M. M. (1975). The riddle of the sphincters. *Gastroenterology, 69,* 249–262.

Schuster, M. M., Hookman, P., Hendrix, T. T., & Mendeloff, A. I. (1965). Simultaneous manometric recording of internal and external anal sphincteric reflexes. *Bulletin of the Johns Hopkins Hospital, 116,* 79–88.

Shepherd, K., Hickstein, R., & Shepherd, R. (1983). Neurogenic fecal incontinence in children with spina bifida: Rectosphincteric responses and evaluation of a physiological rationale for management, including biofeedback conditioning. *Australian Paediatric Journal, 19,* 97–99.

Stass, W. E., & De Nault, P. M. (1973). Bowel control. *American Family Physician, 7,* 90–100.

Wald, A. (1981a). Biofeedback therapy for fecal incontinence. *Annals of Internal Medicine, 95,* 146–149.

Wald, A. (1981b). Use of biofeedback in treatment of fecal incontinence in patients with meningomyelocele. *Pediatrics, 68,* 45–49.

Wald, A. (1983). Biofeedback for neurogenic fecal incontinence: Rectal sensation is a determinant of outcome. *Journal of Pediatric Gastroenterology and Nutrition, 2,* 302–306.

Wald, A., & Tunuguntla, A. K. (1984). Anorectal sensorimotor dysfunction in fecal incontinence and diabetes mellitus. Modification with biofeedback therapy. *New England Journal of Medicine, 310,* 1282–1287.

Whitehead, W. E., Orr, W. C., Engel, B. T., & Schuster, M. M. (1982). External anal sphincter response to rectal distension: Learned response or reflex. *Psychophysiology, 19,* 57–62.

Whitehead, W. E., Parker, L. H., Masek, B. J., Cataldo, M. F., & Freeman, J. M. (1981). Biofeedback treatment of fecal incontinence in patients with myelomeningocele. *Developmental Medicine and Child Neurology, 23,* 313–322.

Whitehead, W. E., & Schuster, M. M. (1983). Manometric and electromyographic techniques for assessment of the anorectal mechanism for continence and defecation. In R. Holzl & W. E. Whitehead (Eds.), *Psychophysiology of the gastrointestinal tract. Experimental and clinical applications* (pp. 311–329). New York: Plenum Press.

III

THE GENITOURINARY SYSTEM

4

The Assessment of Sexual Dysfunctions*

Jerome A. Cerny
Indiana State University

Timothy Bruce
University of Illinois College of Medicine—Peoria

THE CLINICAL ASSESSMENT OF SEXUAL DYSFUNCTIONS

The clinical assessment of sexual dysfunctions is directly related to the availability of a reliable and valid classification system for sexual problems. Such a classification system requires minimally a consensus definition of the problems under consideration, a taxonomy that adequately accounts for the range of defined problems, and a set of normative data that allows the clinician to make appropriate comparisons. The clinician attempting to diagnose and assess patient complaints of difficulties in sexual performance will find little in the scientific and clinical literature that leads to agreement in any of these critical areas. On the other hand, advances in both medical and psychological technologies have pushed forward the frontiers of knowledge in regard to sexual dysfunctions and have provided some useful techniques for the clinical assessment and evaluation of sexual concerns. The purpose of this chapter is to provide an overview of our current state of knowl-

* Preparation of this chapter was partially supported by Indiana State University Faculty Development Grant 48006 to the first author while on sabbatical leave at the Center for Stress and Anxiety Disorders Clinic, State University of New York at Albany.

edge about sexual dysfunctions and the clinical assessment procedures used for the evaluations of such problems.

DEFINITION OF SEXUAL DYSFUNCTION

As Conte (1986) has pointed out, there is no universally accepted definition of what constitutes a sexual dysfunction. For example, Masters, Johnson, and Kolodny (1988) describe sexual dysfunctions as "conditions in which the ordinary physical responses of sexual function are impaired" (p. 499). Conte (1986) restricts the definition of sexual dysfunction to any impairment of the sexual response cycle of an adult man or woman to such an extent that it impairs his or her capacity to achieve satisfactory levels of sexual arousal and/or orgasm. Both definitions recognize the central role of physical sexual responses, namely, vasocongestion of genital tissue. The second definition also allows for subjective dissatisfaction with sexual performance even in the case of actual or potential intact physical responses.

The most recent version of the *Diagnostic and Statistical Manual of Mental Disorders* (DSM-III-R, American Psychiatric Association, 1987) explicitly recognizes the possible independence of subjective and objective evaluations of sexual performance. DSM-III-R states that the essential feature of sexual dysfunctions is "inhibition in the appetitive or psychophysiologic changes that characterize the complete sexual response cycle" (p. 290). The model proposed in this diagnostic manual is one in which sexual behavior is divided into four conceptual phases: An appetitive phase consists of fantasies about sexual activity and a desire to have sexual activity; excitement basically incorporates the vasocongestive changes typically associated with sexual arousal; orgasm is marked by a peaking of sexual pleasure with a concomitant release of sexual tension accompanied by rhythmic contraction of the perineal muscles and pelvic reproductive organs; finally, the resolution phase consists of a sense of general relaxation, well-being, and muscular relaxation. In addition DSM-III-R recognizes that in most cases both subjective evaluations of pleasure or desire will be diminished and there will be a concomitant decrement in objective performance, that is, impairment of the motor responses. In some cases, however, there may be indications of subjective disturbance alone without any objective signs of physical impairment or conversely disruption of the physical responses associated with sexual behavior without any acknowledgment of subjective distress.

Our intent here is not to debate the merits of various definitions of sexual dysfunctions but rather to point out the commonalities. In all of these definitions the physical responses of sexual behavior clearly have a central role. However, for appetitive disorders, the exact relation of physical responses to the appetitive problem remains unclear. Nevertheless, inclusion of appetitive difficulties underscores the importance of psychological, that is, cognitive or subjective evaluations and attitudes toward the physical responses of sexual behavior. That these two sets of response classes may be independent is clearly recognized in the definition proposed in DSM-III-R. Most professionals working with sexual dysfunctions emphasize the interrelatedness of psychological and biological functioning in defining and classifying sexual problems. In fact, perhaps in no other areas of either medicine or psychology is the interaction between biological and psychological determinants more manifest or more widely recognized.

Generally, then, sexual dysfunctions may be broadly defined as psychological or biopsychological disruption of normal sexual behavior. This definition as well as the DSM-III-R definition of sexual dysfunction would preclude those disturbances of sexual responding that are due exclusively to biological problems. Organic problems, however, are not easily differentiated from psychological problems, and sexual adjustment difficulties associated with physical problems often remain after the physical problem is corrected.

CLASSIFICATION OF SEXUAL DYSFUNCTIONS

The classification of sexual dysfunctions, as with the definition of sexual dysfunctions, has no consensus in the professional literature. Several classification and/or diagnostic systems have been proposed. Masters and Johnson (1966, 1970) suggested a diagnostic system based upon their conceptualization of the sexual response cycle. That classification system was incorporated into earlier editions of DSM-III-R. While several other diagnostic systems for the sexual dysfunctions have been proposed (e.g., Graber & Kline-Graber, 1981; Schover, Friedman, Weiler, Heiman, & LoPiccolo, 1982; World Health Organization, 1977), DSM-II-R apparently remains the most popular of the diagnostic classification systems. Consequently, for the purposes of this chapter we follow the classification system used in DSM-III-R, albeit not without some reservation, especially since the reliability and the validity of this diagnostic system has not been satisfactorily demonstrated. DSM-III-R classifies sexual dysfunctions as disorders of sexual desire, sexual arousal, orgasm, sexual pain, and/or other sexual dysfunctions.

Sexual Desire Disorders

There are two sexual desire disorders. *Hypoactive sexual desire disorder* is described as a persistent and recurrent deficiency or absence of sexual fantasy and desire for sexual activity. The clinician is to consider variables such as the patient's age, sex, and life situation in assigning this diagnosis. In addition, the disorder must not occur exclusively during another sexual dysfunction. Low sexual desire is not in and of itself sufficient cause for the diagnosis. The patient must report being distressed by the condition. On the other hand, engaging in sexual behavior does not necessarily preclude this diagnosis, since in some cases biological and sexual responsivity is intact and once initiated, sexual arousal may be experienced. Clinically, hypoactive sexual desire may occur concomitantly with other sexual dysfunctions. While no strong epidemiological studies exist, the prevalence of this disorder is estimated at 20 percent of the total population.

Sexual aversion disorder is a new diagnostic category that did not appear in previous versions of DSM-III. This dysfunction is defined as a persistent or recurrent extreme aversion to, and avoidance of, all or almost all, genital sexual contact with a sexual partner. Sexual aversion disorder is essentially a phobic reaction to genital contact. The epidemiology as well as treatment outcome of this disorder awaits further study.

Sexual Arousal Disorders

In DSM-III (American Psychiatric Association, 1980) male and female sexual arousal disorders were considered under one diagnostic category, namely, inhibited sexual excitement. In DSM-III-R, male and female excitement disorders have been given separate rubrics. *Female sexual arousal disorder* is characterized by partial or complete failure to maintain vaginal lubrication and vasocongestive swelling associated with sexual excitement until the completion of sexual activity *or* the lack of a subjective sense of sexual excitement and pleasure by the woman during sexual behavior. One study (Frank, Anderson, & Rubenstein, 1978) of nonclinical couples reported that 48 percent of their female sample complained of difficulties becoming sexually aroused and 33 percent complained of difficulties maintaining arousal. These relatively high rates of excitement phase problems suggest that the lack of specificity in the definition promotes inflation in these statistics. Methodological problems associated with studying female arousal disorders, for example, a lack of reliable and practical methods for assessing genital vasocongestion also has impaired progress in this area.

The diagnostic criteria for *male erectile disorder* includes partial or complete failure to attain or maintain erection to completion of sexual activity, or a persistent and recurrent lack of subjective sexual excitement and pleasure during sexual activity. Two studies (Frank et al., 1978; Reading & Wiest, 1984) have reported that between 8 percent and 9 percent of their respective nonclinical couples complained of difficulty obtaining and/or maintaining satisfactory erections during sexual activity. These more reasonable figures are in stark contrast to the figures above for female arousal disorder and may likely reflect the difference in specificity of the criteria for the two disorders as well as the availability of methods to quantify the presenting complaint. It should be noted that erectile disorder is somewhat of a misnomer since a fairly large percentage of men assessed for erectile failure manifest significant increase in penile tumescence without penile rigidity sufficient to effect vaginal penetration (Wein, Fishkin, Carpiniello, & Malloy, 1981).

Orgasm Disorders

In *inhibited female orgasm* a woman experiences a persistent or recurrent delay in or absence of orgasm following normal sexual excitement during sexual activity judged to be adequate in focus, intensity, and direction. Some women are able to experience orgasm with noncoital stimulation but not able to reach orgasm during coitus without additional noncoital clitoral stimulation. Such a sexual behavior pattern is considered a normal variation of female sexual responses. In these cases the diagnosis of inhibited female orgasm is not warranted unless the clinician can determine that some kind of distressing psychological inhibition is interfering with coital orgasm. The difficulty in such a judgment is exacerbated by the lack of large sample normative and epidemiological data on typical female sexual responsiveness. Nevertheless, a recent study (Levin & Wagner, 1985) has provided useful information about female orgasm induced by self-stimulation in the laboratory. In this study of adult women, mean orgasm latency was 6.4 minutes (S.D. = 4.3 minutes) with a range of 0.75 to 25 minutes. The mean orgasm duration was measured at 19.9 seconds (S.D. = 12.0 seconds). Of even more interest was the data showing that the subjective estimate of orgasm duration greatly underestimated the objectively measured duration. In addition, subjective evaluations of the orgasms, orgasm latency, or measured orgasm duration were not correlated with vaginal blood flow measures at orgasm.

The above data reaffirm that the concept of orgasm is multidimensional and suggests that giving priority to biological correlates of sexual arousal may not be justified. Orgasm may be best defined not on the basis of any single component associated with sexual arousal but rather as a high, positive correlation among the biological, psychological, and behavioral sexual responses. In addition, the usual estimate that as many as 30 percent of the female population have inhibited female orgasm again makes one question the lack of specificity in the diagnostic criteria which may lead to overinclusiveness.

For males, a persistent or recurrent delay or absence of orgasm following normal sexual excitement and adequate sexual stimulation justifies a diagnosis of *inhibited male orgasm*. This diagnostic category was formerly termed retarded ejaculation. Inhibited male orgasm is usually limited to the inability to reach orgasm in the vagina, since men with this disorder may be able to have orgasm in noncoital activities. Reading and Wiest (1984) found that 16.5 percent of a rather large, nonclinical sample of men living in London reported difficulty achieving climax during intercourse; interestingly, these researchers found that nearly an identical number of men (17.3%) reported having difficulty climaxing during masturbation. These data suggest that for some men inhibited sexual orgasm may be less situation-specific and could be an important marker for a specific subtype of the disorder. In contrast to the above study, Frank et al. (1978) found that only 4 percent of the men in their nonclinical sample reported difficulty ejaculating and none reported an inability to ejaculate. The latter data are more consistent with clinical studies (e.g., Masters & Johnson, 1970) which suggest that inhibited male orgasm is the least common of the clinical disorders. As with other sexual dysfunctions, organic problems (e.g., retrograde ejaculation, retroperitoneal surgery, and drug therapies) have to be ruled out.

The second male organic dysfunction is *premature ejaculation*. We note that while archaic terms like impotence for inhibited male orgasm and frigidity for female inhibited sexual excitement have nearly disappeared from the literature, premature ejaculation has remained. Like the other archaic terms, premature ejaculation carries with it unnecessary and unjustified connotations. We prefer the term rapid ejaculation.

Rapid ejaculation is defined in DSM-III-R as persistent or recurrent ejaculation with minimal sexual stimulation before, upon, or shortly after penetration and before the person wishes it. The diagnostic criteria cautions the clinician to take into account factors such as the patient's age, novelty of the situation, the partner, and frequency of sexual activity. Unfortunately, very little normative data is available on any of these issues. This lacuna is especially troublesome since the estimated rate of this disorder is high and at one time was the most frequent presenting complaint at sexual dysfunction clinics (Kaplan, 1974). Incidence of rapid ejaculation for British men was 37 percent (Reading & Weist, 1984) and 36 percent for an American sample

(Frank et al., 1978). DSM-III-R suggests a 30 percent prevalence rate for the total male population. Again, lack of more complete diagnostic criteria, especially in regard to age parameters, may account for these high prevalence rates.

We have begun a research program in our laboratory to collect normative data on ejaculatory latencies and to test some of the hypotheses proposed to account for rapid ejaculation. For example, in a preliminary study (Cerny, Hutchison, Guido, & Katz, 1988), we have developed a method for assessing ejaculatory latencies in the laboratory using vibrotactile stimulation. Under this highly stimulating yet controlled laboratory situation, the average ejaculatory latency for an unselected group of men was approximately ten minutes.

Using this paradigm we then compared ejaculatory latencies in a group of men who complained about poor ejaculatory control to a normal control group (Cerny & Katz, 1990). Rapid ejaculators had significantly shorter latencies to full erection ($\bar{x}$ = 80.75 seconds) than did the matched normal control group ($\bar{x}$ = 280.10 seconds). In addition, the average orgasm latency for rapid ejaculators ($\bar{x}$ = 4.20 mins) was significantly shorter than for nonrapid ejaculators ($\bar{x}$ = 11.78 mins). Perhaps of more importance is the fact that the rapid ejaculators were less able to withhold ejaculation *after* reaching full erection ($\bar{x}$ = 2.87 mins) than were the normal controls ($\bar{x}$ = 7.11 mins). We use the term *plateau phase tolerance* to describe this phenomenon. These data show that rapid ejaculators can be accurately diagnosed in a laboratory situation. However, neither the rapid ejaculators nor the normal controls were able to demonstrate differential instructional control of the ejaculatory response. This latter result does not support the concept of voluntary ejaculatory control. This preliminary study does, then, suggest that while voluntary control of ejaculation may not be valid, rapid ejaculators do display relatively shorter plateau phase tolerance than nonrapid ejaculators. These data indicate a need to examine erectile and ejaculatory latencies as independent (but probably correlated) phenomena and have led to the introduction of the concept of plateau phase tolerance as a more accurate description of the mechanism involved in rapid ejaculation. Clearly, additional research is needed in this area.

When the next phase of our research program is complete, we hope to be able to specify more clearly the parameters associated with rapid ejaculation. Until such time, clinicians shall have to rely on their clinical experiences and subjective evaluations of the patients problems.

For women there is no sexual dysfunction parallel to rapid ejaculation for men. Although Frank et al. (1978) found that 11 percent of the women in their sample reported reaching orgasm too quickly, these reports were not correlated with degree of sexual satisfaction. Presumably reaching orgasm *too* quickly is not problematic for women; however, in lieu of data, this presumption is at best speculative and may be sexist. Clearly, this area merits some additional research.

Sexual Pain Disorders

The final subclassification of sexual dysfunctions is sexual pain disorders which are carryovers from previous versions of DSM. *Dyspareunia* is characterized as recurrent or persistent pain in either males or females before, during, or after sexual intercourse. The pain is not related to either lack of vaginal lubrication or vaginismus. This syndrome apparently is rare in males but not uncommon among women. This diagnosis should not be given if the pain results exclusively from organic or other psychiatric disorders. While psychological factors often may be involved in dyspareunia, multiple physical problems, for example, skin problems, clitoral irritation, or infections, vaginal, urethral, anal, or other pelvic disorders, diabetes, and medication may all cause the disorder (Masters, Johnson, & Kolodny, 1988).

Vaginismus occurs when a woman experiences involuntary spasms of the perivaginal musculature that disrupts or prevents coitus. While dyspareunia may predispose a woman to vaginismus, organic problems rarely are directly implicated in this disorder (Kolodny, Masters, & Johnson, 1979); nor is vaginismus associated with desire or organic problems since many women with this dysfunction enjoy sex and desire intercourse.

THE DIFFERENTIATION OF PSYCHOGENIC FROM ORGANIC SEXUAL PROBLEMS

A rather large and growing body of research is focused on assessing the relative contributions of organic factors contributing to the etiology of sexual dysfunctions. Early investigators of sexual problems estimated that organic problems occurred relatively infrequently among patients presenting with sexual dysfunctions. Later research, however, (Fisher et al., 1979; Kaya, Moore, & Karacan, 1979) has suggested that 50–60 percent of men diagnosed with psychogenic erectile difficulties, in fact, have an organic condition. Etiological estimates for other sexual disorders are not available. Masters and Johnson (1970) have listed a large number of possible biological problems that could cause erectile dysfunctions, including such factors as congenital abnormalities, cardiac respiratory problems, drug ingestion, endocrine problems, genitourinary problems, hematologic problems, neurologic problems, and several infectious diseases. While most of the available data implicating organic factors in sexual disorders has focused on male sexual dysfunctions, Hatch (1981) has speculated that at least some forms of female arousal dysfunctions may have an organic basis.

The importance of a thorough medical examination in evaluating sexual dysfunctions is obvious. Advances in medical technology have provided the medical practitioner with a formidable and expanding array of tools for the assessment of erectile problems. Besides the physical examination and laboratory studies to evaluate hormonal functioning, medical procedures have been developed to assess both neurological and vascular integrity. Because vascular problems are so often implicated in erectile problems, a number of vascular assessment techniques, each of which provides different information, has captured the efforts of medical researchers. Noninvasive procedures included penile blood pressure, pulse pressure, and penile plethysmography; invasive procedures available for more in depth studies include arteriography, direct flow measures, for example, penile xenon washout, and artificial erections (Virag, Spencer, & Frydman, 1984) produced by infusion of saline. The use of drugs to stimulate artificial erections (Blum, Bahnson, Porter, & Carter, 1985; Virag, 1982) has provided another procedure for assessing penile anatomical integrity. Montague (1982) provides a good review of most of these medical procedures. Except for the physical exam and hormonal studies, these procedures have been limited to the evaluation of erectile problems. The application of similar techniques to etiology in female sexual dysfunctions awaits future research.

As discussed above, DSM-III-R requires that exclusive organic causes be ruled out before a diagnosis of sexual dysfunction is warranted. While theoretically possible, such decisions are rarely practically feasible. Most referrals to sexual disorder clinicians come from primary care physicians, urologists, or gynecologists. When organic causes of the disorder are obvious, these practitioners treat the medical problem themselves. Only when there is doubt about the etiology of the sexual problem are psychological referrals made.

Although there is a dearth of baserate data, it would appear that few sexual problems are exclusively caused by either organic or psychogenic factors. This point is manifest when one considers that 25 percent of surgically successful penile implant patients remain dissatisfied with their sexual functioning (Steege, Stout, & Carson, 1986), suggesting that careful psychological assessment is called for even when organic etiologies are highly probable. Finally, Segraves, Segraves, and Schoenberg (1987) found that the best predictor of organogenic erectile difficulty was the patients' self-report of the presence or absence of early morning erections. In the absence of early morning erections, organic problems should be highly suspect and referral for the proper medical evaluations made.

MECHANISMS OF SEXUAL DISORDERS

The model of sexual dysfunctions that has received the widest acceptance is that proposed by Masters and Johnson (1966, 1970). These authors suggested that fear related to sexual performance is the common, although not the only, mechanism underlying many of the sexual dysfunctions. While performance fears may develop from a wide range of potential personal experiences (e.g., poor sex education, negative attitudes toward sexuality, traumatic or inadequate sexual experiences, etc.), such fears generate apprehension and an anxiety process termed "spectatoring" that are manifested in sexual situations. In spectatoring, the sexually fearful person's attention is redirected from involved processing of sexual foci to critical monitoring of one's own sexual performance from a third-person perspective. Such cognitive processes disrupt the "natural responsivity" (Masters & Johnson, 1970, p. 11) of sexual behavior. Other writers have elaborated upon this basic model (e.g., Kaplan, 1981; Barbach, 1975; Zilbergeld, 1978; Zeiss & Zeiss, 1978), but all have maintained the central role of fears and anxieties related to sexual behavior.

Another anxiety-based model of sexual dysfunction has been proposed by Wolpe (1958, 1978). In this model, fear or anxiety is a learned sympathetic response that interferes with sexual performance. Elimination of the anxiety response should facilitate sexual responding. While the origin of the anxiety response in Wolpe's model does not invoke cognitive variables, it maintains the importance of fear responses.

Barlow (1986) and Beck and Barlow (1984) have suggested a multivariate model of sexual functioning based upon feedback loops. Barlow and his colleagues have pointed out that the "anxiety" construct does not sufficiently account for sexual dysfunction since under some conditions "anxiety" actually facilitates sexual performance. Any model of sexual functioning must account for several generalizations that seem to differentiate sexually functional from sexually dysfunctional individuals. Relative to sexually functional people, dysfunctional adults generally display more negative affect in sexual situations, underreport sexual arousal levels, report less control of sexual arousal, show decrements in sexual performance induced by anxiety and sex related stimuli, but show performance enhancements when distracted by non-sexual-performance related stimuli. Barlow (1986) reviewed the data in support of these conclusions and suggested that inhibited sexual excitement in men and women is a function of a multidimensional process characterized by cognitive interference that is driven by autonomic physiological arousal. According to this model, dysfunctional individuals are distracted by a focus on task irrelevant stimuli. The task irrelevant focus is energized by physiological (autonomic) arousal (presumably from any source but clinically from anxiety) which in turn interferes with sexual behavior. Sexually functional individuals have positive affect and expectancies in anticipation and during sexual situations and focus on the task relevant, erotic cues within this context. This positive cognitive process is also energized by autonomic arousal, but because of the positive focus on erotic cues, sexual performance is enhanced. If cognitive distraction interrupts the dysfunctionals inappropriate attentional focus, sexual performance is enhanced. For functionals, cognitive distraction interrupts the appropriate attentional focus on erotic cues and this distraction leads to performance decrements.

While more complex than presented here and currently limited to erectile problems, the cognitive interference model provides new avenues to explore in both the assessment and treatment of sexual problems. The assessment of affective and cognitive functioning in sexual situations may strengthen treatment protocols and better predict treatment outcome. Should the merits of this model be substantiated, it could suggest entirely new approaches to treatment. For example, anxiety reduction treatments may be contraindicated in at least some cases or types of sexual dysfunctions. In fact, in some cases anxiety induction might be therapeutic. To the extent that sexual dysfunctions can be considered a type of avoidant or phobic social behavior (Beck & Barlow, 1984), exposure treatments and cognitive behavioral treatments might be indicated. For a more detailed review of this model and its implications see Bruce and Barlow (in press).

ASSESSMENT METHODS

As suggested in Barlow's cognitive interference model, evaluation of sexual dysfunctions requires assessment in at least four major systems—namely, affective, behavioral, cognitive, and psychophysiological variables. It is beyond the scope of this chapter to discuss each of these systems in detail. We will, however, provide overviews of the currently available assessment methods in each area and refer readers to more detailed discussions of these methods.

Affective Measures

While dysphoria, anxiety, and sex guilt have long been considered concomitants of sexual dysfunction (Barlow, 1986; Kaplan, 1974; Masters & Johnson, 1970), very little progress has been made either in assessing affective states associated with sexual dysfunctions or in specifying the role of these states in the etiology or treatment of sexual problems. One of the first instruments designed to specifically assess affect among persons with sexual problems was the Derogatis Sexual Functioning Index (DSFI) (Derogatis, 1975; Derogatis & Melisaratos, 1979). Among other areas, this questionnaire includes an Affect Balance Index (ABI) that is the difference between positive and negative mood measured on an adjective checklist. The test-retest reliability of the DSFI seems satisfactory (Derogatis & Melisaranto, 1979). Derogatis and his colleagues (Derogatis & Melisaranto, 1979; Derogatis, Meyer, & Duplin, 1976) have reported that men with psychogenically based erectile problems tend to have slightly more positive ABI than do men with clear organic etiologies. In addition, the ABI reliably discriminates both male and female sexually functional persons from those who are experiencing sexual dysfunctions. Unfortunately others have not been able to replicate these results (Segraves, Schoenberg, Zarins, Knopf, & Camic, 1981).

Using a different mood scale, Kockott, Feil, Revenstorf, Aldenhoff, and Besinger (1980) also found that sexually dysfunctional patients rated themselves more depressed than matched groups of normal controls. Men with erectile difficulties and men with rapid ejaculation also scored significantly higher than sexually functional subjects on anxiety measures. Other psychometric instruments also have been used to assess emotional states and to discriminate psychogenic and organic causes of sexual disorders. The Minnesota Multiphasic Personality Inventory (MMPI) and the California Psychological Inventory (CPI) are two of the most common screening devices. But again the data in support of the utility of these psychometric instruments is equivocal at best (see Conte, 1986, for a cogent review). Mosher's (1966) Sex Guilt subscale has been shown repeatedly to correlate with self-reported sexual behavior, sexual knowledge, and various word association tasks. But with normal subjects we have found that sex guilt scores do not correlate with laboratory measures of penile tumescence (Cerny & Clodfelter, 1980). Morokoff (1985) found that sexually functional women *reported* less sexual arousal in response to erotic stimuli but *showed* significantly higher physiological responses (recorded from a vaginal photoplethysmograph) than did subjects low in sex guilt. Finally, Bruce and Barlow (in press) have reviewed a series of studies that show a relationship between dysphoria and self-estimates of sexual arousal. While the data relating affect to sexual behavior are both scant and inconsistent, we believe that the available data justify continued effort in this direction. Further progress awaits the development of more adequate and specific measures of affect related to sexual disorders.

Psychophysiological Measures

Psychophysiological assessments of sexual disorders usually involve measurement of either penile tumescence or vaginal blood flow in a laboratory while the patient is sleeping or awake.

The assessment of nocturnal penile tumescence (NPT) has received the major research focus. The use of NPT has been limited primarily to differentiating organic from psychogenic erectile problems. Males often experience erections during periods of sleep known as the rapid eye movement (REM) phase. Assuming that psychogenic factors are not operative during sleep periods, it follows that males not displaying the typical NPT pattern have a higher probability of organic etiology. Men with erectile disorders who have the ability to achieve full erection during sleep may suggest a primary role for psychological etiology. NPT usually requires the patient to spend 2–3 nights in a sleep laboratory while penile tumescence, electroencephalograph, and eye movement patterns are recorded. The utility of NPT assessments has been reasonably well documented in the literature (e.g., Karacan et al., 1977, 1978; Leliefeld & Muhr, 1982; Marshall, Surridge, & Delva, 1981; Zuckerman et al., 1985). The NPT methodology, however, is not without problems. Marshall, McGrath, and Schillinger (1983) have pointed out that carefully measuring electroencephalograph and eye movements during sleep is essential during NPT monitoring. Since sleep disorders can influence NPT results, it is necessary to assure that a normal sleep pattern is present. Because of this requirement portable NPT devices that do not have somnography capabilities are highly suspect. Secondly, Wein, Fishkin, Carpiniello, and Malloy (1981) found that a number of NPT patients achieved significant penile expansion without enough penile rigidity to effect vaginal penetration. In addition, Fisher et al. (1979) and Macksgood and James (1983) have found that NPT data were inaccurate or equivocal in 15–28 percent of the patients assessed. When NPT results do suggest organic involvement, it is not possible to specify whether the organic problem is cardiovascular, neurological, endocrine, and so on. In the face of such global results, additional medical and laboratory studies are required. These results have raised serious questions about the general utility of NPT assessments for differential diagnosis of erectile problems. Finally the cost of NPT assessment is not insignificant.

During REM sleep women also show photoplethysmographic changes in vaginal blood flow that approximate the pattern of NPT in males (Abel, Murphy, Becker, & Bitar, 1979). However, to our knowledge this method of assessing female sexual disorders has not been pursued. This lack of effort may be related to the meager reliability and validity data in support of the vaginal blood flow measure as well as considerable controversy over such methodological issues as which blood flow index to use (pulse pressure or blood volume), how to calibrate the probe, how to deal with movement artifacts, and so on (see Conte, 1986, and Heiman, 1976). While other methods to assess physiological changes associated with sexual arousal in women have been proposed (e.g., labia temperature, vaginal temperature changes, pelvic thermography) none has proven any more useful or clinically practical than vaginal photoplethysmography.

A second approach to assessing sexual capacity is to evaluate erectile potential while the patient is awake and attending to erotic stimulation. Sakheim, Barlow, Abrahamson, and Beck (1987) have termed this method waking erectile potential (EPA). Examples of this approach with both women (e.g., Cerny, 1978; Geer & Quartararo, 1976; Hoon, Hoon, & Wincze, 1976) and men (e.g., Beck, Barlow, & Sakheim, 1983; Kockott, Feil, Ferstl, Aldenhoff, & Besinger, 1980; Sakheim et al., 1987) are available in the literature. In terms of global assessments, this method is not only more cost-effective than NPT studies but also has other advantages. For example, it allows evaluation of the patients' affect and cognitions when presented with erotic cues (Sakheim et al., 1987). In addition, it is possible to collect behavioral data as well as physiological data. These advantages are attenuated somewhat by the results of several studies (Laws & Rubin, 1969; Geer & Fuhr, 1976; Rosen, 1973; Henson & Rubin, 1971; Quinsey & Bergerson, 1976; Freund, Chan, & Coulthard, 1979) that show EPA is susceptible to voluntary control and generally affected by cognitive factors such as distraction. However, as proposed in the cognitive inference model, it may be these very factors that are etiologically significant. On the other hand, in cases where the patient can secondarily gain by not becoming aroused, EPA has its limitations. Controlling attention, distraction, expectancies, and other cognitive variables become more important in EPA studies.

Two studies have demonstrated the utility of EPA. Kockott et al. (1980) found that patient groups with diabetes-related erectile insufficiency, psychogenic erectile disorder, and premature ejaculation all differed from control subjects on measures of penile tumescence, systolic blood pressure, GSR fluctuations, erection latency, and erection duration. In addition, organic patients showed minimal changes in penile tumescence and some psychogenic patients showed significant increases in erection while premature ejaculators and control subjects showed no differences in penile responses. Sakheim et al. (1987) also found that self-stimulation during EPA could differentiate psychogenic, organic, and nondysfunctional patients with a 77 percent accuracy rate. Additionally, psychogenic patients underestimated their increases in penile tumescence, while control subjects showed the most accurate estimates of penile tumescence. These data on self-stimulation for penile erection are consistent with a cognitive interference model.

In a direct comparison of NPT with EPA assessment methods, Zuckerman et al. (1985) found significant correlations between NPT and EPA tumescence measures among diabetic and nondiabetic dysfunctions and control subjects. Although the correlations were smaller than one would hope (0.35–0.61), they must be considered in light of the fact that NPT criteria correctly classified only 58% of known dysfunctionals. Taken as whole, these data suggest that EPA, especially if it includes self-stimulation, is a viable alternative to the more costly and time consuming NPT studies. In addition, EPA methodology is such that it could be applied routinely in inpatient clinical assessment practices. Finally, while currently not well developed, similar methodologies could be used to assess other male sexual dysfunctions, for example, rapid ejaculation, as well as female sexual dysfunctions.

Behavioral Measures

The area of assessment that has received the least attention from researchers is, interestingly, behavioral measures of sexual dysfunction. Psychophysiological measures have become the central focus of most sexual dysfunction research, a situation that overlooks the primary importance of motor behavior associated with sexual problems. Early pornography studies (e.g., Brown, Amoroso, Ware, Pruesse, & Pilkey, 1973) used amount of time subjects choose to spend looking at erotic slides as an index of sexual interest, yet this assessment technique has only rarely been employed in clinical studies. Such a procedure may be of special interest in cases of low sexual desire and sexual aversion.

Other behavioral measures may similarly prove to be key elements in understanding and differentiating the various sexual disorders. Presently, the approach to assessment of sexual preference is to present a range of erotic stimuli, including same and opposite sex stimuli, while psychophysiological measures are taken. The assumption is that sexual preference will be manifested in physiological changes and/or self-reports of sexual interest. A more pertinent question may be which type of erotic or nonerotic stimuli does a particular patient *choose* to look at, irrespective of the genital response to that stimulus. Along the same line, one might ask how much effort would a patient expend to view or listen to a particular type of erotic stimulus? These kinds of data may be better predictors not only of sexual interest but also of treatment success. One might even evaluate the ability of clients to terminate an erotic stimulus in the service of controlling a sexual response. With some creative thinking, a rather long list of such measures could be developed.

In our own laboratory we have been developing a behavioral paradigm that takes just such an approach. Bruce, Cerny, and Barlow (1986) questioned whether spectatoring does involve a process of self-monitoring of genital responding as suggested originally by Masters and Johnson (1970). Such a hypothesis raises the possibility that sexually dysfunctional patients may choose to monitor genital responses to the detriment of sexual arousal. Accordingly we developed a paradigm in which males could receive live visual feedback of genital responses while watching preferred erotic stimuli. The feedback was presented for 3 seconds whenever a button was depressed, and there was no limit to the number of times feedback could be requested. We were interested in learning if sexually dysfunctional males requested feedback more often or less often than sexually functional males. The data showed that sexually *functional* males requested feedback significantly more often than did the sexually dysfunctional subjects. While these data are clearly preliminary, they suggest that perhaps men with erectile problems develop a type of avoidance rather than a hypervigilence of genital responding. In any case, the use of this or similar assessment procedures may provide new insights into the mechanisms associated with sexual problems. The basic paradigm described above has already proved useful in assessing the role of cognitive distraction in dysfunctional males. This latter study is described below.

Direct observation of sexual behavior has generally been eschewed because of social taboos or vague appeals to ethical issues. To date neither of these arguments have been particularly convincing. What is clear is that there is little agreement as to what constitutes appropriate observational methods in the study of human sexuality. Some clinicians recommend that for erectile problems routine observation of penile responses (e.g., Karacan, 1978) is an important clinical assessment procedure. Direct observational methods are often used in behavioral tests of sexual deviancies (e.g., Maletzky, 1980). Ethical issues aside, McConaghy (1988) has argued the merits of the potential utility of direct observation of the sexual behavior of dysfunctional patients. It is our position that little progress in this area will accrue until the ethical and social issues are more clearly specified.

Cognitive Assessment

The assessment of cognitive variables associated with sexual dysfunctions has received relatively little attention in the literature in spite of the fact that cognitive factors have been identified as primary variables in the etiology and maintenance of sexual problems. As suggested above, performance expectations, "spectatoring," and cognitive distraction have all been implicated as causes of psychosexual dysfunctions. From a clinical perspective, the clinical interview has been the most frequent method used to assess these cognitive variables. Several good semi-structured formats have been presented in the literature (e.g., Caird & Wincze, 1977; LoPiccolo & Heiman, 1978; Masters & Johnson, 1970; Tollison & Adams, 1979), and McConaghy (1988) has provided a most useful discussion of the merits of clinical interviews for the assessment of sexual problems. In our own laboratory we use a semi-structured interview that is described later in this chapter.

Besides the clinical interview, few methods for assessing the impact of cognitive variables have been developed for clinical assessment situations. Geer and Fuhr (1976) used a laboratory-based dichotic listening paradigm to demonstrate the effects of distraction on sexual arousal, but this procedure has not been used clinically. Others have attempted to access the effects of performance demands on expectations in sexual arousal in laboratory studies with mixed results (Farkas, Sine, & Evans, 1979; Heiman & Rowland, 1983; Lange, Wincze, Zwick, Feldman, & Hughes, 1981; Beck, Barlow, & Sakheim, 1983). While these studies generally show that instructional sets may affect sexual arousal in a laboratory setting, they do not show that these cognitive variables distinguish sexually functional from dysfunctional subjects. Bruce and Barlow (in press) provide a detailed review of this area.

In a current review of cognitive assessment procedures, Parks and Hollon (1988) list 14 different methods that have been used to assess cognitive activity. To our knowledge only three of these methods, namely, thought endorsement (e.g., Abrahamson, Barlow, & Abrahamson, 1989), thought sampling (e.g., Hurlburt, 1980), and thought listing (e.g., Cacioppo & Petty, 1981) have been used to assess cognitive activity associated with sexual arousal. Beck and Barlow (1984) found the use of these cognitive monitoring techniques potentially useful assessment procedures. While many of the other cognitive assessment techniques discussed by Parks and Hollon may hold some potential application for clinical studies of sexual dysfunction, few have been developed for this application.

Another approach to cognitive assessment for sexual problems has focused on the hypothesis that distraction is the cognitive mechanism that mediates the effects of cognitive activity (Barlow, 1986). Using a paradigm first developed by Bruce, Cerny, and Barlow (1986), Abrahamson, Barlow, and Abrahamson (1989) found that video feedback of genital responses elevated penile tumescence of sexually functional subjects relative to a neutral distraction (estimating line lengths). Dysfunctional males, however, showed lower levels of penile tumescence with genital feedback. In addition, dysfunctional subjects reported more negative affect during the genital feedback situation than in the other conditions. This latter again points to the urgent need to develop more reliable and valid affect assessment procedures. Abrahamson et al. (1989) concluded that since sexually functional and dysfunctional males did not differ in the distribution of thought content, they must process the same information in different ways. The dysfunctionals reported more intense thoughts and feelings during the performance-demand feedback. On the other hand, Bruce, Barlow, and Jones (1989) found significant between-group differences in thought content during performance demand and distraction conditions. Thus it appears that a potentially important difference between functional and dysfunctional males may be in the interaction of thought content with the intensity and negative affective tone associated with the thoughts. These data are clearly preliminary, but raise some interesting leads for future research.

EXAMPLE ASSESSMENT OF ERECTILE DYSFUNCTION

Assessment Model

Our assessment of male erectile disorder is guided by the behavioral model discussed above. Affective, behavioral, cognitive, and physiological variables are assessed systematically in an effort to delineate their functional relationship(s) to the target problem (see Adams & Haber, 1984, for a discussion of this type of system as applied in general, and Wincze, 1981 for a specific application to sexual difficulties). We obtain this information through multiple methods, including semi-structured interview, self-monitoring questionnaires and inventories, waking assessment of erectile potential, and physical examination which includes vascular and laboratory studies. The assessment goals are to identify the conditions under which erectile dysfunction occurs and the specific variables that contribute to its etiology and maintenance. The model directly links assessment to treatment in that treatment planning and outcome evaluation are determined by the particular results of the assessment.

Interview

The assessment procedure begins with a diagnostic interview that includes a medical and sexual history as well as a brief screening for other major psychopathology. The following is an outline of the major topic areas covered:

Medical history. The medical history included queries into relevant past or present conditions (e.g., diabetes, heart disease, multiple sclerosis, hypertension); medications (e.g., antihypertensives, psychoactives); surgery (e.g., lumbar sympatectomy, colectomy); radiation therapy; alcohol and tobacco use. Data generated through the interview are combined with information from referral source(s) to complete the history.

Sexual history. The goal of the sexual history is to collect information to help determine if there are sufficient psychological factors to account for the disorder.

The focus of this section of the interview is on problem description and current controlling factors. Discussion covers such areas as definition, onset, and course of the problem; frequency of intercourse and masturbation; use and content of fantasy; sexual behavior in the patient's behavioral repertoire; sexual satisfaction, self or professional treatments; sexual orientation; and current partner relationships. Most of this information can be obtained by asking the client to describe in detail initial and subsequent episodes in which sexual dysfunction has occurred and contrast these occasions to times when the difficulty did not occur.

When investigating a specific instance of sexual interaction among other particulars, the interviewer assists the patient in specifying the behaviors in which the couple engaged, foci of attention, appraisals of verbal and nonverbal communication, and affect experienced as a result of the sexual activity. Asking clients to describe these factors as they occur before (antecedent), during (concurrent), and after (consequent) the sexual activity allows for a more thorough assessment.

Obviously, the above lists of possible problem areas are not exhaustive. Indeed, this point highlights the fact that the specific content of potential controlling variables is varied and depends on what Wincze (1981) has referred to as "the individual processing of factors" (p. 293). Accordingly, an essential aspect of case formulation also involves correlating changes in sexual functioning with context-specific variables, and at the many levels that these relationships can be established (e.g., antecedent, concurrent, and consequent). Examples of some possible content areas common to these variables include apprehensive expectation, negative affect, distracting cognitions, and disruptive physiological activity. Factors bearing close relationship to the onset of the dysfunction are seen as precipitating and often vary from case to case. Commonly reported general precipitants influencing the development of the problem include religious orthodoxy and disturbed interpersonal relationships.

Psychiatric Diagnostic Interview

Finally, screening for relevant psychopathology is conducted. The Psychiatric Diagnostic Interview (Othmer, Penick, & Powell, 1981) is a structured interview that includes history of past psychiatric hospitalization, screens for organic brain syndrome, schizophrenia, affective, anxiety, somatoform, psychophysiological, personality, dissociative, and adjustment disorders as defined by DSM-III criteria.

Questionnaires and inventories. There are many reasons that we include pencil-and-paper assessment tools in our assessment package. Such instruments can sometimes provide more detailed information within certain content areas than is practical by interview alone (e.g., sexual behavior repertoire). Secondly, information gathered from questionnaires can be used to grossly assess the reliability of interview-generated material. The data can also be used to establish baselines helpful in the assessment of therapeutic change. Table 4.1 presents a list of useful scales and the content areas they assess. Additional scales can be used to supplement interview-generated data concerning topic areas not focused directly on sexual concerns, but which may be particularly relevant in specific cases (e.g., assertive-

Table 4.1.
Questionnaires and Inventories Used in the Assessment of Male Erectile Disorder

Sexual Dysfunction: Derogatis Sexual Functioning Inventory (Derogatis, Meyer, & Dupkin, 1976; Derogatis, 1975); Sexual Interaction Inventory (LoPiccolo & Steger, 1974).
Sexual Knowledge: SKAT (Lief & Reed, 1972).
Sexual Anxiety: Sexual Anxiety Inventory (Janda & O'Grady, 1980); Card-Sorting Method, (Caird & Wincze, 1977).
Sexual Attitudes: Sexual Opinion Survey (Fisher & Byrne, 1978a, 1978b).
Sexual Guilt: Mosher Guilt Scale (sex-guilt subscale) (Mosher, 1966).
Relationship Satisfaction: Index of Sexual Satisfaction (Hudson, Harrison, & Crosscup, 1981).

ness, or affective assessment tools). Finally, questionnaires are cost-effective methods of data collection, since most are self-administered.

Physical Examination

The physical examination consists of an assessment of general appearance including height, weight, body type, secondary characteristics, temperature, and respiration. Evaluation of the head, ears, eyes (arcus senilus, vessels, xanthalasma, fundi), neck (thyroid bruits), and heart (auscult) is conducted. Genital examination includes, a check for plaques, fibrosis, phimosis, posthitis, balantis, and testicular abnormality. Rectal examination includes saddle sensation, prostrate, and bulbocavernosus reflex checks.

A noninvasive screening of genital circulation is performed. Blood pressures and peripheral pulses and temperatures are assessed. The mean arterial pressure is calculated by adding 1/3 of the pulse pressure to the diastolic pressure, where pulse pressure is defined as the difference between systolic and diastolic pressures. For example, a patient with a brachial blood pressure of 113/80 mm Hg has a pulse pressure of 33 mm Hg, 1/3 of which is 11. This value added to the diastolic value of 80 yields a mean arterial pressure of 91 mm Hg. Two ratios are calculated from doppler evaluations: penile brachial index (PBI) and the ratio of penile systolic pressure to the mean arterial pressure (PMAI). Unremarkable values for both ratios (approximately .85 for PBI and 1.0 for PMAI) are not viewed as sufficient criteria for vasculogenic rule-out. Both are evaluated in the context of the problem topography. Cases wherein a vascular component is significant receive referral for more invasive assessment (e.g., arteriography).

Laboratory study results have often been completed prior to assessment. Relevant tests include complete blood count, profile I and II, serum testosterones (FSH, LH), serum prolactins, and 3–5 hour glucose tolerance tests.

Waking Assessment of Erectile Potential

This procedure involves the measurement of the sexual response to visual, auditory, and tactile stimulation. During the procedure, the gowned client is seated in a private laboratory room designed to reduce external distractions (e.g., low lighting and a comfortable recliner are provided). After the initial instruction and a period of relaxation, the client views and/or listens to a series of sexually explicit stimuli while his penile circumference is monitored via mechanical and/or mercury strain gauges. Other physiologic indices can be monitored as well. During some trials, continuous measures of subjective states are obtained via client movement of a scaled hand lever (Wincze, Barlow, Qualls, & Steinman, 1979). Post-trial subjective ratings of other variables can also be obtained. In addition, excerpt content can be varied for assessment of erotic cue preferences. Clients can also be asked to manually self-stimulate to fullest erection in response to preferred excerpts and fantasy. The procedure not only allows assessment of erectile potential, but also includes measurement of important information not possible through traditional NPT assessment.

We now present two case studies to illustrate the assessment procedure discussed above. We selected these cases because each represents a rather clear etiological example. Neither case, however, is typical of the cases we assess in our program since most cases are not as clear-cut as these two. With that caveat in mind, we now discuss the cases of Mr. P and Mr. O.

Case study #1. Mr. P is a 26-year-old single, caucasian heterosexual male who complained of erectile problems of 5 years duration. He described the problem as an inability to maintain, and occasionally attain, an erection sufficient for completion of intercourse. He described an intermittent course and stated that penile detumescence had occurred before and after penetration with approximately equal frequency. Mr. P. reported that the problem had occurred on approximately 15 occasions, and with 10 different partners, none of whom were "steady." At the time of assessment, Mr. P did have a girlfriend, but had refrained from sexual contact with her because of "his problem." His frequency of intercourse had decreased steadily since onset. The frequency of masturbation and accompanying fantasy remained steady. He stated that he has been able to consistently attain approximately 100 percent erection during masturbation and while waking in the morning. Finally, he stated that his feelings of sexual arousal (i.e., subjective arousal) during intercourse were low relative to those he experiences during masturbatory fantasy.

Mr. P.'s physical examination showed him to be of normal appearance and in good general health. Upon examination, his abdomen was soft. His liver and spleen were not enlarged. There were no flank masses, and his bladder was not palpable. Examination of the inguinal area revealed no hernias. Genital examination revealed a normal phallus and meatus. Both testicles were descended and normal to palpatation. His prostate was small and benign. Bulbocavernosus reflex was normally active. Femoral pulses were strong and symmetrical. Doppler evaluation revealed that all four vessels could be heard easily, and that both his PBI and PMAI were 1.0. Laboratory studies were negative. During the medical history section of the interview, he reported no surgery and no significant illness or disease. He claimed to be a nonsmoker, and reported occasional alcohol use unrelated to erectile problems.

Given the course, situational specificity of the erectile problem, and a quite unremarkable physical examination, it was not surprising to find that results from the interview revealed a number of probable maintaining factors, as well as a corroborative history. For brevity's sake, only these significant variables are presented below.

During one portion of the interview, Mr. P. described his typical sexual interactions including those of the initial episode. He stated that he had often felt insecure about his abilities to satisfy his partners, and stated that this concern had occupied much of his attention during sexual relations. He described a hypersensitivity to his partner's reactions during sexual relations, and related many examples in which he perceived these reactions to be negative. He described several instances of obtaining partner feedback by inferring her satisfaction through selective attention and misattribution of rather innocuous and irrelevant reactions. He also stated he has experienced embarrassment, anger (toward himself and his partners), and frustration on various occasions following the realization that he could not maintain an erection. He stated that he could typically attain an erection sufficient for penetration during foreplay "directed toward" him; however, when it was "his turn," he typically could not sustain erection. Mr. P's use of fantasy also correlated with this self-defined dichotomization of his foreplay, in that he would fantasize and show erection when he was the role of recipient, but would not when he was the provider. The content of Mr. P's most frequent masturbatory fantasy (one to which he can attain erection) painted a picture of him in the role of his ideal sexual male described below.

Both questionnaire and interview revealed a history of sexual misinformation, the sources of which seem to be peers. The misinformation seemed related to the attributes Mr. P might have used to describe the ideal sexual male: a well-endowed, highly skilled technician who never left a partner unsatisfied. Additionally, Mr. P reported an experience of being ridiculed by friends after they had been told by one of Mr. P's dates that he had ejaculated prematurely during an episode of petting. He described the experience as "extremely embarrassing," and denied it when with these friends. He also stated that fear of rapid ejaculation had been a concern of his during subsequent sexual encounters, including his initial experience with erectile failure.

Finally, Mr. P was able to attain 100 percent erection in response to self-stimulation during the waking assessment. Interestingly, subjective estimates of arousal during some film segments was low relative to degree of erection and corresponded to negative affective ratings. These results confirmed self-report and results from the physical examination showing Mr. P capable of full erection, as well as supporting his self-report of differential subjective arousal.

In sum, Mr. P has developed a pattern of entering sexual situations with apprehensive expectations concerning his sexual "skill" and ability to maintain erection. Beside these antecedents, other factors bearing concurrent functional relation are primarily cognitive as well. They include attention to performance concerns, fear of failure (i.e., both in skills and erection), and misattribution of partner reactions. Consequent variables include emotional responses such as anger, frustration, and embarrassment. Poor sexual communication (i.e., he relies primarily on inference) seems to have precluded address and any chance of resolution of these concerns. The factors are seen to distract Mr. P from foci more conducive to sexual responding. Development of this pattern was supported by a history of misinformation and relevant negative experiences.

Mr. P's current girlfriend was supportive and willing to join him in recommended sex therapy.

Case study #2. Mr. O is a 51-year-old married, Caucasian, heterosexual male who complained of erectile problems of 7 years duration. He described the problem as an increasing difficulty to attain erection sufficient for penetration. He stated that onset was gradual, with steady decreases in erectile potential from episode to episode. He further described the exacerbating course stating that approximately one year ago he had reached the point where his maximum erection was insufficient for penetration (which he described as 50 percent of full erection). Mr. O reported that his maximum erection across situations (e.g., masturbation) has corresponded to his erectile potential during intercourse. For example, he stated that 3 years ago, 70 percent erection was the maximum attained during masturbation, while waking, and during intercourse; whereas, at present, it is 50 percent. He reported no decreases in subjective arousal or overall desire stating, "I feel as turned on as I did 30 years ago, but my penis just won't get hard."

Mr. O's physical examination showed him to be slightly endomorphic and in fair general health. Upon examination, his abdomen was soft. His liver and spleen were not enlarged. There was no flank masses, and his bladder was not palpable. Examination of the inguinal area revealed no hernias. Genital examination revealed a normal phallus and meatus, although slightly cool to the touch. Both testicles were descended and normal to palpatation. His prostrate was small and benign. Bulbocavernosus reflex was normally active. Femoral pulses were moderate and symmetrical. Doppler evaluation revealed that all four vessels could be heard but with difficulty. Mr. O's BPI was .73, and PMAI was .89. Laboratory studies showed elevated cholesterol which was being treated through diet. During the medical history section of the interview, Mr. O reported no surgery and no significant illness or disease. He claimed to be a one-pack per day smoker, and reported occasional alcohol use unrelated to erectile problems.

Mr. O's interview showed an absence of problematic psychological factors. The following excerpts reveal rather functional coping responses: In describing his reactions to a decreasing erectile potential, Mr. O stated that he thought initially the decrease was due to normal aging. Continuing, he described conversations between himself and his wife about the noticeable change in his erection. These talks often took the form of cooperative problem solving. As the course exacerbated, and penetration was becoming more difficult, the couple described engaging in or prolonging alternative forms of sexual expression. Finally, Mr. O had read that assessment and treatment for a condition such as his was available, and decided to seek our help.

When asked why he sought assessment, Mr. O explained that noncoital sex has become as enjoyable to him and his wife as intercourse. However, in consideration of his relatively young age, health, and the availability of effective treatments, he decided to investigate the option of treatment. Indeed, the couple was prepared to return to their previous practices if they decided that the treatment option was not feasible. Although the couple had sought assessment, they seemed to have had no second thoughts in considering no treatment as an option. Sexual history, questionnaire, and inventory results supported the picture of a sexually informed, communicative, and flexible couple.

Finally, Mr. O demonstrated a 50 percent erection in response to viewing films and self-stimulation. Subjective arousal ratings were relatively high given the level of erectile change. These results confirmed self-report and expected erectile capacity given the findings through physical examination of decreased penile blood pressure and flow.

In sum, the onset and maintenance of Mr. O's erectile problem was most likely related to a vascular abnormality. He was referred for further assessment of this component (e.g., arteriography) in preparation for a possible surgical intervention.

REFERENCES

Abel, G. G., Murphy, W., Becker, J., & Bitar, A. (1979). Women's vaginal responses during REM sleep. *Journal of Sex & Marital Therapy, 5,* 5–11.

Abrahamson, D. J., Barlow, D. H., & Abrahamson, L. S. (1989). Differential effects of performance demand and distraction on sexually functional and dysfunctional males. *Journal of Abnormal Psychology, 98,* 241–247.

Adams, H. E., & Haber, J. D. (1984). The classification of abnormal behavior. In H. E. Adams & P. B. Sutker (Eds.), *Comprehensive handbook of psychopathology* (pp. 3–25). New York: Plenum Press.

American Psychiatric Association. (1980). *Diagnostic and statistical manual of mental disorders* (3rd ed.). Washington, DC: Author.

American Psychiatric Association. (1987). *Diagnostic and statistical manual of mental disorders* (3rd ed., revised). Washington, DC: Author.

Barbach, L. G. (1975). *For yourself: The fulfillment of female sexuality.* New York: Doubleday.

Barlow, D. H. (1986). Causes of sexual dysfunction: The role of anxiety and cognitive interference. *Journal of Consulting and Clinical Psychology, 54,* 140–148.

Beck, J. G., & Barlow, D. H. (1984). Current conceptualizations of sexual dysfunctions: A review and an alternative perspective. *Clinical Psychology Review, 4,* 363–378.

Beck, J. G., & Barlow, D. H. (1986). The effects of anxiety and attentional focus on sexual responding—II: Cognitive and affective patterns in erectile dysfunction. *Behaviour Research and Therapy, 24,* 19–26.

Beck, J. G., Barlow, D. H., & Sakheim, D. K. (1983). The effects of attentional focus and partner arousal on sexual responding in functional and dysfunctional men. *Behaviour Research and Therapy, 21,* 1–9.

Blum, M. D., Bahnson, R. R., Porter, T. N., & Carter, M. F. (1985). Effect of local alpha-adrenergic blockade on human penile erection. *The Journal of Urology, 134,* 479–481.

Brown, M., Amoroso, D., Ware, E., Pruesse, M., & Pilkey, D. (1973). Factors affecting viewing time of pornography. *The Journal of Social Psychology, 90,* 125–135.

Bruce, T. J., & Barlow, D. H. (in press). The nature and role of performance anxiety in sexual dysfunction. In H. Leitenberg (Ed.), *Handbook of social and evaluation anxiety* (pp. 357–384). New York: Plenum Press.

Bruce, T. J., Barlow, D. H., & Jones, J. C. (1989, November). *Differential response to distraction of sexually functional and dysfunctional males.* Paper presented at the meeting of the Association for the Advancement of Behavior Therapy, Washington, DC.

Bruce, T. J., Cerny, J. A., & Barlow, D. H. (1986, November). *Spectatoring operationalized: Its influence in sexually functional and dysfunctional men.* Paper presented at the meeting of the Association for the Advancement of Behavior Therapy, Chicago, IL.

Cacioppo, J. T., & Petty, R. E. (1981). Social psychological procedures for cognitive response assessment: The thought listing technique. In T. V. Merluzzi, C. R. Glass, & M. Genest (Eds.), *Cognitive assessment* (pp. 309–342). New York: Guilford Press.

Caird, W., & Wincze, J. P. (1977). *Sex therapy: A behavioral approach.* New York: Harper & Row.

Cerny, J. A. (1978). Biofeedback and the voluntary control of sexual arousal in women. *Behavior Therapy, 9,* 847–855.

Cerny, J. A., & Clodfelter, E. (1980). [The assessment of sexual anxiety]. Unpublished raw data.

Cerny, J. A., & Katz, L. C. (1988, May). *The assessment of ejaculatory latency.* Paper presented at the meeting of the Midwestern Psychological Association, Chicago, IL.

Cerny, J. A., & Katz, L. C. (1990, May). *Differential ejaculatory control in rapid ejaculators and sexually functional men.* Paper presented at the meeting of the Midwestern Psychological Association, Chicago, IL.

Conte, H. R. (1986). Multivariate assessment of sexual dysfunction. *Journal of Consulting and Clinical Psychology, 54,* 149–157.

Derogatis, L. R. (1975). *Derogatis sexual functioning inventory.* Baltimore: Johns Hopkins University.

Derogatis, L. R., & Melisaratos, N. (1979). The DSFI: A multidimensional measure of sexual functioning. *Journal of Sex & Marital Therapy, 5,* 244–281.

Derogatis, L. R., Meyer, J. K., & Dupkin, C. N. (1976). Discrimination of organic versus psychogenic impotence with the DSFI. *Journal of Sex and Marital Therapy, 2,* 229–240.

Farkas, G. M., Sine, L. F., & Evans, I. M. (1979). The effects of distraction, performance demand, stimulus explicitness, and personality on objective and subjective measures of male sexual arousal. *Behaviour Research and Therapy, 17,* 25–32.

Fischer, C., Schiavi, R., Edwards, A., Davis, D. M., Reitman, M., & Fine, J. (1979). Evaluation of nocturnal penile tumescence in the differential diagnosis of sexual impotence. *Archives of General Psychiatry, 36,* 431–437.

Fisher, W. A., & Byrne, D. (1978a). Sex differences in response to erotica? Love versus lust. *Journal of Personality and Social Psychology, 36,* 119–125.

Fisher, W. A., & Byrne, D. (1978b). Individual differences in affective, evaluative, and behavioral responses to an erotic film. *Journal of Applied Social Psychology, 8,* 355–365.

Frank, E., Anderson, C., & Rubenstein, D. (1978). Frequency of sexual dysfunction in "normal couples." *The New England Journal of Medicine, 299,* 111–115.

Freund, K., Chan, S., & Coulthard, R. (1979). Phallometric diagnosis with "Nonadmitters." *Behaviour Research and Therapy, 17,* 451–457.

Geer, J., & Fuhr, R. (1976). Cognitive factors in sexual arousal: The role of distraction. *Journal of Consulting and Clinical Psychology, 44,* 238–243.

Geer, J. H., & Quartararo, J. D. (1976). Vaginal blood volume responses during masturbation. *Archives of Sexual Behavior, 5,* 403–413.

Graber, B., & Kline-Graber, G. (1981). Research criteria for male erectile failure. *Journal of Sex & Marital Therapy, 7,* 37–49.

Hatch, J. P. (1981). Psychophysiological aspects of sexual dysfunction. *Archives of Sexual Behavior, 10,* 49–64.

Heiman, J. R. (1976). Issues in the use of psychophysiology to assess female sexual dysfunction. *Journal of Sex & Marital Therapy, 2,* 197–204.

Heiman, J. R., & Rowland, D. L. (1983). Affective and physiological sexual patterns: The effects of instructions on sexually functional and dysfunctional men. *Journal of Psychosomatic Research, 27,* 105–116.

Henson, D. E., & Rubin, H. B. Voluntary control of eroticism. *Journal of Applied Behavior Analysis, 4,* 37–44.

Hoon, E. F., Hoon, P. W., & Wincze, J. (1976). Physiological assessment of sexual arousal in women. *Psychophysiology, 13,* 196–204.

Hudson, W. W., Harrison, D. F., & Crosscup, P. C. (1981). A short-term scale to measure sexual discord in dyadic relationships. *Journal of Sex Research, 17,* 157–174.

Hurlburt, R. T. (1980). Validation and correlation of thought sampling with retrospective measures. *Cognitive Therapy and Research, 4,* 235–238.

Janda, L. H., & O'Grady, K. E. (1980). Development of a sex anxiety inventory. *Journal of Consulting and Clinical Psychology, 4,* 169–175.

Kaplan, H. S. (1974). *The new sex therapy.* New York: Brunner/Mazel.

Kaplan, H. S. (1981). *The new sex therapy: Active treatment of sexual dysfunctions.* New York: Brunner/Mazel.

Karacan, I. (1978). Advances in the psychophysiological evaluation of male erectile impotence. In J. LoPiccolo & L. LoPiccolo (Eds.), *Handbook of sex therapy* (pp. 137–145). New York: Plenum.

Karacan, I., Salis, P. J., Ware, J. C., Dervert, B., Williams, R. L., Scott, F. B., Attia, S. L., & Bentler, L. E. (1978). Nocturnal penile tumescence and diagnosis in diabetic impotence. *American Journal of Psychiatry, 135,* 191–197.

Karacan, I., Scott, F. B., Salis, P. J., Attia, S. L., Ware, J. C., Altinel, A., & Williams, R. (1977). Nocturnal erections, differential diagnosis of impotence and diabetes. *Biological Psychiatry, 12,* 373–380.

Kaya, N., Moore, C., & Karacan, I. (1979). Nocturnal penile tumescence and its role in impotence. *Psychiatric Annals, 9,* 426–431.

Kockott, G., Feil, W., Fersth, R., Aldenhoff, J., & Besinger, W. (1980). Psychological aspects of male inadequacy: Results of an experimental study. *Archives of Sexual Behavior, 9,* 477–493.

Kockott, G., Feil, W., Revenstorf, D., Aldenhoff, J., & Besinger, U. (1980). Symptomatogy and psychological aspects of male sexual inadequacy: Results of an experimental study. *Archives of Sexual Behavior, 9,* 457–475.

Kolodny, R. C., Masters, W. H., & Johnson, V. E. (1979). *Textbook of sexual medicine.* Boston: Little, Brown.

Lange, J. D., Wincze, J. P., Zwick, W., Feldman, S., & Hughes, K. (1981). Effects of demand for performance, self-monitoring of arousal, and increased sympathetic nervous activity on male erectile response. *Archives of Sexual Behavior, 10,* 443–464.

Laws, D., & Rubin, H. (1969). Instructional control of autonomic sexual response. *Journal of Applied Behavior Analysis, 2,* 93–100.

Leliefeld, H. H. J., & Muhr, S. (1982). Erectile impotence—Clinical experience with the phalloplethysmography. *Urology International, 37,* 257–266.

Levin, R. J., & Wagner, G. (1985). Orgasm in women in the laboratory—Quantitative studies on duration, intensity, latency, and vaginal blood flow. *Archives of Sexual Behavior, 14,* 439–449.

Lief, H., & Reed, D. (1972). *Sexual knowledge and attitude test.* Philadelphia: University of Pennsylvania, Department of Psychiatry.

LoPiccolo, L., & Heiman, J. R. (1978). Sexual assessment and history interview. In J. LoPiccolo & L. LoPiccolo (Eds.), *Handbook of sex therapy* (pp. 103–112). New York: Plenum.

LoPiccolo, J., & Steger, J. C. (1974). The sexual interaction inventory: A new instrument for assessment of sexual dysfunction. *Archives of Sexual Behavior, 2,* 585–595.

Macksgood, M. J., & James, R. E., Jr. (1983). Complete diagnostic evaluation and classification of the impotent male. *Journal of the American Osteopathic Association, 8,* 158–162.

Maletzky, B. M. (1980). Assisted covert sensitization. In D. J. Cox & R. J. Dritzman (Eds.), *Exhibitionism: Description, assessment, and treatment* (pp. 289–293). New York: Garland STPM Press.

Marshall, P., McGrath, P., & Schillinger, J. (1983). Importance of electromyographic data in interpreting nocturnal penile tumescence. *Urology, 22,* 153–156.

Marshall, P., Surridge, D., & Delva, N. (1981). The role of nocturnal penile tumescence in differentiating between organic and psychogenic impotence. The first stage of validation. *Archives of Sexual Behavior, 10,* 1–10.

Masters, W. H., & Johnson, V. E. (1966). *Human sexual response.* Boston: Little, Brown.

Masters. W. H., & Johnson, V. E. (1970). *Human sexual inadequacy.* Boston: Little, Brown.

Masters, W. H., Johnson, V. E., & Kolodny, R. C. (1988). *Human sexuality* (3rd ed.). Glenview, IL: Scott, Foresman.

McConaghy, N. (1988). Sexual dysfunction and deviation. In A. S. Bellack & M. Hersen (Eds.), *Behavioral assessment* (pp. 490–541). New York: Pergamon Press.

Montague, D. K. (1982). The evaluation of the impotent male. In A. H. Bennett (Ed.), *International perspectives in urology* (Vol. 5). Baltimore: Williams & Wilkins.

Morokoff, P. J. (1985). Effects of sex guilt, repression, sexual "arousability," and sexual experience on female sexual arousal during erotica and fantasy. *Journal of Personality and Social Psychology, 49,* 177–187.

Mosher, D. L. (1966). The development and multitrait-multimethod matrix analysis of three measures of three aspects of guilt. *Journal of Consulting Psychology, 30,* 25–29.

Othmer, E., Penick, E., & Powell, B. (1981). *Psychiatric diagnostic interview.* Los Angeles, CA: Western Psychological Services.

Parks, C. W., & Hollon, S. D. (1988). Cognitive assessment. In A. S. Bellack & M. Hersen (Eds.), *Behavioral assessment* (pp. 161–212). New York: Pergamon Press.

Quinsey, V. L., & Bergersen, S. G. (1976). Instructional control of penile circumference in assessments of sexual preference. *Behavior Therapy, 7,* 489–493.

Reading, A. E., & Wiest, W. M. (1984). An analysis of self-reported sexual behavior in a sample of normal males. *Archives of Sexual Behavior, 13,* 69–83.

Rosen, R. C. (1973). Suppression of penile tumescence by instrumental conditioning. *Psychosomatic Medicine, 35,* 509–514.

Sakheim, D. K., Barlow, D. H., Abrahamson, D. J., & Beck, J. G. (1987). Distinguishing between organogenic and psychogenic erectile dysfunction. *Behaviour Research and Therapy, 25,* 379–390.

Schover, L. R., Friedman, J. M., Weiler, S. J., Heiman, J. R., & LoPiccolo, J. (1982). Multiaxial problem-oriented system for sexual dysfunctions. *Archives of General Psychiatry, 39,* 614–619.

Segraves, R. T., Schoenberg, H. W., Zarins, C. K., Knopf, C. K., & Camic, P. (1981). Discrimination of organic versus psychological impotence with DSFI: A failure to replicate. *Journal of Sex & Marital Therapy, 7,* 230–238.

Segraves, K. A., Segraves, R. T., & Schoenberg, H. W. (1987). Use of sexual history to differentiate organic from psychogenic impotence. *Archives of Sexual Behavior, 16,* 127–137.

Steege, J. F., Stout, A. L., & Carson, C. C. (1986). Patient satisfaction in Scott and Small-Carrion penile implant recipients: A study of 52 patients. *Archives of Sexual Behaviour, 15,* 393–399.

Tollison, C. D., & Adams, H. E. (1979). *Sexual disorders: Treatment, therapy, and research.* New York: Gardener Press.

Virag, R. (1982). Intravenous injection of papaverine for erectile failure. *Lancet, 2,* 938.

Virag, R., Spencer, P. P., & Frydman, D. (1984). Artificial erection in diagnosis and treatment of impotence. *Urology, 24,* 157–161.

Wein, A. J., Fishkin, R., Carpiniello, V. L., & Malloy, T. (1981). Expansion without significant rigidity during nocturnal penile tumescence testing: A potential source of misinterpretation. *The Journal of Urology, 126,* 343–344.

Wincze, J. P. (1981). Sexual dysfunction (distress and dissatisfaction). In S. M. Turner, K. S. Calhoun, & H. E. Adams (Eds.), *Handbook of clinical behavior therapy*. New York: Wiley.

Wincze, J. P., Barlow, D. H., Qualls, B., & Steinman, D. (1979, October). *Continuous subjective and physiological measurement of sexual arousal*. Paper presented at the American Association of Sex Educators, Counselors, and Therapists, Charleston, SC.

Wolpe, J. (1958). *Psychotherapy by reciprocal inhibition*. Stanford, CA: Stanford University Press.

Wolpe, J. (1978). Comments on "A test of reciprocal inhibition" by Hoon, Wincze, and Hoon. *Journal of Abnormal Psychology, 87,* 452–454.

World Health Organization. (1977). *International classification of diseases* (9th ed., Vol. 1). Geneva: Author.

Zeiss, R. A., & Zeiss, A. (1978). *Prolong your pleasure*. New York: Pocket Books.

Zilbergeld, B. (1978). *Male sexuality*. New York: Little, Brown.

Zuckerman, M., Ficher, M., Goldman, A., Cohen, S. N., Jacobs, J. A., & Weisberg, M. (1985). Nocturnal penile tumescence and penile responses in the waking state in diabetic and nondiabetic sexual dysfunctionals. *Archives of Sexual Behavior, 14,* 109–129.

5

The Behavioral Management of Sexual Dysfunctions

Walter Vandereycken

Dept. of Psychology
University of Leuven, Belgium

INTRODUCTION

The unscientific popularization of sex therapy and research in the 1970s has led to the common misconception that sexual problems and their management are simple if not simplistic. An overview of the scientific literature as well as some years of clinical experience will suffice, however, to ascertain the complexity of sexual problems. Since so many factors—medical, psychological, and sociocultural—may interplay, professionals nowadays show a growing awareness that sexual dysfunctions require a multidisciplinary approach leading to the development of individually tailored treatment programs (Wincze, 1982). "Sex therapy" is not essentially behavioral, but quite eclectic. Many different activities and techniques have been classified under this title. "Its unchecked growth has generated a number of concerns—e.g., how to distinguish between legitimate sex therapy and quackery; minimum training standards for sex therapists; evidence that sex therapy works. Solutions to such basic problems might be facilitated by a period of assessment, scrutiny and conservatism" (Levine, 1981, p. 429).

Because of the overpopularization of sex therapy, sexual problems are often classified into distinct categories (e.g., anorgasmia, impotence) for which package-like treatment is offered. Moreover, hard-sell advertising has hit the "do-it-yourself" sex therapy market characterized by an incredible proliferation of self-help programs and advice books. The status of these self-help manuals warrants professional concern since current empirical evidence on their efficacy is very limited and falls on the negative side despite the extravagant claims appearing on the book covers (Dow, 1982; Glasgow & Rosen, 1979). It is up to the behavior therapists themselves to create realistic expectancies regarding behavior change programs. Therefore, guided by a "scientist-practitioner" spirit (Barlow, Hayes, & Nelson, 1984), we have chosen to limit our contribution to the discussion of behavioral treatment methods that have achieved an adequate level of validation. Moreover, the discussion will be restricted to "sexual dysfunction," a category of complaints that will be used here in reference to symptoms developed by apparent heterosexuals without obvious gender-identity problems or paraphilias (we will follow the definitions of DSM-III-R: American Psychiatric Association, 1987).

SEX THERAPY AND THE BEHAVIOR THERAPIST

According to Heiman, LoPiccolo, and LoPiccolo (1981), the "behavioral approach" to sexual dysfunctions refers to "a type of therapy in which the therapist actively and directly educates the patient about sexual physiology and sexual techniques, restructures maladaptive behavior patterns and cognitions regarding sexuality, and uses anxiety-reduction and skill-training techniques to improve the patient's functioning" (p. 594). This description, however, is focused too much on the type of techniques a therapist applies. Instead, we are more inclined to endorse Brady's (1976) conceptualization, which views behavior therapy or modification as an approach to problems that make extensive use of the findings of empirical behavioral science. The behavioral approach consists largely of testing clinical hypotheses by changing behavioral and environmental variables that are thought to be functionally related to the patient's difficulties. An approach to a sexual problem—the so-called "sex therapy"—is behavioral to the extent that the functional analysis is multivariate and empirical, and that the treatment consists of the systematic application of learning principles to modify (segments of) behaviors that are functionally linked to the patient's sexual performance (Brady, 1976).

Annon's four-level PLISSIT model (Annon, 1981; Annon & Robinson, 1980) emphasizes the different levels of treatment for sexual dysfunctions: Permission-Limited Information-Specific Suggestions-Intensive Therapy. Since each level requires increasing amounts of knowledge, training, and skills on the part of the clinician, such a model allows practitioners to treat clients up to their level of competence or comfort, and make a referral elsewhere if necessary. The PLISSIT model is aimed at providing a framework for discrimination between problems that require intensive specialized therapy and those that respond to brief and less complex interventions. In fact, Annon and Robinson (1980) underscore that the latter should be tried first before involving clients in expensive, long-term treatment programs.

The major weakness of this model is its conceptualization of the treatment process as applying step by step a series of techniques of a gradually increasing complexity. This risk of reducing treatment to a kind of "psychotechnology" is equally present in Lazarus's (1981) BASIC ID model upon which a multimodal sex therapy is proposed that makes use of behavioral, affective, sensory, imagery, cognitive, and interpersonal strategies. Both Annon and Lazarus seem to overlook that even the "psychotechnologist" has to recognize the relationship between the "technology" and the "person" of the therapist, that is to take into account those therapist factors that influence the process and outcome of treatment, and cut across specific schools, professions, and techniques. Although this aspect has, for the most part, been ignored in the behavior therapy literature, therapists must realize that relationship variables do interact with techniques to effect outcome (Sweet, 1984).

Especially sex therapists should be aware of the influence of their own ideas and experiences as to "normal " sexual functioning.

> In the therapy of sexual dysfunction, patients are helped to define what sexuality is. Some years ago sex was mainly seen as coitus and orgasm through coital stimulation. Now, it seems, feeling is very dominant in defining sex. Undoubtedly there will be new definitions. These definitions, although propagated with pleasurable promises, take control over the lives of many people. Most therapists are as much under the control of these various definitions as are their patients. Therapists seem to know what sex is, but like their patients they do not know why they themselves behave sexually. (Everaerd, 1982, p. 170)

In a similar sense, therapists are influenced by the Zeitgeist—the prevailing sociocultural norms and ideals—while defining the goals of their treatment: Should we change sexual performance, sexualized feelings, or sexual contact within a broader interpersonal context?

THE CRUX OF THE TREATMENT

The essence of the behavioral management of sexual dysfunctions, as crystalized in the well-known Masters and Johnson (1970) approach, is a combination of "doing" and "understanding": getting patients to try things and helping them to understand the difficulties they have in carrying them out. The framework and structure of therapy can be summarized as follows (Bancroft, 1983):

1. Set appropriate behavioral assignments ("homework").
2. Examine the patient's attempts to carry out those assignments.
3. Identify those obstacles (attitudes, fears, feelings) that underlie the difficulties encountered.
4. Help the patient to modify or reduce those obstacles so that the behaviors can be carried out successfully.
5. Set the next appropriate behavioral assignments. Etcetera.

The strength of this approach lies in the *combination of behavioral change and discovery*: The setting of target behaviors is a rapidly effective way of uncovering the crucial interpersonal or intrapersonal problems that underlie eventual obstacles and have, therefore, to be dealt with. This implies that therapy is no mere matter of applying techniques.

The experienced therapist knows that sex therapy requires much more than just prescribing the "right" technique. Very often it is not the therapist's technical knowledge but psychotherapeutic skills that will be tested at different stages of the treatment when difficulties are encountered in carrying out specific behavioral tasks. Time and again, the therapist will have to (a) facilitate the patient's understanding of the specific difficulties encountered, and (b) take active steps to help the patient resolve those difficulties by (1) making explicit the patient's commitment to specific changes, (2) confronting the patient with a particular resistance or lack of compliance, (3) fitting appropriate behavioral steps to the actual situation, (4) facilitating the expression and communication of affect (Bancroft, 1983).

Regarding the specific Masters and Johnson techniques, one may doubt the necessity for interventions such as the ban on intercourse, sensate focus exercises, and the woman-above position, but the value of these prescriptions has not been studied in a systematic way. There is more research evidence for casting doubt on the insistence of Masters and Johnson (1970) on certain aspects of the therapeutic format such as the use of a male and female co-therapy team (Libman, Fichten, & Brender, 1985). Though there exists some controversy about the value of several "essential ingredients" of the Masters and Johnson approach (see, for example, Zilbergeld & Evans, 1980), this does not mean that these techniques are superfluous or ineffective. Other approaches, however, appear to produce similar results (Friedman, Weiler, LoPiccolo, & Hogan, 1982; LoPiccolo & Stock, 1986; Marks, 1981).

It is assumed that *anxiety reduction* is the essential effective factor in the Masters and Johnson approach and that such an anxiety reduction in sexually dysfunctional people can be successfully achieved by other therapeutic techniques (Crowe, Gillan, & Golombok, 1981; Beck & Barlow, 1984). But, as Mathews (1982) remarked, Masters and Johnson's guided practice appears to produce more change than imaginal desensitization, and this change has more to do with increases in enjoyment and arousability than with anxiety reduction. Hence, the change occurring in successful behavioral sex therapy, following the Masters and Johnson model, do not seem to fit any simple model of anxiety reduction. It remains possible, however, that increases in sexual arousal are secondary to a reduction of anxiety associated with sexual performance, brought about by the "in vivo exposure" element in guided practice. "Alternatively a more general reduction in sexual anxiety might be relevant only in a subgroup of clients in whom the sexual dysfunction is of a phobic sort, while in others anxiety is less relevant" (Mathews, 1982, p. 158).

Within the theoretical framework on sexual dysfunction, most conceptual accounts emphasize cognitive aspects of anxiety (e.g., worries over sexual performance, fears over loss of control) without specifying how anxiety blocks sexual functioning since it has also been shown to facilitate sexual arousal (Beck & Barlow, 1984; Norton & Jehu, 1984). In clinical reports, the role of *distracting cognitions* is underlined as a factor which may hamper normal sexual functioning, that is, especially interfering with sexual arousal (Kaplan, 1974). A special type of distracting cognitive process would be the direction of the individual's focus of attention during sexual interaction: focusing upon oneself versus focusing upon one's partner. Self-focus is viewed then as potentially distracting through a process of "spectatoring" (Masters & Johnson, 1970) which involves the focus upon one's own reactions during a sexual encounter from a objective "outsider" perspective. It is assumed to increase performance fears and self-evaluation, especially in males, dissociating subjective sexual thoughts and feelings from sexual activity. When sex therapists recommend to focus upon the partner's responses during sexual interaction, this seems to interfere with the frequently employed technique of sensate focus which directs the client's attention to his or her own sensations during sexual encounter. The coexistence of these techniques, both of which have been reported as clinically effective, clouds a clear conceptualization of the role of attentional focus in sexual dysfunction (Beck, Barlow, & Sakheim, 1983).

Existing treatments for sexual dysfunction, when successful, may achieve their results by intervening in a complex cognitive process involving attentional focus, partner-arousal level, and cognitive labeling (particularly negative self-fulfilling expectancies). This implies that therapeutic interventions, however effective they may be in specific problems, might block a client's sexual functioning—instead of facilitating change—through a process of negative distracting thoughts. For example,

> It is possible that when asked to attend to partner-arousal cues and when these cues indicate high levels of arousal, a demand for performance is created. For men with a sexual history of problematic erectile functioning, this situation may be perceived as one in which they "have to" perform satisfactorily to please their partner. Given a history of erectile difficulties, this demand may create a self-fulfilling prophecy wherein pressure to perform decreases arousal, possibly through a process which distracts the individual from more arousing, erotic cognitions. This process further confirms the expectation for failure. (Beck et al., 1983, p. 6)

These warnings seem justified by the finding that sexually dysfunctional men appear to show greater psychological distress and awareness of a variety of physiological responses, as well as more negative and fewer positive cognitive-affective states. And, as expected, these dysfunctional men show less penile tumescence and lower subjective sexual arousal under performance demand instructions (Heiman & Rowland, 1983). Moreover, another study demonstrated that focus on excitement of the partner suppresses the sexual response in dysfunctional men, as compared with focus on ones own excitement (Sakheim, Barlow, Beck, & Abrahamson, 1984).

Generally speaking, sex therapy (especially in male dysfunctionals) aims at reducing avoidance of sexual interaction and sexual stimulation. Many patients, however, are not avoiding sexual encounter but defending themselves against any *emotional involvement*. So, the crucial factor may be that they are avoiding intimacy. Or, as Everaerd (1982) points out, a number of males are "untouchable": They avoid every stimulating type of touch from their partners which could possibly result in a display of feeling. "It seems that different complaints correlate with different coping styles. Premature ejaculators are coping with threats in sexual interactions by avoiding intimate interaction. Retarded ejaculators on the contrary often engage in intimate interactions with their partners but control the situation by being very active towards their partners" (Everaerd, 1982, p. 166). Maybe this has also to do with other interpersonal dynamics in heterosexual relationships such as the power balance between the partners. Though males may fantasize about female desire and initiative, they might feel not at ease with an "active" partner: Overt desire can be interpreted as sexual "demand" eliciting performance anxiety or fear of being "out of control" in the male. So, sex therapists must be aware of the fact that even simple "homework" instructions may disrupt an interactional equilibrium. This brings us to the important question of whether sex therapy can really work without influencing the relationship dynamics involved.

TREATING THE SEX OR THE RELATIONSHIP?

Behavior therapists have often been—and still are—criticized for being too wedded to the "prima facie" problems (here the sexual complaints) that the client brings to therapy, while ignoring "underlying determinants" which might be directly responsible for eliciting or maintaining the manifest behavior. A behaviorally oriented clinician is often faced with the question of whether symptomatic behavior appears to be functionally autonomous or whether it appears to be shaped by other aspects of the patient's intra- and interpersonal organization. The answer to this question will be decisive as to the choice of the therapeutic strategy, that is, whether to treat the presenting problem directly or to treat other aspects of the patient's behavior in order to solve that particular problem. This indication dilemma—direct versus indirect or "central" versus "peripheral" approaches (Wilder, 1983)—is particularly important when opposing sex therapy and marital therapy.

For some people, the complexity of sexual problems resembles the complexity of interpersonal relationships (Hinde, 1978) of which they are an epiphenomenon. Even the fact of asking help for a sexual dysfunction may be part of that complexity. Bancroft (1983) remarked that some couples find it easier to present with a sexual problem, which they see as a physical illness, than to admit they have interpersonal difficulties. In spite of the obvious importance of these interpersonal factors to common sexual problems, the (medical) sexology literature and especially the sex therapy movement has tended to focus almost exclusively on genital or orgasmic responses and their disturbances. Another source of unjustified narrowing of the clinical scope is the misleading tendency to see sexual problems as either psychologically or physically determined. Even if we can identify specific psychological or physiological determinants, we have to place these factors into the "psychosomatic circle of sex" (Bancroft, 1983). Breaking into this circle at specific points enables us to identify particular types of problems or pathology which become only meaningful figures when placed against the background of a biopsychosocial perspective.

The *interface between marital adjustment and sexual (dys)functioning* has been a controversial issue for several years. Some therapists view sexual inadequacy as the overt manifestation of underlying relationship problems while others state that couples may exhibit sexual dysfunction in the context of a satisfactory overall relationship. According to some studies in this area, sexual functioning and marital relation factors may operate independently of one another (Hartman, 1980a, 1980b). Nevertheless, some findings indicate that there is a certain level of mutual commitment in a couple necessary for a successful sex therapy (Hartman & Daly, 1983; Roffe & Britt, 1981). Or, as Talmadge and Talmadge (1985) put it: The emotional relatedness of the couple is the core of relational sexuality.

However, the clinical decision as to whether a couple should receive sex therapy, marital therapy, or some combination of both (either sequentially or concurrently) is rather complex. When some studies have found no significant difference between sex therapy and marital therapy for sexual dysfunction (e.g., Crowe et al., 1981), conclusions are still difficult to draw because one may claim that in each type of conjoint sex therapy relationship factors are dealt with, be it in a direct or an indirect way. Whatever the explanation, it seems that sex therapy may help both sexual and marital problems, whereas marital therapy alone has a smaller impact on sexual dysfunctions though it may improve general aspects of sexual interaction (Bennun, Rust, & Golombok, 1985; Everaerd & Dekker, 1981; O'Leary & Arias, 1983). But the primary factor that determines whether or not a couple will evidence a positive response to sex therapy is the degree of motivation to improve the relationship shown by each of the partners. Marital distress is a moderator of couples' response to sex therapy to such an extent that treatment effects are partially predictable from certain features of marital (dis)satisfaction existing prior to treatment (Snyder & Berg, 1983b). In case of relationship problems, restoring a couple's capacity for affectionate cooperation may set the stage for subsequent improvement in sexual functioning with more specific sex therapy (Hartman & Daly, 1983). When treatment leads to increased satisfaction about sexual and nonsexual interaction with the partner, this improvement may remain fairly stable at long-term (5 to 8 years) follow-up (Dekker & Everaerd, 1983).

Strikingly enough, there exists only poor literature on integrating the technology of sex therapy and marital therapy (Appelt, 1984; Melman & Jacobson, 1984). According to Johnson (1983), the artificial dichotomy between marital and sexual problems is one of the peculiar idiosyncracies of our field. "A truly integrative relationship therapy avoids artificial dichotomies. Clearly, marital and sex therapy investigators must combine their efforts, so that the treatments described and evaluated in the literature correspond more closely to the complexities and realities of clinical practice" (Jacobson, 1983, p. 93). In everyday practice, academic discussions between sex therapists and marital therapists become irrelevant when taking into account the following consideration: Since mostly sexual satisfaction arises from a couple's collaborative experience as a unit, in case of sexual dysfunction both suffer a significant loss in sexual gratification regardless of which individual is designated as dysfunctional (Derogatis & Meyer, 1979). For both males and females seeking sex therapy, important determinants of sexual distress include the partner's lack of response to sexual requests, infrequent intercourse, lack of affection for the partner, and the absence of specific sexual dysfunctions in oneself. In addition, males' sexual dissatisfaction seems to be strongly influenced by their wives' failure to reach orgasm, whereas wives are more responsive to concerns regarding their own sexual adequacy (Snyder & Berg, 1983a). But a successful outcome in an individual sex therapy does not necessarily improve the (dis)satisfaction or interpersonal attitude of the partner: In some couples, when one partner clearly "wins," the other "loses," and all this at the expense of their relationship (Clement & Pfäfflin, 1980; Dickes & Strauss, 1980; Payn & Wakefield, 1982). So, even when one favors an individual approach, it is better to know—and thus assess—the quality of the marital relation before starting a sex therapy (Berg & Snyder, 1981; Watters, Askwitch, Cohen, & Lamont, 1985).

Masters and Johnson (1970) postulated greater effectiveness of a *dual-sex cotherapy team* over a single therapist. Such teamwork is said to prevent sex-role bias problems, dilute transferential conflicts, reduce resistances, and allow experiential understanding of both members of the patient couple. But, also in the light of what has been discussed so far, has the advantage of a dual-sex cotherapy team been proven? Like Crowe et al. (1981)—and with similar results—Clement and Schmidt (1983) studied couples suffering from sexual dysfunction, who were treated with three different formats: (a) two therapists, long-term treatment; (b) one therapist, long-term treatment; and (c) two therapists, intensive treatment. The analysis of outcome data showed no significant differences between one versus two therapists. A slight trend for better results from long-term as compared to intensive therapy was no longer evident at one-year follow-up. The authors conclude that the success of couple therapy is rather independent of the format. A similar conclusion may be drawn from the study by LoPiccolo, Heiman, Hogan, and Roberts (1985) who also found that, in cases treated by single therapists, a matching of sex of therapist with sex of the dysfunctional member of the patient couple did not lead to better outcome. In other words, the available research data show no obvious advantage for the dual-therapist team, though it may be useful in cases where the main obstacles to progress arise from severe marital conflict (Mathews, 1982).

THERAPEUTIC VARIATIONS ON A SEX THEME

Sex therapy is no longer a particular set of specific prescriptions but a direct and directive approach to the treatment of sexual problems. Instead of being characterized by a standard treatment package à la Masters & Johnson or Kaplan, its central configuration—though translated in an amalgam of techniques—is consistently and persistently symptom-focused, task-oriented, and time-limited, based on the assumption that sexual (dys)functioning is essentially (mis)learned and that therapy is aimed at removing the psychosocial roadblocks which impede the normal expression of sex as a natural human function (Rosenbaum, 1985). According to the needs of the sexually dysfunctional individual or couple, today's therapists try to blend together several therapeutic elements. Although the choice of strategies varies according to the therapist's own preferences (clinical experience and theoretical bias), the management of sexual dysfunctions usually includes some common ingredients. The basic rationale of the therapy can mostly be summarized as ensuring the dominance of positive sexual arousal over (performance) anxiety. Depending on the emphasis upon the first or second factor, the following methods are frequently used in some kind of combination:

For *decreasing sexual anxiety*, a series of "nondemand" procedures may be applied:

- deemphasis on sexual intercourse (temporary ban on coitus)
- relaxation training
- imaginal or in vivo desensitization
- sensate focus accentuating nonsexual touching and exploring
- graded (noncoital) contact and stimulation.

For *increasing sexual arousal*, several "excitement-awareness" procedures may be utilized:

- development of sexual fantasy and imagery
- body awareness and self-exploitation
- directed masturbation or self-stimulation (vibrator)
- (super)stimulation by partner
- role play of (exaggerated) orgasm

Usually therapists prefer to manage the problem in such a way that the interactional dimension of sexuality is also brought into focus by involving the partner (if there is any), directly or indirectly, in the treatment process. Moreover, in each case the therapist must be aware of the possible need for sexual education and information as well as of the importance of changing negative or unrealistic attitudes towards sexuality and restructuring irrational beliefs or myths about sex. Both the format and content of therapy may vary a lot following the principle that the therapist's strategy must be flexible enough to fit the (changing) attitudes of all parties involved. With regard to the chief complaint (we will briefly discuss the major sexual dysfunctions as defined in DSM-III-R), some therapeutic procedures seem to have a special value as pivotal intervention within the general framework described so far.

Functional Vaginismus and Dyspareunia

The vaginismic response to sexual activity is an involuntary spastic contraction of the circumvaginal musculature caused by fear of penetration, usually reinforced by pain experiences resulting from attempts to force the penis into the vagina. Though the classic imaginal desensitization procedure may be helpful, most therapists prefer in vivo desensitization, namely progressive dilation of the vagina (e.g., by insertion of fingers or a series of gradually larger dilators) often combined with the acquisition of voluntary control over the vaginal muscles through relaxation and contraction (Fertel, 1977, Leiblum, Pervin, & Campbell, 1980). The essential factor in the treatment of vaginismic response to sexual activity is the step-by-step progression under the woman's own control (therefore intercourse will be usually attempted in the "women-above" position). The same rule applies to the management of functional dyspareunia, that is, pain during intercourse from any source other than vaginismus but without actual physical lesion causing pain (Steege, 1984). If the coital pain is due to a lack of lubrication (without organic reasons) the dysfunction must be viewed primarily as a symptom of inhibited sexual excitement, and treated accordingly. As in the case of vaginismic women, traumatic and relational factors must be taken into consideration whenever coital discomfort is a persisting complaint (Lazarus, 1980).

Premature Ejaculation

In the case of premature ejaculation the individual complains of recurrent and persistent lack of reasonable voluntary control of ejaculation and orgasm during sexual activity. As for the opposite dysfunction, retarded ejaculation (see inhibited male orgasm), the problem is in fact one of unsatisfactory timing of ejaculation, and as such it is essentially a complaint based upon the subjective dissatisfaction of the patient and/or his partner (Vandereycken, 1986). Kaplan (1974) theorized that the failure in self-control to avoid rapid ejaculation is caused by the patient's poor perception of his own level of sexual arousal, although there is little research evidence to support this hypothesis (Spiess, Geer, & O'Donahue, 1984). Anyway, one may consider rapid ejaculation as a common reaction in young males who then progressively learn to control their ejaculation—through a natural learning process—by growing sexual experience. This probably explains why premature ejaculation is the most frequent complaint in males but, at the same time, thought of as one of the easiest to treat (though the long-term results of treatment may be not always so successful; see Kilmann & Auerbach, 1979). The therapy emphasizes reduction of performance anxiety (see procedures mentioned above) and, most typically, involves discrimination learning to enhance self-control over the ejaculatory response (Perelman, 1980; Zilbergeld, 1978). For this purpose, the pause procedure or stop-start technique is usually prescribed: It includes gradually increasing stimulation of the penis (by the patient and/or the partner) until high arousal near to the point of ejaculation is reached. This implies that the patient focuses on his own sensations and that he has to stop or signal his partner to cease stimulation when he feels he is close to the threshold for inevitable ejaculation. After a pause for arousal to subside, the same procedure is repeated and a similar progressive approximation procedure must be applied when attempting intercourse (intravaginal stimulation). In conjunction with this stop-start method, Masters and Johnson (1970) have advised the "squeeze" technique: When the patient feels he is about to ejaculate, the partner squeezes the head of the penis just below the coronal ridge. This would inhibit the ejaculatory reflex, but we have no real understanding why it works (LoPiccolo & Stock, 1986).

Inhibited Male Orgasm

This dysfunction is characterized by a recurrent and persistent delay or absence of ejaculation following an adequate phase of sexual excitement. Functional ejaculatory inhibition may be found in varying degrees, representing a spectrum of severity which ranges from involuntarily delayed ejaculation (retarded ejaculation) to total ejaculatory inability (absence of ejaculation). The most difficult to treat are those cases with a complete failure to ejaculate under any circumstances, either by masturbation or during intercourse; the intensity of sexual excitement is never high enough in order to reach conscious ejaculation (Vandereycken, 1986). Usually, however, the ejaculatory failure is situational, that is, the man can ejaculate when masturbating on his own. Various theoretical formulations of ejaculatory inhibition have been proposed (Munjack & Kanno, 1979; Shull & Sprenkle, 1980). The classic approach—desensitization and successive approximation—relies on a discriminative learning model: The individual has learned to reach orgasm in the particular stimulus condition of solitary sexual activity, but with a failure to transfer the sexual response to an interpersonal situation (Dow, 1981; Libman, Brender, Burstein, & Hodgins, 1984). Beside reduction of performance anxiety, treatment usually emphasizes increasing sexual stimulation (see techniques mentioned above). Sex therapists most commonly recommend the application of highly intensive extravaginal stimulation to the penis by a cooperative partner. The man is encouraged to ejaculate progressively closer to his partner's body or the partner is asked to maximize extravaginal stimulation, then suddenly switching to intromission near the point of ejaculatory inevitabiity. However, compared to other male sexual dysfunctions, the success rate of this standard approach is generally lower. This may be ascribed to the use of a strategy which might put a performance pressure on those individuals whose dysfunction reflects either a more general sexual inhibition (aversive conditioning or lack of sexual education) or a specifically interpersonal inhibition. Regarding the latter possibility, Apfelbaum (1980) considers the ejaculatory failure as a partner-specific desire problem in males with a rather "autosexual" orientation. Whatever the explanation, this dysfunction underlines that not all (heterosexual) men answer to the expectation of "normal" sexual performance, that is, considering erection as a surefire sign of arousal, intercourse as a self-evidently pleasant activity, and ejaculation as a definite proof of satisfaction.

Inhibited Female Orgasm

Orgasmic dysfunction is one of the most common sexual complaints in women but in many cases it concerns only a secondary or situational lack of orgasmic responsivity. These women can experience orgasm but are dissatisfied about its frequency or circumstances of occurrence, especially the difficulty of reaching orgasm during intercourse. Primary anorgasmia, on the contrary, refers to women who have never experienced orgasm through any means. In these cases, treatment is usually started on an individual basis: The woman concerned is taught how to overcome her sexual anxiety or inhibition (Andersen, 1983). When anxiety is thought to play a central role in the dysfunction, systematic desensitization may be useful, involving relaxation, imaginal presentation of a hierarchy of feared situations, and graduated in vivo tests (solitary and then interactional sexual activity in real life). Another more straightforward behavioral approach is directed masturbation which, instead of anxiety reduction, emphasizes the importance of self-exploration in order to improve one's own sexual skills. It involves a series of self-examination exercises to discover pleasurable whole-body and genital sensations which are then intensified by one's own manual stimulation (eventually including the use of a vibrator). Both individual-oriented forms of therapy—systematic desensitization and directed masturbation—may be combined and, usually, their effects are transferred to an interpersonal situation by progressively involving the partner into sexual interaction (e.g., by means of a sensate focus program). There is no clear-cut support for the usefulness of Kegel's exercises, that is, systematic strengthening of the pubococcygeal muscle supposed to increase sexual responsiveness and orgasmic potential in women (Trudel & Saint-Laurent, 1983). Though there is insufficient investigation of the various components in the aforementioned treatment packages for primary anorgasmia (Adkins & Jehu, 1985; Nairne & Hemsley, 1983), similar therapeutic strategies are said to be effective in secondary or situational orgasmic dysfunction but again without solid research evidence about the factors contributing to treatment effectiveness (LoPiccolo & Stock, 1986). The basic problem here is how to transfer the orgasmic capacity from the solitary situation of self-stimulation to partner-related sexual activities while considering the fact that orgasm during intercourse may be an unrealistic goal for many women. Whether a woman can experience orgasm with her partner during intercourse probably depends less on "technical" aspects (sexual skills) than on the quality of the relationship (De Bruyn, 1982). Becoming orgasmic by manual (self)stimulation, on the other hand, is a reasonable and reachable goal, and essentially a matter of self-management (Morokoff & LoPiccolo, 1982). In these cases, group therapy is a valuable alternative (Barbach, 1980) though it is premature to make any conclusive statements regarding the relative efficacy of group versus individual treatment formats (Mills & Kilmann, 1982).

Inhibited Sexual Excitement

An inhibition in the excitement stage of the sexual response cycle is manifested by a failure to attain or maintain the physiological changes accompanying sexual arousal: erection in males, vaginal lubrication and swelling in females. Impaired sexual arousal is a relatively uncommon problem in premenopausal women in the absence of inhibited sexual desire. In men, however, erectile dysfunction is a very frequent complaint showing how vulnerable the erectile response may be to psychological influences (particularly anxiety), and to physical disorders and side effects of drugs, including alcohol (Hawton, 1985). The concept of "psychogenic impotence" is misleading especially for overlooking physiological pathology involved in a considerable proportion of erectile dysfunctions (Spark, White, & Connolly, 1980). The either/or categorization of erectile failure being organic or psychogenic should be abandoned since it often concerns a combination of etiological factors (Williams, 1985). A similar danger of overestimating the physiological basis of erectile dysfunctions is quite evident when looking at the suddenly growing interest in physical treatments (prosthetic implants, vascular surgery, hormonal therapy). If a man is hormonally within the normal range, administration of testosterone may only have a placebo effect (Bancroft, 1984). It is also time to qualify the overenthusiasm about the implantation of sophisticated penile prostheses: sex therapists, urologists, and vascular surgeons should combine their skills to develop comprehensive multidisciplinary evaluation and treatment plans (Schover & von Eschenbach, 1985). Behavior sex therapy still is the treatment of choice for the vast majority of males showing erectile problems during sexual activity. If a careful screening is carried out, selecting cases of erectile failure without (occult) physiological disorders or important interpersonal problems, treatment of the couple according to an anxiety reduction approach à la Masters and Johnson (see above) is quite effective (LoPiccolo, 1985) with the restriction that, in the long run, these men generally report significant improvement in their ability to maintain erections during intercourse but may still complain of insufficient erection prior to coitus (DeAmicis, Goldberg, LoPiccolo, Friedman, & Davies, 1985). For men without partner, both individual and group treatment may be tried involving cognitive therapy (rational emotive therapy), masturbation exercises, and social skills training (Dekker, Dronkers, & Staffeleu, 1985).

Inhibited Sexual Desire

An impairment of the desire phase of the sexual response cycle may vary from low sexual interest to strong sexual aversion. Often it is presented as a desire discrepancy referring to a conflicting difference in the frequency with which two partners want to have sex (Zilbergeld & Ellison, 1980). As a descriptive term, the notion of "libido" should be abandoned because of its psychoanalytic connotations. Since Kaplan's (1979) appealing work, sex therapists have increasingly recognized the prevalence of desire phase disorders as if in recent years clinical problems have shifted toward the basic factors that give start to sexual interaction (Rosenbaum, 1985). This might be linked with the common failure of standard sex therapy to raise sexual desire probably because its manifestations (both in "normal" and "abnormal" forms) are the least "behavioral," that is, observable and quantifiable, compared to other stages of the sexual response. Sexual desire is essentially an experiential dimension of human beings sexualizing their interactions. It is a complex phenomenon produced by the interplay of biologic drive, psychologic motivation, and cognitive aspiration (Levine, 1984). The recent seemingly effective attempts to treat sexual desire problems integrate an amalgam of experiential, cognitive, and behavioral techniques (Friedman & Hogan, 1985; LoPiccolo, 1980; McCarthy, 1984; Schover & LoPiccolo, 1982). Very often the desire disorder is rooted in the dynamics of the couple relationship and may express a lack of intimacy. It is important to explore and increase the partners' attraction, communication, and emotional expression. Insight in the interactional aspects of the problem sets the stage for further interventions such as sensory awareness exercises, cognitive restructuring, and various ingredients of standard sex therapy. Understanding and treating inhibited sexual desire is the greatest challenge for today's sex therapists. Its complexity certainly requires a multidimensional approach.

Sexual Dysfunctions in the Physically Disabled

When sexual difficulties occur in association with physical disabilities (brain trauma, spinal cord injury, diabetes, tumors, etc.) both organic and behavioral dysfunctions are usually present. Though the primary sexual problem is mostly of physical origin, important behavioral dysfunctions may occur as secondary components resulting from: preexisting psychosocial influences and attitudes regarding sexuality, in addition to mechanisms of personal devaluation (desexualization: the "sexless invalid") and fears about the primary organic disorder. Treatment of these problems is best accomplished by a health care team that can combine a special knowledge of the medical-physical modalities with experience in counseling techniques and behavioral approaches (see Griffith & Trieschmann, 1983). It is within a multidisciplinary management team that the best decisions can be made with respect to special interventions such as the application of drug therapy, specific surgery, penile prostheses, and adaptive devices. If treatment is purely "instrumental," however, it may "disable" the person in a psychological way: He or she is reduced to a dysfunctional machine that has to be "repaired." Therefore, regardless of their psychological inspiration, therapeutic approaches along the lines suggested in the previous paragraphs can be very beneficial for people with sexual problems resulting from physical impairment.

EVALUATION AND CONCLUSION

According to Cole (1985), the idea that human sex behavior is easily modifiable must be viewed, unfortunately, as a myth. Sexual problems present the therapist with one of the most complex scenarios the caring professions have to face. In contrast with the initial enthusiasm, sex therapy proved to have its intrinsic limitations. Failure to recognize this leads to the methods of sex therapy, which have much to offer, becoming devalued. The management of sexual difficulties requires a flexible approach to problem solving and a reappraisal of the fundamental issues involved, so that realistic goals can be defined (Cole, 1985). Many therapists, however, still try to avoid the reality that all things are not possible. They keep on seeking safety and self-confidence in the development of a sophisticated "psychotechnology." Two trends seem to emerge in the field of sex therapy (Vandereycken, 1982): The "*narrow-spectrum*" therapists show a tendency to apply a standard format to a wide variety of patients (e.g., a modified Masters

& Johnson approach) while the "*broad-spectrum*" therapists tend to jump from one technique toward another or essentially always presume underlying intrapsychic or interpersonal problems that should be brought into the therapeutic focus. So the therapists risk either to become too restrictive in rigidly applying a standard method, or they may conceal their therapeutic impotence behind a pseudoflexibility by applying an impressive variety of techniques without any leading strategy. Finally, they may be tempted to broaden the therapeutic scope in such a way as to move the treatment goal ever further from the original symptom or complaint which concerned a sexual function (Vandereycken, 1982).

The evaluation of sex therapy shares many of the aims and problems common to psychotherapy research in general (Milne & Cordle, 1984). The central question still is: What treatment by whom is most effective for a given client with a specific dysfunction under certain circumstances (Hoon, Krop, & Wincze, 1984)? But in the area of sex therapy, anecdotal case reports and uncontrolled research are the rule rather than the exception. In order to replace single-case studies and to avoid the methodological shortcomings of the Masters and Johnson research (Zilbergeld & Evans, 1980), treatment outcome studies should utilize factorial designs to include (Hogan, 1978); client variables (e.g., type of dysfunction, type of marital problems); treatment components (e.g., masturbation, sensate focus); and mode of therapy (e.g., individual, group, conjoint). To these variables, Hoon et al. (1984) recommend adding therapist characteristics, including gender. Recent studies on prognostic factors in sex therapy (Hawton & Catalan, 1986; Whitehead & Mathews, 1986) seem to show that client variables are among the most important factors related to successful outcome, in particular: sexual attitudes, the quality of the general relationship, and the clients' motivation. Regarding the latter, an important therapeutic skill might be difficult to measure. Indeed, resistance or lack of cooperation is a major obstacle to therapeutic progress: "It is tempting to hypothesize that it is precisely with the inescapably real and difficult problem of patient resistance to treatment that well-trained, experienced therapists might demonstrate their mettle" (Wilson, 1982, p. 546).

Though some conclusions are tentative due to the uneven nature of available research evidence, Wilson's (1982) sketch of the *current status of behavioral sex therapy* is rather positive. From a practitioner's point of view, we wish to emphasize the following conclusions:

1. Behavioral procedures which reduce sexual anxiety and increase sexual responsiveness are effective for specific forms of sexual

dysfunctions (e.g., orgasmic difficulties in women, premature ejaculation and erectile failure in men).
2. The cost-effectiveness ratio of sex therapy is evident when judged on the short term, but more compelling evidence on the long-term efficacy is needed.
3. For optimal efficacy, behavioral sex therapy should be used flexibly, tailoring the treatment to the individual's (couple's) particular problem. Hence, multifaceted treatment programs (including both sexual and nonsexual methods) are often required.
4. Though many couples need a mixture of marital therapy and sex therapy, numerous couples can be treated by interventions focused on their sexual interaction.
5. More attention should be paid to treatment formats in terms of maximizing adherence to therapeutic directives and coping constructively with inevitable "crisis-points" in the therapy.

Three major issues should be mentioned here in order to shade their rather optimistic view on sex therapy. First of all, very little is known about the natural history of sexual dysfunctions. There is minimal information concerning the frequency of *spontaneous remission*. Both from a clinical and theoretical viewpoint it would be useful to know which cases would resolve themselves simply with the passage of time. Recent reports suggest that one can anticipate approximately 15–30 percent of men with erectile disorders to have spontaneous remission of symptoms without therapy (Segraves, Camic, & Ivanoff, 1985). Hence, spontaneous remission may account for the variability in reported treatment outcomes especially in centers employing stringent screening criteria. The second point concerns the already mentioned *shift to sexual desire problems*, which appear to show a particular resistance toward sustained behavioral change (De Amicis et al., 1985). Together with growing experience in the field of sex therapy, views on what is called "sexual response" have changed over the last decade (Everaerd, 1983). Desire and emotional satisfaction as components of this response have been emphasized more than ever and present a challenge to sex therapists who in the tradition of Masters and Johnson (1970) have almost exclusively focused their efforts on the arousal and orgasm components of sexual response. This shift in attention seems to be related to some sociocultural changes, particularly the feminist movement that has questioned the "orgasm-through-coitus" criterion of treatment success (Everaerd, 1983). Finally, the third issue concerning the *use of nonprofessionals* is a controversial one. Already in the introduction of this chapter, we expressed some skepticism with regard to the popular self-help literature. But, on the other hand, behavior modification currently defends a self-management approach to treatment assuming an active participant role of the client. In sex therapy the application of self-management principles became a central part of the treatment strategy (Morokoff & LoPiccolo, 1982). The growing popularity of group therapies (as well as self-help groups) and the frequent involvement of the nondysfunctional partner into a conjoint treatment raise the question of whether effective management of sexual problems cannot be carried out by nonprofessionals. If it is true that paraprofessionals can be trained to produce results similar to those of professional therapists (Brown & Bollinger, 1985), it is time to set up comparative research on this matter.

One cannot discuss sexuality without being influenced by personal values and societal norms. The same applies, *a fortiori*, to the evaluation of sex therapy. Should it be judged according to the capacity to restore the target symptoms (the reversal of a sexual deficit or the unblocking of an inhibition in a naturally occurring sexual response) or its capacity to resolve all major problems supposed to be linked with the development and maintenance of a sexual complaint? There is no easy answer to this crucial question. "Here is the dilemma. If the criterion of effectiveness is too narraow—e.g., simply erectile function—sex therapy will be erroneously rated as highly effective. If the criterion is too broad—e.g., capacity to make patients subjectively normal—the power of sex therapy will be unappreciated" (Levine, 1981, p. 432). But even narrowly defined, is the assessment of treatment success or failure not as simple as it looks? Adequate evaluation of treatment outcome must include multiple subjective and objective measures, but this basic methodologic principle is neglected in the vast majority of outcome studies (Wilson, 1982).

Levine (1981) summarized the actual state of the art as follows:

> The appearance of sex therapy has been associated with a number of positive changes in the mental health professions: new clinical services, often to individuals who previously would not have sought help; graduate and postgraduate educational programs in sexuality; public discussion of many sexual issues; stimulation of research. . . . There are three major clinical dangers of sex therapy: its naive application to unskillfully selected patients; the assumption that any specific dysfunction can best be treated by a specifix sex therapy; therapists who violate the ethical guidelines for dealing with patients. (p. 439)

Twenty years after the pionering work of Masters and Johnson (1970) the learning theory model is still a useful paradigm, that is, an inspiring approach to research and therapy. We have abandoned the era of techniques which were routinely applied as medical prescriptions. Sex therapy is no standard method but a directive treatment strategy that takes into account the significance of intra- and/or interpersonal factors and realizes the importance of the therapeutic relationship as a vehicle of a change process.

REFERENCES

Adkins, E., & Jehu, D. (1985). Analysis of a treatment program for primary orgasmic dysfunction. *Behaviour Research and Therapy, 23,* 119–126.

American Psychiatric Association. (1987). *Diagnostic and Statistical Manual of Mental Disorders (DSM-III-R).* Washington, DC: Author.

Andersen, B. L. (1983). Primary orgasmic dysfunction: Diagnostic considerations and review of treatment. *Psychological Bulletin, 93,* 105–136.

Annon, J. S. (1981). PLISSIT therapy. In R. J. Corsini (Ed.), *Handbook of innovative psychotherapies* (pp. 626–639). New York: John Wiley.

Annon, J. S., & Robinson, C. H. (1980). Treatment of common male and female sexual concerns. In J. M. Ferguson & C. B. Taylor (Eds.), *The comprehensive handbook of behavioral medicine* (Vol. 1, pp. 273–296). Jamaica, NY: Spectrum.

Apfelbaum, B. (1980). The diagnosis and treatment of retarded ejaculation. In S. R. Leiblum & L. A. Pervin (Eds.), *Principles and practice of sex therapy* (pp. 263–296). New York: Guilford Press.

Appelt, H. (1984). Sexual dysfunction and partnership. In K. Hahlweg & N. S. Jacobson (Eds.), *Marital interaction: Analysis and modification* (pp. 387–295). New York: Guilford Press.

Arentewicz, G., & Schmidt, G. (1983). *The treatment of sexual disorders: Concepts and techniques of couple therapy.* New York: Basic Books.

Bancroft, J. (1983). *Human sexuality and its problems.* New York-London: Churchill-Livingstone.

Bancroft, J. (1984). Hormones and human sexual behavior. *Journal of Sex and Marital Therapy, 10,* 3–22.

Barbach, L. (1980). Group treatment of anorgasmic women. In S. R. Leiblum & L. A. Pervin (Eds.), *Principles and practice of sex therapy* (pp. 107–146). New York: Guilford Press.

Barlow, D. H., Hayes, S. C., & Nelson, R. O. (1984). *The scientist practitioner.* New York: Pergamon Press.

Beck, J. G., & Barlow, D. H. (1984). Current conceptualizations of sexual dysfunction: A review and an alternative perspective. *Clinical Psychology Review, 4,* 363–378.

Beck, J. G., Barlow, D. H., & Sakheim, D. K. (1983). The effects of attentional focus and partner arousal on sexual responding in functional and dysfunctional men. *Behaviour Research and Therapy, 11,* 1–8.

Becker, J. V., & Skinner, L. J. (1983). Sexual dysfunction. In M. Hersen (Ed.), *Outpatient behavior therapy* (pp. 203–228). New York: Grune & Stratton.

Bennun, I., Rust, J., & Golombok, S. (1985). The effects of marital therapy on sexual satisfaction. *Scandinavian Journal of Behaviour Therapy, 14*, 65–72.

Berg, P., & Snyder, D. K. (1981). Differential diagnosis of marital and sexual distress. *Journal of Sex and Marital Therapy, 7*, 290–295.

Brady, J. P. (1976). Behavior therapy and sex therapy. *American Journal of Psychiatry, 133*, 896–899.

Brown, P. T., & Bollinger, C. (1985). Training non-professionals in the treatment of sexual dysfunction with special reference to the training of marriage guidance counsellors. *British Journal of Medical Psychology, 58*, 257–265.

Chesney, A. P., Blakeney, P. E., Chan, F. A., & Cole, C. M. (1981). The impact of sex therapy on sexual behaviors and marital communication. *Journal of Sex and Marital Therapy, 7*, 131–140.

Clement, U., & Pfäfflin, F. (1980). Changes in personality scores among couples subsequent to sex therapy. *Archives of Sexual Behavior, 9*, 235–244.

Clement, U., & Schmidt, G. (1983). The outcome of couple therapy for sexual dysfunctions using three different formats. *Journal of Sex and Marital Therapy, 9*, 67–78.

Cole, M. (1985). Sex therapy — A critical appraisal. *British Journal of Psychiatry, 147*, 337–351.

Cooper, A. J. (1981). Short-term treatment in sexual dysfunction: A review. *Comprehensive Psychiatry, 22*, 206–217.

Crowe, M. J., Gillan, P., & Golombok, S. (1981). Form and content in the conjoint treatment of sexual dysfunction: A controlled study. *Behaviour Research and Therapy, 19*, 47–54.

Crown, S., & D'Ardenne, P. (1982). Symposium on sexual dysfunction: Controversies, methods, results. *British Journal of Psychiatry, 140*, 70–77.

De Amicis, L. A., Goldberg, D. C., LoPiccolo, J., Friedman, J., & Davies, L. (1985). Clinical follow-up of couples treated for sexual dysfunction. *Archives of Sexual Behavior, 14*, 467–489.

De Bruyn, G. (1982). From masturbation to orgasm with a partner: How some women bridge the gap and why others don't. *Journal of Sex and Marital Therapy, 8*, 151–161.

Dekker, J., Dronkers, J., & Staffeleu, J. (1985). Treatment of sexual dysfunctions in male-only groups. *Journal of Sex and Marital Therapy, 11*, 80–90.

Dekker, J., & Everaerd, W. (1983). A long-term follow-up study of couples treated for sexual dysfunctions. *Journal of Sex and Marital Therapy, 9*, 99–113.

Derogatis, L. R., & Meyer, J. K. (1979). The invested partner in sexual disorders: A profile. *American Journal of Psychiatry, 136*, 1545–1549.

Dickes, K., & Strauss, D. (1980). Adverse reaction of the apparently healthy partner in response to improvement in the overtly dysfunctional partner. *Journal of Sex and Marital Therapy, 6*, 109–115.

Dow, M. G. T. (1981). Retarded ejaculation as a function of non-aversion conditioning and discrimination. *Journal of Sex and Marital Therapy, 7*, 49–53.

Dow, M. G. T. (1982). Behavioral bibliotherapy. In C. J. Main (Ed.), *Clinical psychology and medicine: A behavioral perspective* (pp. 177–203). New York: Plenum Press.

Everaerd, W. (1982). Current research on sexual dysfunction. In J. Boulougouris (Ed.), *Learning theory approaches to psychiatry* (pp. 165–170). New York: John Wiley.

Everaerd, W. (1983). Failure in treating sexual dysfunctions. In E. B. Foa & P. M. G. Emmelkamp (Eds.), *Failures in behavior therapy* (pp. 392–405). New York: John Wiley.

Everaerd, W., & Dekker, J. (1981. A comparison of sex therapy and communication therapy. *Journal of Sex and Marital Therapy, 7*, 278–289.

Fertel, N. S. (1977). Vaginismus: A review. *Journal of Sex and Marital Therapy, 3*, 113–121.

Ficher, I. V., & Eisenstein, T. (1985). Current approaches in sex therapy. In M. Ficher, R. E. Fishkin, & J. A. Jacobs (Eds.), *Sexual arousal* (pp. 142–156). Springfield, IL: Charles C. Thomas.

Friedman, J. M., & Hogan, D. R. (1985). Sexual dysfunction: Low sexual desire. In D. H. Barlow (Ed.), *Clinical handbook of psychological disorders* (pp. 417–461). New York: Guilford Press.

Friedman, J. M., Weiler, S. J., LoPiccolo, J., & Hogan, D. R. (1982). Sexual dysfunctions and their treatment: Current status. In A. S. Bellack, M. Hersen & A. E. Kazdin (Eds.), *International handbook of behavior modification and therapy* (pp. 653–682). New York: Plenum Press.

Glasgow, R. E., & Rosen, G. M. (1979). Self-help behavior therapy manuals. *Clinical Behavior Therapy Review, 1*(1), 1–20.

Griffith, E. R., & Trieschmann, R. B. (1983). Sexual dysfunctions in the physically ill and disabled. In C. C. Nadelson & D. B. Marcotte (Eds.), *Treatment interventions in human sexuality* (pp. 241–277). New York: Plenum Press.

Hartman, L. M. (1980a). The interface between sexual dysfunction and marital conflict. *American Journal of Psychiatry, 137*, 576–579.

Hartman, L. M. (1980b). Relationship factors and sexual dysfunction. *Canadian Journal of Psychiatry, 25*, 560–563.

Hartman, L. M. (1983). Effects of sex and marital therapy on sexual interaction and marital happiness. *Journal of Sex and Marital Therapy, 9*, 137–151.

Hartman, L. M., & Daly, E. M. (1983). Relationship factors in the treatment of sexual dysfunction. *Behaviour Research and Therapy, 21*, 153–160.

Hawton, K. (1982). The behavioural treatment of sexual dysfunction. *British Journal of Psychiatry, 140*, 94–101.

Hawton, K. (1985). *Sex therapy. A practical guide.* Oxford New York: Oxford University Press.

Hawton, K., & Catalan, J. (1986). Prognostic factors in sex therapy. *Behaviour Research and Therapy, 24*, 377–385.

Heiman, J. R., LoPiccolo, L., & LoPiccolo, J. (1981). The treatment of sexual dysfunction. In A. S. Gurman & D. P. Kniskern (Eds.), *Handbook of family therapy* (pp. 592–627). New York: Brunner/Mazel.

Heiman, J. R., & Rowland, D. L. (1983). Affective and physiological sexual response patterns: The effects of instructions on sexually functional and dysfunctional men. *Journal of Psychosomatic Research, 27*, 105–116.

Hinde, R. A. (1978). Interpersonal relationships: In quest of a science. *Psychological Medicine, 8*, 373–386.

Hogan, D. R. (1978). The effectiveness of sex therapy: A review of the literature. In J. LoPiccolo & L. LoPiccolo (Eds.), *Handbook of sex therapy* (pp. 57–84). New York: Plenum Press.

Hoon, E. F., Krop, H. D., & Wincze, J. P. (1984). Sexuality. In E. A. Blechman (Ed.), *Behavior modification with women* (pp. 113–142). New York: Guilford Press.

Jacobson, N. S. (1983). Clinical innovations in behavioral marital therapy. In K. D. Craig & R. J. McMahon (Eds.), *Advances in clinical behavior therapy* (pp. 74–98). New York: Brunner/Mazel.

Jehu, D. (1984). Clinical practice in behavioral treatment for sexual dysfunction. In C. M. Franks (Ed.), *New Developments in behavior therapy* (pp. 231–279). New York: Haworth Press.

Kaplan, H. S. (1974). *The new sex therapy*. New York: Brunner/Mazel.

Kaplan, H. S. (1979). *Disorders of sexual desire*. New York: Brunner/Mazel.

Kilmann, P. R., & Auerbach, R. (1979). Treatments of premature ejaculation and psychogenic impotence. *Archives of Sexual Behavior, 8*, 81–100.

Krane, R. J., Siroky, M. B., & Goldstein, I. (1983). *Male sexual dysfunction*. Boston: Little, Brown.

Lazarus, A. A. (1980). Psychological treatment of dyspareunia. In S. R. Leiblum & L. A. Pervin (Eds.), *Principles and practice of sex therapy* (pp. 147–166). New York: Guilford Press.

Lazarus, A. A. (1981). *The practice of multimodal therapy*. New York: McGraw-Hill.

Leiblum, S. R., Pervin, L. A., & Campbell, E. A. (1980). The treatment of vaginismus. In S. R. Leiblum & L. A. Pervin (Eds.), *Principles and practice of sex therapy* (pp. 167–192). New York: Guilford Press.

Levine, S. B. (1981). Overview of sex therapy. In G. P. Sholevar (Ed.), *The handbook of marriage and marital therapy* (pp. 417–441). New York: Spectrum Publications.

Levine, S. B. (1984). An essay on the nature of sexual desire. *Journal of Sex and Marital Therapy, 10*, 83–86.

Libman, E., Fichten, C. S., & Brender, W. (1985). The role of therapeutic format in the treatment of sexual dysfunction: A review. *Clinical Psychology Review, 5*, 103–117.

Libman, E., Brender, W., Burstein, R., & Hodgins, S. (1984). Ejaculatory incompetence: A theoretical formulation and case illustration. *Journal of Behavior Therapy and Experimental Psychiatry, 15*, 127–131.

LoPiccolo, J. (1985). Diagnosis and treatment of male sexual dysfunction. *Journal of Sex and Marital Therapy, 11*, 215–230.

LoPiccolo, J., Heiman, J. R., Hogan, D. R., & Roberts, C. W. (1985). Effectiveness of single therapists versus cotherapy teams in sex therapy. *Journal of Consulting and Clinical Psychology, 53*, 287–294.

LoPiccolo, J., & Stock, W. E. (1986). Treatment of sexual dysfunction. *Journal of Consulting and Clinical Psychology, 54*, 158–167.

LoPiccolo, L. (1980). Low sexual desire. In S. R. Leiblum & L. A. Pervin (Eds.), *Principles and practice of sex therapy* (pp. 29–64). New York: Guilford Press.

Marks, I. M. (1981). Review of behavioral psychotherapy. II. Sexual disorders. *American Journal of Psychiatry, 138*, 750–757.

Masters, W. H., & Johnson, V. E. (1970). *Human sexual inadequacy*. Boston: Little, Brown.

Mathews, A. (1982). Treatment of female sexual dysfunction. In J. Boulougouris (Ed.), *Learning theory approaches to psychiatry* (pp. 157–163). New York: Wiley.

Mathews, A. (1983). Progress in the treatment of female sexual dysfunction. *Journal of Psychosomatic Research, 27*, 165–173.

McCarthy, B. W. (1984). Strategies and techniques for the treatment of inhibited sexual desire. *Journal of Sex and Marital Therapy, 10*, 97–104.

Melman, K. N., & Jacobson, N. S. (1984). The integration of behavioral marital therapy and sex therapy. In M. L. Aronson & L. R. Wolberg (Eds.), *Group and family therapy 1983—An overview*. New York: Brunner/Mazel.

Mills, K. H., & Kilmann, P. R. (1982). Group treatment of sexual dysfunctions: A methodological review of the outcome literature. *Journal of Sex and Marital Therapy, 8*, 259–296.

Milne, D., & Cordle, C. (1984). Evaluating sex therapy. *British Journal of Sexual Medicine, 11*, 110–114.

Morokoff, P. J., & LoPiccolo, J. (1982). Self-management in the treatment of sexual dysfunction. In P. Karoly & F. H. Kanfer (Eds.), *Self-management and behavior change* (pp. 489–521). New York: Pergamon Press.

Munjack, D. J., & Kanno, P. H. (1979). Retarded ejaculation: A review. *Archives of Sexual Behavior, 8*, 139–150.

Nairne, K. D., & Hemsley, D. R. (1983). The use of directed masturbation training in the treatment of primary anorgasmia. *British Journal of Clinical Psychology, 22*, 283–294.

Norton, G. R., & Jehu, D. (1984). The role of anxiety in sexual dysfunctions: A review. *Archives of Sexual Behavior, 13*, 165–183.

O'Leary, K. D., & Arias, I. (1983). The influence of marital therapy on sexual satisfaction. *Journal of Sex and Marital Therapy, 9*, 171–181.

Payn, N., & Wakefield, J. (1982). The effect of group treatment of primary orgasmic dysfunction on the marital relationship. *Journal of Sex and Marital Therapy, 8*, 135–150.

Perelman, M. A. (1980). Treatment of premature ejaculation. In S. R. Leiblum & L. A. Pervin (Eds.), *Principles and practice of sex therapy* (pp. 199–233). New York: Guilford Press.

Roffe, M. W., & Britt, B. (1981). A typology of marital interaction for sexually dysfunctional couples. *Journal of Sex and Marital Therapy, 7*, 207–222.

Rosenbaum, M. B. (1985). Sex therapy today. *Bulletin of the Menninger Clinic, 49*, 270–279.

Sakheim, D. K., Barlow, D. H., Beck, J. G., & Abrahamson, D. J. (1984). The effect of an increased awareness of erectile cues on sexual arousal. *Behaviour Research and Therapy, 22*, 151–158.

Schover, L. R., & LoPiccolo, J. (1982). Treatment effectiveness for dysfunctions of sexual desire. *Journal of Sex and Marital Therapy, 8*, 179–197.

Schover, L. R., & von Eschenbach, A. C. (1985). Sex therapy and the penile prosthesis: A synthesis. *Journal of Sex and Marital Therapy, 11*, 57–66.

Segraves, R. T., Camic, P., & Ivanoff, J. (1985). Spontaneous remission in erectile dysfunction: A partial replication. *Behaviour Research and Therapy, 23*, 203–204.

Shull, G. R., & Sprenkle, D. H. (1980). Retarded ejaculation: Reconceptualization and implications for treatment. *Journal of Sex and Marital Therapy, 6*, 234–246.

Snyder, B. K., & Berg, P. (1983a). Determinants of sexual dissatisfaction in sexually distressed couples. *Archives of Sexual Behavior, 12*, 237–242.

Snyder, B. K., & Berg, P. (1983b). Predicting couples' response to brief directive sex therapy. *Journal of Sex and Marital Therapy, 9*, 114–120.

Spark, R. F., White, R. A., & Connolly, P. B. (1980). Impotence is not always psychogenic. *Journal of the American Medical Association, 243*, 750–755.

Spiess, W. F., Geer, J. H., & O'Donohue, W. T. (1984). Premature ejaculation: Investigation of factors in ejaculatory latency. *Journal of Abnormal Psychology, 93*, 242–245.

Steege, J. F. (1984). Dyspareunia and vaginismus. *Clinics in Obstetrics and gynecology, 27*, 750–759.

Sweet, A. A. (1984). The therapeutic relationship in behavior therapy. *Clinical Psychology Review, 4*, 253–272.

Talmadge, W. C., & Talmadge, L. D. (1985). A transactional perspective on the treatment of sexual dysfunctions. In L. L'Abate (Ed.), *The handbook of family psychology and therapy* (pp. 1107–1127). Homewood, IL: Dorsey Press.

Trudel, G., & Saint-Laurent, S. (1983). A comparison between the effects of Kegel's exercises and a combination of sexual awareness relaxation and breathing on situational orgasmic dysfunction in women. *Journal of Sex and Marital Therapy, 9*, 203–209.

Vandereycken, W. (1982). Paradoxical strategies in a blocked sex therapy. *American Journal of Psychotherapy, 36*, 103–108.

Vandereycken, W. (1986). Towards a better delineation of ejaculatory disorders. *Acta Psychiatrica Belgica, 86*, 57–63.

Watters, W. W., Askwitch, J., Cohen, M., & Lamont, J. A. (1985). An assessment approach to couples with sexual problems. *Canadian Journal of Psychiatry, 30*, 2–11.

Whitehead, A., & Mathews, A. (1986). Factors related to successful outcome in the treatment of sexually unresponsive women. *Psychological Medicine, 16*, 373–378.

Wilder, S. (1983). Indications for central and peripheral approaches to presenting problems: A case of sexual impotence. In H. Fensterheim & H. I. Glazer (Eds.), *Behavioral psychotherapy* (pp. 171–185). New York: Brunner/Mazel.

Williams, W. (1985). Psychogenic erectile impotence: A useful or a misleading concept? *Australian and New Zealand Journal of Psychiatry, 19*, 77–82.

Wilson, G. T. (1982). Adult disorders. In G. T. Wilson & C. M. Franks (Eds.), *Contemporary behavior therapy* (pp. 539–552). New York: Guilford Press.

Wincze, J. P. (1981). Sexual dysfunction (distress and dissatisfaction). In S. M. Turner, K. S. Calhoun & H. E. Adams (Eds.), *Handbook of clinical behavior therapy* (pp. 290–317). New York: Wiley.

Wincze, J. P. (1982). Assessment of sexual disorders. *Behavioral Assessment, 4*, 257–271.

Zilbergeld, B. (1978). *Male sexuality*. Boston: Little, Brown.

Zilbergeld, B., & Ellison, C. R. (1980). Desire discrepancies and arousal problems in sex therapy. In S. R. Leiblum & L. A. Pervin (Eds.), *Principles and practice of sex therapy* (pp. 65–101). New York: Guilford Press.

Zilbergeld, B., & Evans, M. (1980, August). The inadequacy of Masters and Johnson. *Psychology Today*, pp. 29–43.

6

Premenstrual Syndrome

Carol Morse
Lorraine Dennerstein

Key Centre for Women's Health in Society
University of Melbourne
Carlton, 3053, Victoria, Australia

Obvious events of the human menstrual cycle are hormonal fluctuations, ovulation, both local and systemic metabolic changes, and menstruation. The less obvious events of this cycle are the wide range of physical, behavioral, affective, and cognitive variables which are reported to change with each discrete cycle phase. Premenstrual syndrome is the name given to this collection of complex symptom clusters which appear to arise from an interaction of physiological, psychological, and sociocultural sources (Dennerstein & Burrows, 1979; Green & Dalton, 1963).

These symptoms become manifest predominantly in the late luteal phase, often severely incapacitating women at work and in their social lives. Dramatic relief from symptoms usually occurs at, or during, the menstrual flow. This condition of psychophysical changes is the most common endocrine disorder universally reported (Rouse, 1978), but, to date, has no known single etiology nor cultural specificity (Snowden & Christian, 1982).

Different methods of investigation have arisen from the multifactorial composition and varying magnitude of symptoms. This has resulted in a confusing set of definitions, estimates of incidence, and management strategies. Today, workers in the related disciplines of psychology, psychiatry, and gynecology recognize that menstrual-related complaints comprise two main patterns. "True" premenstrual syndrome appears in the late luteal phase during the seven to ten days prior to menses, is relieved at or during menstruation, and at least one week in every cycle is symptom-free. Menstrual distress is the name given to similar symptoms that are present throughout the cycle and worsen during the luteal phase (Dalton, 1980). It is important on methodological grounds to maintain this distinction in order to limit the possibility of contamination of findings and treatment efforts.

Reports of menstrual-cycle-related problems of women have been known since ancient times but the contemporary view of premenstrual syndrome (PMS) arose from a description attributed to Frank (1931). He described a condition observed in a large group of women who persistently presented for help, as "premenstrual tension." This condition was characterized by "feelings of indescribable tension" during seven to ten days prior to menstruation, of "unrest, irritability . . . desires to find relief by foolish and ill-considered actions." These descriptive symptoms were clearly of a psychological nature and provided many of the most distinctive complaints for which women, then and now, continue to seek help. In addition, symptoms of endocrinologic and autonomic disturbances are also reported, most notably of nostalgia, lethargy, body swelling, pain, and disruption of information-processing capacities. These psychophysical complaints together form the multiple symptom complex regarded as premenstrual syndrome.

From a variety of studies the incidence of the condition ranges from 29–96 percent depending on the timing of measurements and the characteristics of the subjects under study. Many early estimates were derived from retrospective studies before recognition was accorded to the unreliability of recalled events. The PMS incidence rates of general practice attenders in Britain were reported as 29 percent (Appleby, 1960), 25 percent (Kessel & Coppen, 1963), and 75 percent (Clare, 1977); of factory workers in America as 36 percent (Bickers & Woods, 1951); of hospital personnel and students in Britain as 33 percent (Sutherland & Stewart, 1965); of American women as 96 percent (Pennington, 1957); of wives of American university graduates as 52 percent (Moos, 1969); and of French women in a community sample as 64 percent (Van Keep & Lehert, 1981). The apparent increase in prevalance of PMS over the years may be reflecting the confusion of approaches to symptom recognition as well as an increased demand from women for symptom investigation and treatment.

PHYSICAL SYMPTOMS IN PMS

Pain

Women who experience premenstrual syndrome, menstrual distress, or dysmennorrhoea may report pain experiences at certain phases of the premenstrual cycle. In PMS, the pain is described as dull and aching in the lower pelvic region, may radiate to the lower lumbar spine, and be relieved during the menstrual flow. In menstrual distress, pain experiences are reportedly present from ovulation and intensify premenstrually in the abdominal region, spreading to include the lower back and upper thighs at and during menstruation. Dysmennorrhoea (menstrual pain) is reported to affect about half of the young female population aged under 25 years, and is experienced as spasmodic episodes of abdominal pain during menstruation (Dalton, 1968; Dennerstein, Burrows, Cox, & Wood, 1978).

The most commonly used self-report measure of menstrual-cycle-related symptoms is the Menstrual Distress Questionnaire (MDQ) Moos, 1969). This has a "pain" subscale which includes muscle stiffness, headache, cramps, backache, fatigue, and general aches and pains. Thus, more than the discrete pain experiences emanating from the recognizable distinct conditions above may be reported on the MDQ by treatment seekers in particular. Evidence for and against significant phase fluctuations on the pain subscale have been reported and it is possible that more than one subtype of premenstrual syndrome exists (Moos & Leiderman, 1981). Variations in pain experiences have been reported to occur in relation to other characteristics. Timonen and Procope (1971) studied Finnish female university students and found significant diferences in reported severity of premenstrual and menstrual low-back pain between gymnasts, athletes, and students from faculties other than physical education. Female athletes reported a lower magnitude of low-back pain than the gymnasts did and this was attributed to the greater perfusion of oxygenated blood circulation which occurred from sustained effort on the sports field. Interestingly, both premenstrual and menstrual pelvic pain was not positively influenced by the practice of sports although both groups of physical education students reported a lower rate of pelvic pain than students from other faculties. These researchers suggested that pelvic pain seems to be connected with increased stimulation of α - receptors in the myometrium which results from overflow of prostaglandins into the circulation. Users of tobacco and or alcohol tend to have an equally high incidence of menstrual pelvic pain (Timonen & Procope, 1971; Dennerstein et al., 1978). This finding may indicate a direct causal effect of a noxious substance on body biochemistry, or may reflect a third underlying causal characteristic, notably, a certain personality type which predisposes a woman to become a tobacco or alcohol user and therefore to be at risk for increased menstrual pain experiences. Further individual differences in menstrual-cycle-related pain are reported by Sheldrake and McCormack (1976) who surveyed the entire female population at a Scottish university enrolled for the 1974–75 academic year. They found that the "more expressive" arts students reported most symptoms of all, and that backache was reported more often by later-born than by first-born or only-born women. What is not clear from these interesting studies is the method used for collecting the data. Moos (1969) developed two forms of the MDQ: Form A, a retrospective scale of symptoms from the last menses, and Form T (Today), which seeks symptom reports from the present time experience. Significant differences have been reported, particularly on pain, water retention, and negative affect subscales, between retrospective and current reporting of symptoms (Rouse, 1978). Parlee (1974) has suggested that retrospective reports reflect more a measure of stereotypic beliefs and experiences than true symptom levels. Other researchers have found that pain reports showed a distinct cycle phase relationship on both daily and retrospective recordings although other symptoms (water retention, swelling, moods) were not consistent on both reports (Englander-Golden, Whitmore, & Dienstbier, 1978).

Headache

The incidence of premenstrual and menstrual headaches is common and may vary in intensity from a mild ache which may be relieved by rest or mild analgesia, to one which persists for many hours as a full migraine experience which responds only to narcotic injections. Headache poses a classification problem and some writers (e.g., Sheldrake & Cormack, 1976) question whether this symptom is to be regarded as physical or nonphysical. Clearly there are elements of both. Headaches tend to be reported as more severe menstrually (Short, 1972) and are often related to usage of the contraceptive pill in the early months although long-term users report headaches as an infrequent problem. This may be because recurring headaches will cause women to give up using a specific pill or any pill, so that long-term users are likely to be pain-free and therefore more comfortable. Headache reporting was found to be greatest in women who are younger by seven years or more to another sibling, more frequent in later-born than first-born or only-born, and related to a cycle length of less than 30 days (Sheldrake & McCormack, 1976). Sports participants report a significantly lower incidence of headache at both the premenstrual and menstrual phase than nonactive women and the use of tobacco seems not to produce any adverse effect (Timonen & Procope, 1971). Rather, these researchers proposed that headache develops from vasoconstriction in the brain in response to stress-related excess catecholamine release. This partly explains the ambiguous classification of the symptom as physical or emotional and suggests that headache may develop as a secondary symptom to other aspects of PMS. Thus, increased oxygenation from sustained and frequent physical activity appears to directly benefit the brain and enables it to overcome increased peripheral resistance that may have resulted from nervous tension.

It is important to clearly differentiate headache types during initial assessment. True migraine experiences must be identified from tension headaches. As some patients present with "mixed" types, careful baseline recordings are imperative. Migraines which occur in relation to the menstrual cycle tend to appear a day or two prior to menses and persist during menstruation. They tend to be unresponsive to common analgesia or usual migraine medications and sufferers frequently report that relief is obtained only from narcotic agents. This provides a problem for regular use and many women suffer extreme distress when narcotics are witheld on the grounds of potential addiction by zealous medical practitioners. Although the etiology of menstrual migraine is unconfirmed, Somerville's (1972a) hypothesis is impressive. He reported that the dramatic premenstrual drop in estrogen triggered migraine attacks in susceptible women. These painful experiences could be overcome by maintaining high plasma estradiol levels with injections of estradiol valerate. As migraines generally cease during pregnancy (Somerville, 1972b), this improvement may be due to the suppression of fluctuations in sex hormone levels which, for the time being, cease to effect the vasomotor responses of the crainal arteries. Much work remains to be done on this interesting related condition.

Water Retention

A second subscale on the MDQ is concerned with water retention and is composed of items incorporating weight gain, skin disorders, painful breasts, and swelling of the abdomen, ankles, and sometimes the fingers or face. Perhaps because of the broad multiple character of this subscale significant phase-related effects have been reported (e.g., Wilcoxon, Schrader, & Sherif, 1976). Although objective measures of water retention have failed to support this finding (Janowsky, Berens, & Davis, 1973), self-reports of weight changes through edema and swelling have been reported to occur at all phases of the cycle by various studies so it has been difficult to identify an exact causative factor. High levels of estrogen reportedly cause an increased permeability of capillary walls which would lead to accumulation of water in the interstitial spaces (Wong, Freedman, Levan, Hyman, & Quilligan, 1972). As estrogen levels peak at midcycle and fluctuate during the luteal phase, the experience of water changes could be expected to occur postovulation. However, the majority of PMS sufferers report water retention predominantly in the late luteal or premenstrual phase. This could suggest that estrogen levels may be ineffectively opposed by progesterone. In fact, Wong et al. (1972) found that PMS complainants did show a fluid increase that was three times greater than a control group, together with limited filtration rate and blood flow. Unfortunately, numbers were very small and this work does not appear to have been clinically replicated.

Autonomic Reactivity

Premenstrual autonomic reactivity is estimated on the MDQ by reports of dizziness or faintness, cold sweats, nausea or vomiting, and hot flushes. Moos (1969) admitted that these symptoms were less frequently reported in the literature but "appear to make good sense" (p. 392). In fact, the inclusion of hot flushes, in particular, is of dubious value when applied to women under 40 years of age as this symptom is regarded firmly as one more truly indicative of menopause. Yet younger women will report this symptom but such a report should be considered together with information on anxiety level and tendency towards social desirability response bias.

Autonomic activation was described as one of three sources of arousal by Lacey (1967) together with behavioral and cortical activation. Asso (1978) reviewed relationships to cycle phase. In general, there appears to be some evidence for increased levels of autonomic reactivity premenstrually, although there are problems with several studies regarding the exact time frame in the cycle when measures have been taken. Some studies which showed no change (e.g., Zimmerman & Parlee, 1973; Little & Zahn, 1974) were criticized for their use of single autonomic indices (skin conductance, heart rate). A study by

Wineman (1971) which found significant changes had utilized multiple sympathetic indices. Her findings showed lower SNS activity during the high levels of estrogen in the first half of the cycle, and high SNS activity during the luteal phase of progesterone dominance. Little and Zahn (1974) used medroxyprogesterone acetate (Provera) 10 mg daily on male subjects and found a significant rise in temperature, reaction time, and decreases in skin conductance. These changes were obtained from synthetic substances that may not mimic naturally occurring progesterone in normally cycling women. Asso and Braier (1982) investigated levels of changes in both central and autonomic system activity using objective and self-report measures at intermenstrual and premenstrual phases. They found the two systems varied independently of each other at each of the two phases of the cycle. Cortical activation was higher intermenstrually; autonomic activation was higher premenstrually. However, the findings were not entirely clear and only three of thirteen indices were positively correlated at the premenstrual phase. Measures of cortical activation still suffer from difficulties arising from the indices chosen for estimation which have shown equivocal results in the past (see Asso, 1978). Strauss and Appelt (1983) attempted to assess pre- and postmenstrual autonomic reactivity by using an auditory conditioning procedure during stress (cold pressor test and mental arithmetic). None of the differences between cycle phases were significant and a general decrease in autonomic reactivity was noted from the first to the second measurement. This reduction would seem to indicate habituation to the tasks which were, of necessity, quite artificial. Neither of the subject groups were PMS-complainants so it is difficult to judge whether an altered reactivity pattern would be found in a clinical group. Certainly the meaning of the tests involved could be expected to play a part in effecting changes in activation or not. At present, the evidence for physical changes in PMS is uncertain regarding whether they occur as a primary reaction or secondary response to some other mediating factor. There is clinical evidence that physical symptoms are a distinct part of the syndrome but as yet, it is unknown whether they occur as cause or effect.

AFFECTIVE CHANGES IN PMS

Changes in emotions and feelings of women have been reported to occur in relation to different phases of the menstrual cycle since ancient times in many cultures. Feelings of well-being (confidence, competence, and contentment) have been reported to predominate during the follicular phase, but the luteal phase, particular the late luteal or premenstrual days, has become identified with negative moods of anxiety, depression, irritability, hostility, and tension (Ivey & Bardwick, 1968; Parlee, 1973). In Western cultures, studies have reported irritability as the predominant premenstrual negative affect (see Taylor, 1979; Watts, Dennerstein, & Horne, 1980; Van Keep & Lehert, 1981; Dennerstein et al., 1985); with feelings of tension, anxiety, and depression occurring at a lowered frequency.

Many early studies during the last two decades utilized volunteer subjects drawn from young adult women undergoing university education. Findings showed that the premenstrual phase was predictably the time of elevated negative moods, loss of competence and coping, in addition to physical symptoms (Ivey & Bardwick, 1968; Wetzel, Reich, McClure, & Wald, 1975; May, 1976). There were several methodological problems with these and similar investigations that attempted to identify menstrual-cycle-related affective fluctuations. These were that (a) the sample selected was unrepresentative of the broader population at large, (b) many of these studies used retrospective reports which were not confirmed by daily records nor at interviews on "present-state" symptoms, (c) age range and socioeconomic group were too narrow, (d) it was not clear whether these subjects regarded their premenstrual experiences as "normal" or "problematic" and whether they sought help or not. When attempts were made to improve the methodology, studies of nontreatment seekers tended to find no relationships between moods, hormone levels, and cycle phase (Abplanalp, Rose, Donnelly, & Livingston-Vaughan, 1979; Lahmeyer, Miller, & DeLeon-Jones, 1982). However, Woods (1985) suggested that those certain women who could be described as fulfilling a "traditional feminine role" tended to regard the whole menstrual process as more debilitating than nontraditional women do. She further reports that negative affect and premenstrual symptoms interact particularly within a person who experiences a stressful social setting. This has been discussed at length in a recent paper (Morse & Dennerstein, 1986).

Later studies have looked at affective change in different groups of women. Findings have shown that adolescents aged 14–15 years showed no significant phase-related differences in anxiety or depression as negative affect scores on the MDQ were elevated most during the menstrual phase (Golub & Harrington, 1981). Negative affects in women aged 45 or older may be confounded by perimenopausal changes even though menstrual cycles may still be regular. Affective symptoms are reported by many women (Van Keep & Lehert, 1981) but only on detailed inspection is it shown whether changes are in relation with the phases of the cycle or at various times throughout the month. For this reason, one of the cornerstones of differential diagnosis is based on the cyclical apearance of negative moods to a marked degree during the premenstrual week in particular. Not only may noncomplainers be separated out from treatment seekers, but true premenstrual syndrome sufferers can be identified from those who suffer from menstrual distress syndrome.

An increase in psychiatric admissions of women during the premenstrual phase has been reported by Dalton (1964). It seems that premenstrual hormonal changes may precipitate bipolar affective disorders in some women who are predisposed or known sufferers. This was shown by Abramowitz, Baker, and Fleischer (1982) who found that 69 percent of depressed patients were admitted in the eight paramenstrual days. A study by McClure, Reich, and Wetzel (1971), who investigated 56 women calling a suicide prevention center, also found that women placed more calls to the center, or made more suicide attempts in the premenstrual phase rather than at any other time of the cycle. Wetzel, Reich, McClure, and Wald (1975) found no relationship between suicide and cycle phase, although attempts to suicide were significantly more likely in the second half of the cycle.

Some studies during the last five years have compared findings from women seeking treatment for PMS with those who do not. In a study by Sanders, Warner, Backstrom, and Bancroft (1983), moods and physical symptoms were found to change clearly in both groups through different cycle phases, showing increasing negative experiences in the late luteal phase. The extent of negative symptoms varied between individuals, but as a group, the women with PMS reported adverse moods and physical symptoms earlier in the cycle and to a greater extent than the controls, although the degree of mood change was not related to hormone concentration levels in another group.

There is little doubt that affective symptoms do fluctuate across the menstrual cycle and that a large number of women are severely troubled by these experiences. Although the incidence of negative mood reports varies between 38 and 71 percent across different cultures (Snowden & Christian, 1982), this difference may arise from the cultural relevance that is accorded specific symptoms. The issue of cultural relativity in symptom recognition is an interesting one that does not appear to have received a great deal of attention. It is possible that hormonal and biological variables differ between women of different races and cultures as Brown (1955) has suggested. A cross-cultural study by Janiger, Riffenburgh, and Kersh (1972) who gathered symptom reports from women of the West Coast of America, Apache Indians, Greeks, Turks, Japanese, and Nigerians found that each cultural group differed from the others in the frequency and magnitude of distress attributed to each of 33 premenstrual symptoms. Turkish women reported the greatest total amount of premenstrual distress and Japanese women reported the least. The characteristics of the "worst" six symptoms also differed for each group. West Coast Americans reported all psychological symptoms, Greek women reported all physical symptoms, and the remaining four racial groups reported a mixture of both physical and nonphysical symptoms. Almost all of the Nigerian women reported headache and nausea as their worst symptoms whereas the frequency of these two complaints was much lower in the other four groups. These discrepant findings are intriguing and seem to suggest that premenstrual experiences are indeed different for women of separate cultures. If a cultural factor does operate it may determine which particular symptom clusters are given attention and which are ignored. Although it seems logical to conclude that a disorder of a given system should be identifiable by the same set of symptoms in the same cluster and thus arise from a common cause, this would be cast in doubt if women from the Orient, the Africian continent, and the West all report different symptom clusters. This not only would appear to exclude there being only one discrete causative factor which can account for the wide array of symptoms (e.g., hormonal imbalance), but also the argument is strengthened for the existence of more than one premenstrual syndrome (Moos & Leiderman, 1978).

At present, this much is clear. Almost all women are aware of mood changes in themselves which may or may not coincide with certain cycle phases. Not all women regard these changes as problematic, perhaps because the magnitude of change is minimal or because some women provide different attributions for such experiences (Van Keep & Lehert, 1981). Other women experience severe distress for one or more weeks in almost every cycle and they seek help for this. The following section examines early and contemporary theories of causation of premenstrual syndrome.

THEORIES OF CAUSATION

Biological Theories

Premenstrual syndrome has been described as the most common minor endocrine disorder (Benedek-Jaszmann, 1979), although in some contemporary circles there are recommendations that the syndrome be included in the DSM-III classification as an affective neurosis. Since

Frank's initial description a major attention has been focused on the ovarian hormones as the causative factors. Frank suggested that excess estrogen was at fault and attempted symptom resolution through chemical or surgical obliteration of the ovaries. Unfortunately, symptoms tended to persist or return after treatment so this method was abandoned. The view of progesterone deficiency as the causative factor has been proposed for the last two decades by several workers, in particular, by Dalton (1964). This view supports and extends Frank's estrogen dominance theory when too little progesterone will provide ineffective opposition to estrogen during the second half of the cycle. This suggests that the affective, behavioral, and physiological symptoms all appear in response to a flooding by estrogen which develops during the luteal phase. Dalton's (1964) view of estrogen-progesterone ratio imbalance has resulted in treatments to boost progesterone levels and she has been the major advocate of this hormone therapy (1971, 1978). However, other workers have been unable to replicate her reported treatment effects. Several double-blind trials of synthetic progsterone with placebo have failed to show beneficial effects for the active substance (see Sampson, 1981), although a recent double-blind study of oral micronized progesterone did produce symptom improvement during the active treatment phase (Dennerstein et al., 1985). Other workers have supported the progesterone deficiency theory as being due to excess prolactin (McNatty, Sawers, & McNeilly, 1974). In some women, the prolactin levels do not drop at the beginning of the premenstrual phase but remain elevated until menses ensues. This is hypothesized to result in depressed progesterone levels and unopposed estrogens. This adds a third factor to the hormone ratio imbalance theories where the same set of symptoms may be produced by excess estrogens with normal progesterone; by normal estrogen with progesterone deficiency, or through normal estrogen with reduced progesterone due to excess prolactin. The curent strong support for ovarian estrogen dominance as the symptom-provocative factor is supported by Backstrom, Sanders, Leask, Davidson, Warner, and Bancroft (1983) because of "the close relationship between symptoms and the ovarian cycle." This prevailing view is an attempt to explain both central dysfunctional elements (moods, information-processing capacities) and systemic effects (behavior change, swelling, pain) by merely a peripheral (ovarian) source of disruption. This position would seem to echo that of Frank's of 50 years ago and, in the light of current psychosomatic theory, would appear to be too simplistic a model to fully account for the complex set of interacting symptoms in premenstrual syndrome (Morse & Dennerstein, 1986).

Considerable research attention has been given to understanding depression in PMS. High levels of plasma monamine oxidase (MAO) activity was proposed as the triggering factor in producing depression by Grant and Pryce-Davies (1968), through its action on sensitive cortical centers. Increased MAO levels during the premenstruum have been demonstrated by Klaiber, Kobayashi, Broverman, and Hall (1971) although other workers (e.g., Belmaker, Murphy, Wyatt, & Loriaux 1974) demonstrated peak MAO activity midcycle and lowest levels at the premenstruum. This reversed pattern has also been shown in premenstrual primates (Redmond, Murphy, Baulu, Ziegler, & Lake 1975). Other workers have been concerned with the renin-angiotension-aldosterone system as the trigger for premenstrual depression (Janowsky et al., 1973) through direct actions on the nervous system. However, as the renin-angiotension-aldosterone levels drop abruptly up to six days prior to menses, it seems unlikely to be able to explain premenstrual depression that persists and intensifies until relief during menstruation (Steiner & Carroll, 1977). Depression is reported also in anovulatory cycles which do not show changes in the renin-angiotension-aldosterone system (Adamopoulos, Loraine, Lunn, Coppen, & Daly 1972). This point would seem to add further to the estrogen-dominance theory (Backstrom, Sanders, Leask, Davidson, Warner, & Bancroft, 1983), particularly when severe premenstrual symptoms coincide with high estrogen levels in the late luteal phase of −4 to −1 day from menses (Munday, Brush, & Taylor 1981). Although increased levels of irritability were reported by Cullberg (1972), and of anxiety by Backstrom and Carstensen (1974), and of both irritability and depression by Munday et al. (1977), it has been proposed by Steiner and Carroll (1977) that two separate subcategories of PMS may operate. One is premenstrual irritability-anxiety due to estrogen-dominance (and progesterone lack) and the other is premenstrual depression in response to raised MAO activity stimulated by progestogenic activity. These interesting speculations seem, however, to rely on tenuous grounds as in some women, all of these negative affects are reported and it is difficult to explain, in hormonal terms, how both sets of ovarian abberations may coexist. An additional intriguing point for consideration is that widespread acceptance is found for positive well-balanced moods during the first half of the cycle when estrogen is approaching its peak and is unopposed by progesterone. Yet during the second half of the cycle high levels of estrogen that are inefficiently balanced by sufficient progesterone are presumably responsible for the onset of negative affects, notably irritability and anxiety, and perhaps depression too.

One explanation to account for this apparent inconsistency may be that ovarian hormones do trigger adverse feelings and behaviors through a delayed (lagged) effect. This has been reported by Dennerstein, Spencer-Gardner, Brown, Smith, and Burrows (1984), who found maximal concordance was achieved between estrogen levels and pregnanediol, irritability, and swelling with a time delay of about seven days. Although the authors cautioned against the outright acceptance of a time-lagged effect as clear evidence of steroidal causation of certain premenstrual symptoms, the implications are compelling. One theory of lagged effects in the development of depression proposed by Stone (1983) is that increased biological demands arising from prolonged stress may outstrip the output of noradrenergic receptors resulting in a depletion of serotonin or norepinephrine or both that results in changed moods and behaviors.

The existing biological theories of causation are complex, confusing, and, as yet, inconclusive. A great deal of effort has also been invested in identifying the sociopsychological characteristics of PMS-complainants and these will now be reviewed.

Psychological theories

From Frank's (1931) earliest description of the syndrome, several writers have identified PMS complainants as neurotic, anxious, introverted, with an entrenched feminine sex-role identification, low self-esteem, negative attitudes to sexuality and menstruation, high dependency and low autonomy (Rees, 1953; Coppen & Kessel, 1963; Berry & McGuire, 1972; May, 1976; Watts et al., 1980). It is likely that PMS sufferers may be differentially identifiable from nonsufferers on the basis of these static personality variables alone. Other researchers have found an absence of significantly related psychological factors and premenstrual symptoms in women who do not regard their menstrual cycles as problematic (Golub, 1976; Abplanalp et al., 1979; Lahmeyer et al., 1982; Woods, 1985). This discrepancy of findings appears to support the concept of premenstrual complaints as having a constitutional basis, or that certain women are predisposed (psychologically vulnerable) to developing symptoms at a certain time. Specific enquiries have focused on the social conditions operating to affect girls' attitudes towards the whole menstrual process from menarche on. Much importance has been attached to inadequate maternal preparation for menarche (Koff, Rierdan, & Sheingold, 1982) especially where only menstrual hygiene considerations were addressed by most mothers with some relating the physiology of the menstrual process to pregnancy, and none at all who discussed changes in moods and feelings in relation to different cycle phases (Bloch, 1978). The role played by superstitious folkloric beliefs and practices of male relatives, mothers, and society in general has been proposed by Parlee (1973) as contributing to subsequent negative menstrual attitudes through social learning from significant female relatives resulting in the emergence of premenstrual symptoms in adulthood (Clarke & Ruble, 1978).

Stress

Many publications on menstruation refer to stress effects playing a role in the etiology and maintenance of symptoms. Interestingly, the stress literature involving females tends not to refer to the effect of menstruation, indicating perhaps both a lack of awareness of the cyclic variations in feelings and abilities reported by women as well as an absence of importance being attributed to the menstrual cycle as a variable to be considered. The concept of stress is nebulous and suffers from a lack of clear definitional criteria. The term has been used to denote both stimulus and response and, until recent years (e.g. Mackay, Cox, Burrows, & Lazzerini 1978) has suffered from a paucity of well-validated psychometric instruments. In the PMS literature, stress is more usually referred to as a stimulus which arises from some external source (e.g., marital, occupational, parenting role) to result in negative moods and disrupted behaviors which escalate premenstrually because of the interaction of the stress with the ovarian hormones' natural effects. The assumption that follows from this perspective would be that an amelioration of the stressful environmental condition should lower premenstrual symptoms to more manageable levels. This has been found to be the case, for many women in an undesirable marriage, for example, have reported a resolution of premenstrual symptoms once the stressful problem has alleviated or been resolved. An alternative view of stress has been proposed as a negative expectance set arising from the anticipation of an unpleasant premenstrual experience, which raises anxiety levels and results in feelings of tension, depression, and irritability. This view proposes a learned association between cycle phase, negative attributions, and emotional disruption. Some studies have sought to show that experimental manipulation of subjects' beliefs and expectations are related to reports of greater magnitude of symptoms if they are informed that menstruation is imminent (e.g., Golub, 1976). These findings suggest that demand characteristics of the situation, whether of clinical patients or of volunteer subjects may determine a variety of premenstrual symptoms that are culturally determined and of inflated estimates (Ruble, 1977; Sommer, 1978). However, the premenstrual symptoms per se may not be assumed to be the result of psychosocial stress alone for every woman; individual aspects must always be considered. These perspectives do suggest the powerful role played by each woman's belief system and this factor is of paramount importance for treatment effects. Overall, although the research on stress and the menstrual cycle is sparse, comparative data from animal studies have shown impressive effects on reproductive processes from environmental influences (Sommer, 1978). Human observations, though less well documented, do support the notion of stress-induced gonadotropin dysfunction (Reichlin, 1979), particularly in instances of prolonged or chronic psychosocial difficulties (e.g., personality, interpersonal problems; Sommer, 1978).

Cognitions

Popular beliefs support the notion that performance capacities and intellectual abilities of women fluctuate with the phases of the menstrual cycle. The usual view is that capacities peak around midcycle and wane dramatically in the premenstrual days. This notion is fiercely rejected by feminists and women's groups, who view this as political propaganda designed to keep women out of responsible and demanding positions in society and the workplace. Many women, and their partners also, who seek treatment at specialist clinics for PMS, do report cyclical effects on concentration capacities, memory, decision making, attention, verbal abilities (e.g., conversing on the telephone), as well as in fine cognitive-motor skills such as typing. Awareness of cognitive factors is tied in inextricably with changed self-concepts of efficacy and well-being, which together with negative moods, as both cause and effect, form at least three-quarters of the symptom complex of PMS.

The notion of a hormonal basis as causal entity of cognitive changes has a longstanding tradition and emanates from the early views of Dalton (1960, 1968) to Ivey and Bardwick (1968) and Graham and Glasser (1985). The theory that has been proposed to explain these cyclical fluctuations is ascribed to Broverman, Klaiber, Kabayashi, & Vogel (1968) who proposed that females are superior to males on "overlearned" tasks (e.g., typing) and inferior on perceptual restructuring tasks, because of the regular female hormonal changes. High estrogen levels appear to facilitate overlearned "automatic" tasks via adrenergic stimulation, and low estrogen-high progesterone levels facilitate perceptual restructuring tasks, while inhibiting behaviors. This theory suggests a differential optimal effect for certain abilities during different halves of the menstrual cycle. However, a comprehensive review by Sommer (1981) of 35 independent studies from 1958 to 1979 found that only 14 of these supported an hypothesis of perimenstrual debilitation, and several of these were of dubious methodological rigor so that subsequent replications failed to support these findings.

In general, reported cognitive changes tend to be discrete small alterations to sensory capacities which are not of global intellectual capacity and abilities. Some studies have found that women make increased compensatory efforts under difficult or stressed conditions related to the perimenstrual phase (e.g., Rodin, 1976) yet the popular belief persists that women's abilities are at risk to the hormonal effects of the menstrual cycle.

It seems that two distinct populations are under scrutiny and perhaps being confounded. On the one hand there are women who seek help and treatment for PMS who consistently and ubiquitously report cognitive changes in capabilities and schemata; on the other side, there are samples of women, students, volunteers, nonseekers of treatment with and without premenstrual symptoms, who under careful experimental conditions, fail to show conclusive evidence of these deficits. It seems possible that these two populations may be very different in hormonal status and/or cognitive style. While distinct hormonal dysfunction is established in very few cases the way seems clear to focus on the cognitive style of treatment seekers.

In a discussion paper by Morse and Dennerstein (1986), it is proposed that PMS complainants exhibit the style of cognitive processing that Beck and Emery (1985) have described as a generalized anxiety disorder. High levels of anxiety in PMS complainants have been recognized for many years, although only regarded as an accepted but static personality variable. Morse and Dennerstein take a psychosomatic view and suggest that the heightened level of anxiety pervades the whole cognitive style of the individual to influence her perception, thinking, feeling, and behaviors that become centered around the menstrual cycle. Past genetic and/or constitutional factors contribute to a raised vulnerability in the organ system which succumbs to felt-effects from adverse environmental conditions at a later date. The woman, predisposed over time to regard both her internal and external environments as arenas of threat, responds with impaired coping strategies and lowered frustration tolerance, to result in reporting of symptoms, increased emotional distress, and ineffectual behaviors for the management of self and others. This view of PMS as an instance of disturbed environment-person-organ-behaviors supports both current thinking of psychosomatic disease (see Reiser, 1975) and cybernetic theory in which disease is regarded as the natural outcome of a disregulation between positive and negative feedbacks that cause the system in question to lose control and become disordered (Schwartz, 1979).

TREATMENT

Many management strategies have been proposed and tried over as many years and uncontrolled studies have reported success in symptom reduction. These various approaches tend to reflect the view of PMS that is supported by the practitioner because carefully controlled studies with stringent methodology generally do not result in satisfying replications.

Progesterone Hormones

Hormone therapy has a long history of use reflecting the substantial support given to the biological theory of progesterone estrogen imbalance. Dalton has been a major advocate of progesterone therapy for over 20 years, but recent careful double-blind studies have not been able to show results that favored the active substance (see Sampson, 1979) when synthetic progestins were used. A pure oral micronized progesterone did prove to have an advantageous effect over placebo (Dennerstein et al., 1985) and this work warrants further replication efforts. Some women report fewer symptoms on progesterone-only contraceptive pills, while others have noticed an increase in symptoms, particularly of negative moods, irrespective of the type of pill used, (Cullberg, 1972; Smith, 1975).

Bromocriptine

The use of this drug, a dopamine receptor agonist, has been proposed because it inhibits prolactin secretion which has been implicated as a cause of lowered progesterone. Significant elevations of prolactin have not been established beyond that of upper normal ranges although some PMS-complainants have shown greater levels than controls during the luteal phase (see Andersch et al., 1978). Doses above 2.5 mg are reported to result in nausea, vomiting, and headache although careful buildup of tolerance over days has been more acceptable. Physical symptoms of breast soreness, weight gain, and irritability may respond although tension and depression do not.

Pyridoxine

The use of Vitamin B6 has gained widespread popularity among both clinicians and sufferers. There is easy access to this substance via health food shops and reports of high-dose toxicity through self-medication have percolated through the scientific literature. Careful double-blind studies with PMS complainants (e.g., Stokes & Mendels, 1972) have failed to show a significant difference, but other studies with a volunteer sample (e.g., Abraham & Hargrove, 1980) have. Many women are staunch supports of this substance in spite of alternate evidence and would not dream (not dare) of going without it.

Psychotropic Drugs

Lithium. The most commonly reported symptoms of irritability, mood swings, and depression in PMS appeared to mimic changes found in patients with affective disorders that had responded to lithium medication. Lithium treatment given to PMS complainants in uncontrolled case studies have shown some success (e.g., DeLeon-Jones, Val, & Herts, 1982), but controlled double-blind trials did not find a superior effect over placebo (Mattson & Schoul, 1974; Steiner et al., 1980).

Alprazolam. A majority of PMS complainants are found to have raised scores of trait anxiety and report feelings of tension, anxiety, and cognitive-behavioral deficits during the late luteal phase. Current trials of alprazolam are under way in major centers. Alprazolam is and has been found to have a superior effect over both placebo and diazepam in the treatment of phobic disorders and generalized anxiety disorders. However, preliminary data from a current study by the authors of a double-blind study of alprazolam, using up to 4 mg daily, found no distinct differences between alprazolam or placebo in reducing premenstrual symptoms, including state-anxiety measured on the Spielberger STAI (Spielberger, Gorsuch, & Lushene, 1970).

Placebo

From a variety of double-blind studies many subjects have responded more to placebo than to the active substance. While this attests to the lack of clinical efficacy of many proposed substances, it is also taken to mean that reports of improvement on placebo attests to the subject's own psychological system of belief, expectation, and compliance. The finding that a proportion of women are placebo responders has prompted researchers to explore psychological theories of etiology as viable alternatives to the possible biological causation. This would appear to be a restricted view that seeks to divide the individual into body or mind just when an integrated approach, which considers the interactive contributions from both, is required. In addition, research into placebo response per se is limited and, to date, poorly understood. It appears that responsiveness to placebo is based on several things—past experiences of treatment effectiveness, commitment to drug use as therapy, and personal variables (age, long-suffering, somatization of stress, hypersensitivity to stress, external locus of control). In addition, Levine et al. (1978) claim that placebo-induced analgesia is mediated by endorphin mechanisms and that positive effects correlate positively with anxiety and depression (Elton, Stanley, & Burrows, 1983). This might indicate that the use of placebo in double-blind studies is a misplaced confidence through an a priori acceptance that placebo is "next to nothing." Reiser (1982) suggests that placebo is a potentially powerful therapeutic aide which currently suffers from a derogative and misapplied use.

Educational Self-Management

Since PMS began to figure in the popular consciousness due to increased media presentations, many women both self-diagnose and self-manage their symptoms for varying lengths of time before seeking help. Even when they do attend a specialist practitioner or center, they may disappear from treatment for a while and reappear a year or two later having explored some new approach they had heard of. Many of these efforts incorporate attempts at stress management through relaxation, yoga, meditation, aerobic gymnastics, jogging, and diets. Clinicians also advocate many of these self-help tasks and recommend "taking things easy" during the premenstrual week. Some women, with admirable determination, do manage to do just that by deliberately avoiding activities and demands, and reorganizing necessary chores with others. Many women try and fail at this task of increased self-discipline and greater assertiveness and then become more distressed at their "failure" which reduces tolerance levels still further. In the event of finding your best efforts working against you, motivation evaporates, attempts are given up, and it seems clear that only specialist professional help can provide the answer.

Cognitive Therapy

It has become increasingly evident that cognitive factors play a large part in producing and sustaining premenstrual symptoms. In view of the rapid development of cognitive therapies during the last 10 years which have shown consistently good results with a wide variety of quite intractible disorders, the limited application of this type of psychotherapy to premenstrual syndrome is somewhat surprising. A pilot study carried out during the last two years by Morse and Dennerstein (1986) provided an elective cognitive-behavioral therapy to 11 women already receiving medication with oral micronized progesterone. The drug treatment had been given for at least two months prior to the addition of cognitive therapy. The specially designed cognitive program was structured around a rational-emotive framework to address faulty self-statements, illogical inferences, and irrational beliefs. Progressive relaxation techniques were taught to the subjects and stress inoculation procedures were introduced. At the end of 10 weeks both drug and cognitive therapies were withdrawn.

Assessment Pretest. Before treatment began subjects were informed at an initial briefing session of the aims of the treatment program. A number of psychological measures were administered as pretests at this time. The personality of subjects was measured by the Eysenck Personality Questionnaire (EPQ) (Eysenck & Eysenck, 1980) and information was obtained on levels of psychoticism, extraversion, and neuroticism. The Cognitive Failures Questionnaire (CFQ) (Broadbent, Cooper, Fitzgerald, & Parkes, 1980) measured loss of cognitive effectiveness through absentmindedness, concentration and memory loss, attention loss, clumsiness, decision-making impairment, disorganization, and irritability. Subjects also completed the Menstrual Distress Questionaire (MDQ) (Moos, 1969) which provided information concerning physical symptoms and mood during a menstrual cycle including pain, concentration loss, behavior change, ANS reaction, water retention, negative affect, and well-being. Subjects were asked to report on symptoms experienced that day, that is, a "present" state was elicited, rather than retrospective reports related to the most recent premenstrual experience, which has usually been the practice reported in the literature. Subjects were also instructed in how to complete daily self-report charts, on a 5-point scale, of the severity of ten PMS-related symptoms (restlessness, irritability, breast soreness, depression, aggression, tiredness, well-being, swelling, sexual interest, irritability). Subjects were asked to complete daily rating charts of

PMS-related symptoms for one complete menstrual cycle before the beginning of treatment. Daily self-ratings were continued throughout the 10 weeks of the combined programs. Short-term followup at 12 weeks showed that physical symptoms had worsened after treatment cessation but psychological symptoms (negative moods) had continued to improve over the break from treatment. At long-term follow-up 12 months later, although both symptom categories showed some deterioration over time, their mean levels were improved over pretreatment levels. None of the subjects had returned to medications nor did they regard their paramenstrual symptoms as problematic. This study is a fresh treatment approach which is encouraging. However, outcome must be viewed cautiously until further work has been done as so many other treatment attempts have also initially seemed promising. It remains to be seen whether cognitive therapy alone is adequate to reduce premenstrual symptoms or whether the main power lies in the combination of medication with psychotherapy.

SUMMARY

Premenstrual syndrome has a long history in at least contemporary times, as well as further back into ancient times. It is today recognized as a complex interactive disorder, of psychosomatic characteristics, that necessarily incorporates biological, psychological, and environmental components. Many efforts have gone into identifying the main causative factor. Various biological theories have been proposed, from an initial peripheralist view of ovarian hormone disturbance, towards, lately, an increasingly centralist view of hypothalamic-pituitary dysfunction. At present, no one theory has been convincingly established and accepted. Certain personality variables have been identified in PMS complainants, and specific environmental influences have been found to be implicated in contributing to negative attitudes towards the menstrual process. Treatment efforts have engaged a wide variety of drugs, nondrug substances, behavioral practices, and nonspecific counseling. Many of these have shown initial success that has subsequently failed under further replication and more stringent methodology. Until recently, theories and management practices have reflected a duality in approach, with mind and body dealt with as almost separate entities. During the next few years a convergence of the psychic and somatic elements of this complex disorder by researchers and clinicians may prove to be the optimal direction to take.

REFERENCES

Abplanalp, J., Rose, R. M., Donnelly, A. F., & Livingston-Vaughan, L. (1979). Psychoendocrinology of the menstrual cycle: II. The relationship between enjoyment of activities, moods and reproductive hormones. *Psychosom. Med, 41* (8), 605–615.

Abraham, G. E., & Hargrove, J. T. (1980). Effect of vitamin B6 on premenstrual symptomatology in women with premenstrual tension syndromes: A double-blind cross-over study. *Infertility, 3*, 155–161.

Abramowit, E. S., Baker, A. H., & Fleischer, D. F. (1982). Onset of depressive psychiatric crises and the menstrual cycle. *American Journal of Psychiatry, 139*, 475–478.

Adamopoulos, D. A., Loraine, J. A., Lunn, S. F., Coppen, A. H., & Daly, R. J. (1972). Endocrine profiles in premenstrual tension. *Clinical Endocrinology, 1*, 283–292.

Andersch, B., Hahn, L., Wendestam, C., Ohman, R., & Abrahamsson, L. (1978). Treatment of premenstrual tension syndrome. *Acta Endocrinologica, Suppl. 216*, 165–174.

Appleby, B. P. (1960). A study of premenstrual tension in general practice. *British Medical Journal, i*, 391–393.

Asso, D. (1978). Levels of arousal in the premenstrual phase. *British Journal of Social Clinical Psychology, 17*, 47–55.

Asso, D. & Braier, J. R. (1982). Changes with the menstrual cycle in psychophysiological and self-report measures of activation. *Biological Psychiatry, 15*, 95–107.

Backstrom, T., & Carstensen, H. (1974). Estrogen and progesterone in plasma in relation to premenstrual tension. *Journal of Steroid Biochemistry, 5*, 257–260.

Backstrom, T., Sanders, D., Leask, R., Davidson, D., Warner, P., & Bancroft, J. (1983). Mood, sexuality, hormones and the menstrual cycle: II. Hormone levels and their relationship to the premenstrual syndrome. *Psychosomatic Medicine, 45*, 503–507.

Beck, A. T., & Emery, G. (1985). Anxiety disorders and phobias: A cognitive perspective. New York: Basic Books.

Belmaker, R. H., Murphy, D. L., Wyatt, R. J., & Loriaux, D. L. (1974). Human platelet monoamine oxidase changes during the menstrual cycle. *Archives of General Psychiatry, 31*, 553–556.

Benedek-Jaszmann, L. J. (1979). Premenstrual Tension Syndrome: A new hypothesis for its cause and treatment. In L. Carena & L. Zichella (Eds.), *Emotion and Reproduction Vol. 20A, Proceedings of Serono Symposia* (pp. 190–203). New York: Academic Press.

Berry, C., & McGuire, F. L. (1972). Menstrual distress and acceptance of the female role. *American Journal of Obstetrics and Gynecology, 114*, 83–87.

Bickers, W., & Woods, M. (1951). Premenstrual tension: Rational treatment. *Texas Reports on Biological Medicine, 9*, 406–419.

Bloch, D. (1978). Sex education practices of mothers. *Journal of Sexual Education Therapy, 4*, 7–12.

Broadbent, D. E., Cooper, P. F., Fitzgerald, P., & Parkes, K. R. (1982). The Cognitive Failures Questionnaire and its correlates. *British Journal of Clinical Psychology, 21* (1), 1–16.

Broverman, D. M., Klaiber, E. L., Kabayashi, Y., & Vogel, W. (1968). Roles of activation and inhibition in sex differences in cognitive abilities. *Psychological Review, 75*, 23–50.

Brown, J. B. (1955). Urinary excretion of oestrogens during the menstrual cycle. *Lancet, 268*, 320–323.

Clare, A. W. (1977). Psychological problems of women complaining of premenstrual symptoms. *Current Medical Research & Opinion, 4* (4), 23–28.

Clarke, A. E., & Ruble, D. N. (1978). Young adolescents beliefs concerning menstruation. *Child Development 49*, 231–234.

Coppen, A., & Kessel, N. (1963). Menstruation and personality. *British Journal of Psychiatry, 109*, 711–721.

Cullberg, J. (1972). Mood changes and menstrual symptoms with different gestagen/estrogen combinations. *Acta Psychiatrica Scandanavica*, Suppl. 236.

Dalton, K. (1980). Progesterone, fluid, and electrolytes in premenstrual syndrome, *British Medical Journal 281*, 61.

Dalton, K. (1968). Menstruation and examinations. *Lancet, 2*, 1386–1388.

Dalton, K. (1964) *The premenstrual syndrome*. London: Heinemann.

Dalton, K. (1960). Effect of menstruation on schoolgirls' weekly work. *British Medical Journal 1*, 326–328.

DeLeon-Jones, F. A., Val, E., & Herts, C. (1982). MHPG excretion and lithium treatment during premenstrual tension syndrome: A case report. *American Journal of Psychiatry, 139*, 950–952.

Dennerstein, L. & Burrows, G. D. (1979). Affect and the menstrual cycle. *Journal of Affective Disorders, 1*, 77–92.

Dennerstein, L., Burrows, G. D., Cox, L., & Wood, C. (1978). *Gynecology, sex and psyche*. Australia: Melbourne University Press.

Dennerstein, L., Spencer-Gardner, C., Brown, J. B., Smith, M. A., & Burrows, G. D. (1984). Premenstrual tension—hormonal profiles. *Journal of Psychosomatic Obstetrics & Gynecology, 3*, 37–51.

Dennerstein, L., Spencer-Gardner, C., Gotts, G., Brown, J. B., Smith, M. A., Burrows, G. D. (1985, June). Progesterone and the premenstrual syndrome: A double blind crossover trial. *British Medical Journal*, ii, 1617–1621.

Dennerstein, L. (1983). Spencer-Gardner, C., Gotts, G., Brown, J., Smith, M., & Burrows, G. The menstrual cycle - correlating biological and psychological changes. In M. deSenarclens (Ed.), *The young woman. Proceedings of the 7th International Congress of Psychosomatic O. & G.* Dublin, Ireland.

Diamond, S. B., Rubinstein, A. A., Dunner, D. L., & Fieve, R. R. (1976). Menstrual problems in women with primary affective illness. *Comp. Psychiatry, 17* (4), 541–548.

Elton, D., Stanley, G., & Burrows, G. D. (1983). The psychology of pain. Amsterdam: Elsevier/North-Holland.

Englander-Golden, P., Whitmore, M. R., & Dienstbier, R. A. (1978). Menstrual cycle as forms of study and self reports of mood and behavior. *Motivation and Emotion, 2*, 75–81.

Eysenck, H. J., & Eysenck, S. B. G. (1975). *Manual of the Eysenck Personality Questionnaire*. London: Hodden & Stoughton.

Frank, R. T. (1931). Hormonal causes of premenstrual tension. *Archives Neurological Psychiatry 26*, 1053–1057.

Golub, S. (1976). The effect of premenstrual anxiety and depression on cognitive function. *Journal of Personality & Social Psychology, 34*, 99–104.

Golub, S., & Harrington, D. M. (1981). Premenstrual and menstrual mood changes in adolescent women. *Journal of Personal Social Psychology, 41* (5), 961–965.

Graham, E. A., & Glasser, M. (1985). Relationship of pregnanediol level to cognitive behaviour and moods. *Psychosomatic Medicine, 47*, 126–33.

Grant, E. C. G., & Pryse-Davies, J. (1968). Effects of oral contraceptives on depressed mood changes and on endometrial monoamine oxidase and phosphatases. *British Medical Journal, iii*, 777–780.

Greene, R., & Dalton, K. (1963). The premenstrual syndrome. *British Medical Journal, i*, 1007–1015.

Ivey, M. E., & Bardwick, J. M. (1968). Patterns of affective fluctuation in the menstrual cycle. *Psychosomatic Medicine 30*(3), 336–345.

Janiger, O., Riffenburgh, R., Kersh, R. (1972). Cross-cultural study of premenstrual symptoms. *Psychosomatics, 13*, 226–235.

Janowsky, D. S., Berens, S. C. & Davis, J. M. (1973). Correlations between mood, weight and electrolytes during the menstrual cycle: A renin-angiotensin-aldosterone hypothesis of premenstrual tension. *Psychosomatic Medicine, 35*, 143–154.

Kessel, N., & Coppen, A. (1963). The prevalence of common menstrual symptoms. *Lancet, iii*, 61–64.

Klaiber, E. L., Kobayashi, Y., Broverman, D. M., & Hall, F. (1971). Plasma Monoumine Oxidase activity in regularly menstruating women and in amennorheic women receiving cyclic treatment with estrogens and a progetin. *Journal of Clinical Endocrinological Metabolism, 33*, 630–637.

Koff, E., Rierdan, J., & Sheingold, K. (1982). Memories of menarche: Age, preparation and prior knowledge as determinants of initial menstrual experience. *Journal of Youth & Adolescence 11*(1), 1–9.

Lacey, J. I. (1957). Somatic response patterning and stress: Some revisions of activation theory. In M. H. Appley & R. Turnbull (Eds.), *Psychological stress*. New York: Appleton.

Lahmeyer, H. W., Miller, M., & DeLeon-Jones, F. (1982). Anxiety and mood fluctuations during the normal menstrual cycle. *Psychsomatic. Medicine, 44* (2), 183–194.

Levine, J. D., Gordon, N. C., & Fields, H. L. (1978). The mechanisms of placebo analgesia. *Lancet, 2*, 654–657.

Little, B., & Zahn, T. (1974). Changes in mood and autonomic functioning during the menstrual cycle. *Psychophysiology, 11*, 579–590.

Mackay, C., Cox, T., Burrows, G., & Lazzerini, T. (1978). An inventory for the measurement of self reported stress and arousal. *British Journal of Social and Clinical Psychology 17*, 283–284.

Mattson, B., & Schoultz, B. A comparison between lithium, placebo and a diuretic in premenstrual tension. *Acta Psychiatrica Scandanavica, 255*, 75–84.

May, R. R. (1976). Moodshifts and the menstrual cycle. *Journal of Psychosomatic Research, 20*, 125–130.

McClure, J. N., Reich, T., & Wetzel, R. D. (1971). Premenstrual symptoms as an indicator of biopolar affective disorder. *British Journal of Psychiatry, 119*, 527–28.

McNatty, K. P., Sawers, R. S., & McNeilly, A. S. (1974). A possible role for prolactin in control of steroid secretion by the human graafian follicle. *Nature, 250*, 653–655.

Moos, R. H. (1969). Typology of menstrual cycle symptoms. *American Journal of Obstetrics and Gynecology, 103*, 390–402.

Moos, R. H., & Leiderman, D. B. (1978). Towards a menstrual cycle symptom typology. *Journal of Psychosomatic Research, 22*, 31–40.

Morse, C. A., & Dennerstein, L. (1986). The role of cognitions and affects in PMS—a transactional analysis.

Munday, M. R., Brush, M. G., & Taylor, R. W. (1981). Correlations between progesterone, oestradiol and aldosterone levels in the premenstrual syndrome. *Clinical Endocrinology, 14*, 1–9.

Parlee, M. B. (1973). The premenstrual syndrome. *Psychological Bulletin, 80*, 454–465.

Parlee, M. B. (1974). Stereotypic beliefs about menstruation. *Psychosomatic Medicine, 36* (3), 229–240.

Pennington, V. M. (1957). Meprobamate (Miltown) in premenstrual tension. *Journal of The American Medical Association, 164*, 638–640.

Redmond, D. E., Murphy, D. L., Baulu, J., Ziegler, M. G., & Lake, C. R. (1975). Menstrual cycle and ovarian hormone effects on plasma and platelet monoamine oxidase (MAO) and plasma dopamine—beta-hydroxylase (DBH) activities in the rhesus monkey. *Psychosomatic Medicine, 37*, 417–428.

Rees, W. L. (1953). The premenstrual tension syndrome and its treatment. *British Medical Journal, 1*, 1014, 1016.

Reichlin, S. (1979, June). The role of stress in female reproductive dysfunction. *Journal of Human Stress, 5* (2), 38–45.

Reiser, M. F. (1975). Changing theoretical concepts in psychosomatic medicine. In M. F. Reiser (Ed.), *American handbook of psychiatry* (Vol. 4). New York: Basic Books.

Reiser, M. F., & Leigh, H. (1982). A general systems taxonomy for psychological defense mechanisms. *Journal of Psychosomatic Research, 26*(1), 73–76.

Rodin, J. (1976). Menstruation, reattribution and competence. *Journal of Personal & Social Psychology, 33*(3), 345–353.
Rouse, P. (1978). Premenstrual tension: A study using the Moos Menstrual Distress Questionnaire. *Journal of Psychosomatic Research, 22,* 215–222.
Ruble, D. N. (1977). Premenstrual symptoms—a reinterpretation. *Science, 197,* 291–292.
Russell, G. F. M. (1972). Premenstrual tension and "psychogenic" amennorrhoea: Psycho-physical interactions. *Psychosomatic Research, 16,* 279–287.
Sampson, G. A. (1979). Premenstrual syndrome: A Double-blind controlled trial of progesterone and placebo. *British Journal of Psychiatry, 135,* 209–215.
Sampson, G. A., & Prescott, P. (1981). The assessment of the symptoms of premenstrual syndrome and their response to therapy. *British Journal of Psychiatry, 138,* 399–405.
Sanders, D., Warner, P., Backstrom, T., & Bancroft, J. (1983). Mood, sexuality, hormones and the menstrual cycle. I: Changes in mood and physical state: Description of subjects and methods. II: Hormone levels and relationship to the premenstrual syndrome. *Psychosomatic Medicine, 45*(6), 487–501 (I): 503–507 (II).
Schwartz, G. (1979). The brain as a health and care system. In G. C. Stone, F. Cohen, & N. E. Adler (Eds.), *Health psychology: A handbook* (pp. 549–572). Jossey-Bass.
Sheldrake, P., & McCormack, M. (Eds.), (1976). Variations in menstrual cycle symptom reporting. *Journal of Psychosomatic Research, 20,* 169–177.
Short, R. (1972, May). The control of menstruation. *British Journal of Hospital Medicine, 7,* 552–555.
Smith, S. L. (1975). Mood and the menstrual cycle. In J. Sachar (Ed.), *Topics in psychoneuroendocrinology.* Grune and Stratton.
Snowden, R., & Christian, B. (Eds.). (1982). *Patterns and perceptions of menstruation. WHO Report.* 1982. New York: St. Martin's Press.
Somerville, B. W. (1972a). The role of estradiol withdrawal in the aetiology of menstrual migraine. *Neurology, 22,* 355–365.
Somerville, B. W. (1972b). A study of migraine in pregnancy. *Neurology, 22,* 824–828.
Sommer, B. (1982). Cognitive behaviour and the menstrual cycle. In R. C. Friedman (Ed.), *Behavior and the menstrual cycle.* New York: Dekker.
Sommer, B. (1978). Stress and menstrual distress. *Journal of Human Stress, 4,* 41–47.
Spielberger, C. D., Gorsuch, R. L., & Lushene, R. (1970). *Manual for the State-Trait Anxiety Inventory (STAI).* Consulting Psychologists Press.
Steiner, M., & Carroll, B. J. (1977). The psychobiology of premenstrual dysphoria: Review of theories and treatments. *Psychoneuroendocrinology, 2,* 321–335.
Steiner, M., Haskett, R. F., Osmun, J. D., & Carroll, R. J. (1980). Treatment of premenstrual tension with lithium carbonate: A pilot study. *Acta Psychiatrica Scandanavica, 61,* 96–102.

Stokes, J., & Mendels, J. (1972). Pyridoxine and premenstrual tension. *Lancet, 1*, 117-118.

Stone, E. A. (1983). Problems with current catecholamine hypothesis of antidepressant agents: Speculations leading to a new hypothesis. *The Brain & Behaviour Sciences, 6*, 535–577.

Strauss, B., & Appelt, H. (1983). Psychological concomitants of the menstrual cycle: a prospective longitudinal approach. *Journal of Psychosomatic Obstetrics and Gynecology, 2–4,* 215–220.

Sutherland, H., & Stewart, I. (1965). A critical analysis of the premenstrual syndrome. *Lancet, i*, 1180–1183.

Taylor, J. W. (1979). The timing of menstrual related symptoms assessed by a daily symptom rating scale. *Acta Psychiatrica Scandanavica, 60*, 87–90.

Timonen, S., & Procope, B. J. (1971). Premenstrual syndrome and physical exercise. *Acta Obstetrica & Gynaecologica Scandanavia, 50*, 33–37.

Van Keep, P.A., & Lehert, P. (1981). The premenstrual syndrome: An exercise in epidemiological and statistical exercise. In P. A. Van Keep & W. H. Utian (Eds.), *The premenstrual syndrome* (pp. 1–9). Lancaster, England: MTP Press.

Watts, S., Dennerstein, L., & Horne, D. de L. (1980). The premenstrual syndrome. *Journal of Affective Disorders, 2*, 257–266.

Wetzel, R. D., Reich, T., McClure, J. N., & Wald, J. A. (1975). Premenstrual affective syndrome and affective disorders. *British Journal of Psychiatry, 127*, 279–281.

Wilcoxon, L. A., Schrader, S. L., & Sherif, C. W. (1976). Daily self reports on activities, life events, moods, and somatic change during the menstrual cycle. *Psychosomatic Medicine, 38*(6), 399–417.

Wineman, E. W. (1971). Autonomic balance changes during the human menstrual cycle. *Psychophysiology, 8*, 1–6.

Woods, N. F. (1985). Relationship of socialisation and stress to perimenstrual symptoms, disability and menstrual attitudes. *Nursing Research, 34*(3) 145–149.

Wong, W. H., Freedman, R. L., Levan, N. E., Hyman, C., & Quilligan, E. J. (1972). Changes in the capillary filtration coefficient of cutaneous vessels in women with premenstrual tension. *American Journal of Obstetrics and Gynecology, 114*, 950–953.

Zimmerman, E., & Parlee, M. B. (1973). Behavioural changes associated with the menstrual cycle: An experimental investigation. *Journal of Applied Social Psychology, 3* (4), 335–344.

7

The Behavioral Management of Nocturnal Enuresis

Jeffrey Bollard

Department of Psychiatry
Adelaide Children's Hospital Inc.
Adelaide, South Australia

T. Nettelbeck

Department of Psychology
University of Adelaide
Adelaide, South Australia

INTRODUCTION

Problems of Definition

The term *enuresis* refers to persistent, involuntary passing of urine, beyond an age by which most children have acquired normal bladder control. Wetting can occur during sleep (nocturnal enuresis or bedwetting), during the day (diurnal enuresis), or during both. Used without specifying time, the term enuresis usually refers to bedwetting, presumably because this is a more common problem than daytime wetting.

This chapter focuses primarily on functional nocturnal enuresis in children who have essentially normal intelligence. For discussion of the treatment of enuresis among intellectually disabled children the reader is referred to Azrin and Foxx (1971), Azrin, Sneed, and Foxx (1973), Bettison (1978, in press), Rentfrow and Rentfrow (1969), and Smith (1981). Although diurnal enuresis is a significant problem that may require treatment, it has attracted surprisingly little research interest when compared to the attention given to bedwetting. For more comprehensive descriptions of the management of diurnal enuresis, the reader is directed to Bettison (1979) and to Azrin and Foxx (1974).

Functional nocturnal enuresis is generally defined as persistent nighttime bedwetting in the absence of neurologic or urologic pathology. As Lovibond and Coote (1970) have emphasized, any more specific definition necessarily involves a number of arbitrary features. Thus, there is no particular age at which normal children achieve nocturnal control of micturition although, according to physiological evidence, control can be established by 3 to 4 years of age (Campbell, 1970; Muellner 1960a, 1960b). Incidence of bedwetting decreases steadily from infancy but a small proportion of people continue to wet the bed into their teens and even into adulthood. Furthermore, the accepted age for continence at night varies both between communities and between social classes within communities. For example, nocturnal enuresis appears to be more prevalent in the United States and Australia than in the United Kingdom and Sweden (Oppel, Harper, & Rider, 1968) and in several countries it has been found more frequently among children from working class homes than among children of middle-class parents (Douglas & Blomfield, 1958; Miller, Court, Walton, & Knox, 1960; Stein & Susser, 1967). There is no firm concensus concerning the minimum frequency of bedwetting for a child to be regarded as enuretic. Patterns of bedwetting are highly variable, with some children wetting the bed several times each night, some wetting only occasionally, and still others wetting heavily but sporadically. Further, two types of enuresis have sometimes been suggested, based on the child's history of bedwetting. The "primary" or lifelong enuretic has never demonstrated complete control over nocturnal micturition. The "secondary" or "acquired" enuretic has experienced a significant period of nocturnal continence (usually for a minimum of 6 months) prior to reverting to regular nighttime wetting. Some writers (e.g., Kolvin & Taunch, 1973) have argued for this distinction, based on the hypothesis that secondary enuresis has a mainly psychogenic basis, whereas primary enuresis is thought to be caused by maturational delay and/or faulty learning. However, to date, there is little evidence that this distinction has prognostic validity (Doleys, 1977; Lovibond, 1964; Sacks & De Leon, 1973).

Incidence

There are substantial difficulties in estimating prevalence of bedwetting and even in technologically advanced countries reliable data for the general population have only recently become available. A summary of epidemiological studies by De Jonge (1973) revealed wide variability in the population of children regarded as enuretic at various ages. Disparity arises, firstly, because of the lack of an agreed definition in terms of minimum frequency of wetting. Some authors (Hallgren, 1956; Notschaele, 1964; Oppel et al., 1968) have accepted a minimum of one wet bed per month, while others (Blomfield & Douglas, 1956; Martin, 1966) have required at least two wet nights per week. Secondly, the method of investigation has varied with different surveys. Incidence data have been collected by personal interview (Blomfield & Douglas, 1965; De Jonge, 1969; Martin, 1966; Oppel et al., 1968), by questionnaire (Hallgren, 1956), and by retrospective questioning (Thorne, 1944). Thirdly, the populations sampled have varied widely, for example, from wartime military recruits (Levine, 1943; Thorne, 1944), to peacetime conscripts (Bieger, 1954), to all children born during a specified time (Blomfield & Douglas, 1956).

Despite such difficulties, studies employing a criterion of at least one wet night per month highlight several important trends with respect to incidence (De Jonge, 1973). Although bedwetting is a common problem during childhood, even by the end of the first year of life perhaps about 7 percent of children have achieved nocturnal continence (Hawkins, 1962) Incidence of bedwetting drops rapidly to about 20 percent of 3-year-olds, 15 percent of 5-year-olds, 5 percent of 10-year-olds, and 2–3 percent of teenagers, reaching an apparent asymptote by adulthood. Throughout, incidence is somewhat higher among males than females, the ratio being approximately 3:2. These estimates have been confirmed for several different economically developed countries and may be regarded as representative.

THE PHYSIOLOGY OF MICTURITION

The Mechanism of Micturition

As illustrated in Figure 7.1, the urinary bladder comprises two principal parts: (a) the *detrusor muscle* in the main body of the organ, and (b) the *trigone*, a muscular mass near the mouth of the bladder through

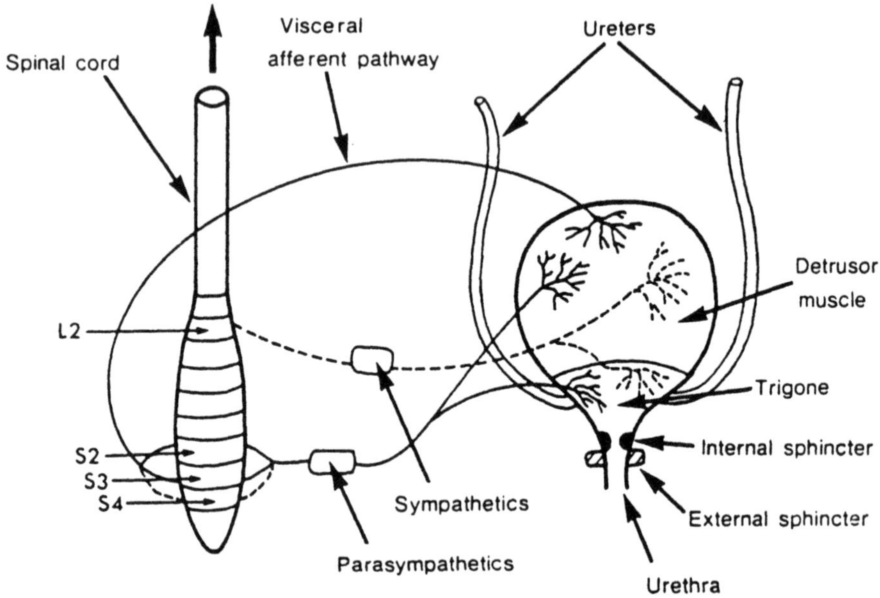

FIGURE 7.1. The urinary bladder and its innervation (from Guyton, 1966, p. 528).

which pass both *ureters* (the tubes conveying urine from each kidney to the bladder) and the *urethra* (the canal through which urine is discharged). The trigonal muscle embraces the *internal sphincter* of the bladder, below which the urethra passes through the *external sphincter* of the bladder.

The act of micturition is described here as a relatively simple reflex although it is actually a complex response resulting from an integrated chain of reflexes. As urine passes through the ureters to the bladder the detrusor muscle tone is repeatedly adjusted, thereby allowing larger volumes of urine to be stored with little increase to internal pressure. A normal adult can store up to about 200 ml of urine before pressure increases significantly. However, with further distension, nervous impulses arising from stimulation of the sensory end organs in the bladder wall trigger reflex micturition. This involves strong rhythmical contractions of the detrusor, relaxation of the internal sphincter followed by relaxation of the external sphincter and, ultimately, the passing of urine.

The Development of Bladder Control

Detailed accounts of the development of bladder control are to be found in Meadow (1970), Muellner (1960a, 1960b), and Yates (1970, pp. 82–86). Infants begin life with a small bladder capacity and frequent reflex voiding in response to bladder distension. As the parasympathetic nervous system matures, most children between 1 and 2 years of age learn to perceive stimulation from increasing bladder tension. This improving awareness is accompanied by the ability to "hold" urine for a brief time after the sensation of a full bladder has been perceived and bladder capacity therefore increases. By 3 years of age most children have learned to hold urine for a considerable time when the bladder is full, by voluntarily tensing the perineal muscles in the crotch, thereby raising the bladder neck and tightening the internal sphincter. With increasing bladder capacity the frequency of voiding drops and a larger volume is passed. Between 3 and 4 years of age the ability to start the urine flow from a full bladder is typically achieved, by combining the pushing down of the thoracic wall and tightening the abdominal muscles. By about 4 years of age most children can also stop the urinary stream at will. Full continence is commonly developed at about 6 years of age, when the ability to start the urinary stream at almost any degree of bladder filling is mastered. Toilet training is complete when the child learns to initiate micturition only in appropriate places.

For nocturnal continence the child must transfer inhibitory control over micturition to the sleeping state. Normally, this is achieved by 3 to 4 years when, as a consequence of increased functional bladder capacity together with the reduced level of urine production during sleep, the child can retain urine throughout the hours of sleep. However, if bladder pressure exceeds the limits of compensatory adjustment in the detrusor during sleep, feedback stimuli from the filling bladder wakes the child before the micturitional reflex is triggered (Lovibond & Coote, 1970).

Pathophysiology of the Genitourinary System

Enuresis due to organic disease is rare but for any child presenting with enuresis organic disease must be excluded before the functional nature of the disorder can be accepted. Incontinence may be associated with spina bifida or other neurological disorders like nocturnal epilepsy. Neurogenic bladders that never fill because of poor resistance at the urethra are almost always associated with other somatic neurological signs, such as perineal anesthesia, and absent or poor rectal tone, impaired bowel control, and disturbances in gait. A condition in which a ureter is in an abnormal position may produce dribbling incontinence, despite normal micturition at regular intervals, and obstruction to the bladder outlet or urethra may result in overflow incontinence. Also, enuresis may occur in association with urinary tract infections. It may be secondary to the excessive production of urine (polyuria) caused by diabetes mellitus, diabetes insipidus, or renal tubular defects. The likelihood of association with organic disease is increased if diurnal enuresis is also present.

THEORIES AND TREATMENT OF ENURESIS

Many different and contradictory explanations about the nature and etiology of nocturnal enuresis have been advanced and the array of available remedies is likewise wide, since usually the form of treatment recommended reflects theoretical orientation concerning etiology. Nonetheless, in broad terms theoretical explanations and associated treatments falls into three main categories: psychodynamic theories favoring treatment by psychotherapy; physiological theories associated with some form of medical intervention; and behavioral theories and treatments. Each of these categories is discussed in turn in the sections that follow.

Psychodynamic Theories and Treatment

One implication that follows from the proposition that enuresis is a surface indicator of an underlying emotional disturbance is that a representative sample of enuretic children should evidence a substantially greater degree of emotional maladjustment than a group of nonenuretics matched for age, IQ, educational level, socioeconomic status, and other relevant descriptor variables. This association remains uncertain, however, despite considerable research. The problem is that while general population surveys such as the Isle of Wight Investigation (Rutter, Yule, & Graham, 1973) and the National Child Development Study (Essen & Peckham, 1976) have indicated an association between enuresis and psychological disorders, particularly the common neurotic and conduct disorders, these surveys have also made it abundantly clear that the vast majority of enuretic children are actually well-adjusted and free from other problems affecting their behavior. Comparative studies of the personalities of enuretics and nonenuretics have indicated similar results (Collins, 1973; Lickorish, 1964; Lovibond, 1964). Although the relationship between enuresis and psychological disorders is somewhat stronger in the case of secondary enuresis (McGee, Mackinson, Williams, Simpson, & Silva, 1984), or when bedwetting is accompanied by diurnal enuresis (Hallgren, 1956), and enuretic children referred to child guidance clinics are more likely to be psychologically disturbed (Hallgren, 1957), even so, the majority of enuretic children are free from other behavioral difficulties.

Even when an enuretic child displays signs of emotional disturbance, these are not proof of a psychogenic origin since the disturbance may be secondary to the enuresis itself. Lovibond (1964), for example, has pointed out that persistent enuresis can result in social limitations and consequences that could upset the child. Thus, a necessary condition which must be met to support a psychogenic explanation is that the postulated stress or conflict should have preceded or coincided with the onset of acquired enuresis, or in the case of primary enuresis, have been operating at a time when the child would normally have been becoming dry. To date, however, the evidence is not clear on this point.

A second implication of a psychodynamic orientation is consistent with psychoanalytic views about symptom substitution. The psychodynamic position has generally been that direct treatment of the symptom itself is both futile and undesirable, since this strategy does not deal with the underlying emotional disturbance—which remains, in effect, the real problem. Psychoanalytic theorists insist that it can be dangerous to eliminate enuresis directly, since underlying anxieties may be exacerbated, producing some other serious disturbance. However, Lovibond (1964) has insisted that eradicating bedwetting could be beneficial to overall psychological health, consistent with his opinion that prolonged enuresis may result in psychological disturbance. The evidence has clearly supported Lovibond; elimination of nocturnal enuresis following direct treatment has been shown to be at least psychologically benign and more often beneficial when compared with alternative forms of treatment (Baker, 1969; Collins, 1973; Dische, Yule, Corbett, & Hand, 1983; Sacks, De Leon, & Blackman, 1974; Shaffer, 1973). Even when direct treatment of bedwetting has not been successful, parents have generally not reported additional symptoms (Collins, 1973).

A third important implication of the psychodynamic position is that some form of psychotherapy must be the treatment of choice because it is only in this way that the fundamental emotional disorder causing enuresis can be removed. Because of the wide range of theoretical perspectives within the psychodynamic framework, there is no unitary form of psychotherapy applied to the treatment of enuresis but alternative procedures have in common the aim that the enuretic child and/or the childs' parents can learn to identify the nature of underlying anxieties by exploring relevant life experiences thoroughly under the guidance of a skilled therapist. However, research evaluating this assertion has tended not to support it. When reviewing the literature on the efficacy of different forms of treatment, Behrle, Elkin, and Laybourne (1956) and Lovibond (1964) found so few adequately reported studies of psychotherapy with reasonably large groups of enuretics that no firm conclusions regarding this type of treatment could be drawn. A similar assertion was made more recently by Kolvin and Taunch (1973) and Baller (1975).

Two studies have reported evidence for the ineffectiveness of psychotherapy as a method of treating bedwetting (De Leon & Mandell, 1966; Werry & Cohrssen, 1965). Subjects in the Werry and Cohrssen study were primary nocturnal enuretics aged about 10 years, with a wetting frequency of at least 1 wet bed per week. Parents of children in a no-treatment control group ($n = 27$) were told that they would be contacted after 4 months to check progress. A psychotherapy group ($n = 21$) received 6 to 8 sessions of psychodynamically-oriented therapy supplemented by suggestion and encouragement over a period of 4 months. The third group ($n = 22$) were treated in their own homes using a bell-and-pad apparatus[1] until the child had been dry for at least 1 month, or until 4 months of treatment had elapsed. After an initial interview no contact was made with the parents of children in this group apart from an occasional telephone call. At the end of 4 months all parents were telephoned and asked to report on the child's bedwetting frequency during the preceding months. Results showed that the behavioral treatment resulted in a significantly higher rate of improvement than either psychotherapy or no-treatment, both of these being ineffective.

These results were subsequently supported by De Leon and Mandell (1966), using a similar design to that in the Werry and Cohrssen study. Subjects were allocated to one of three groups: no-treatment, psychotherapy, and conditioning involving a bell-and-pad procedure. At the end of the 90-day experimental period, psychotherapy was shown to be ineffective in eliminating bedwetting compared with no-treatment, whereas conditioning resulted in a significantly higher success rate. As De Leon and Mandell (1966) were careful to point out, there are many parameters not yet explored, such as the form of the therapy, the number of therapeutic sessions, the interval between sessions, and individual differences among therapists as to skills and experience. Nevertheless, these two studies do not support psychotherapy as an effective treatment when compared with the conditioning treatment.

Physiological Theories and Treatment

A number of physiological theories have been proposed to account for nocturnal enuresis and these are discussed in the sections that follow. In broad terms, such theories attribute a failure to develop control of

[1] The bell-and-pad method is described fully later in this chapter.

micturition to either (a) immaturity of central nervous system (CNS) connections governing bladder control, (b) immaturity of the bladder, resulting in reduced functional capacity, or (c) profoundly deep sleep or faulty sleep-arousal mechanisms.

Immaturity of the central nervous system. Many authors subscribe to the view that enuresis results from immaturity of neurophysiological structures subserving bladder control and that age is the best cure for enuresis (Barbour, Borland, Boyd, Oppe, & Miller, 1963; Bakwin & Bakwin, 1972; Illingworth, 1968). Evidence supporting maturational disorder is derived from a variety of sources. Firstly there is the strong tendency to spontaneous improvement in bedwetting with increasing age, already noted earlier. Secondly, evidence for the relative somatic immaturity of bedwetters is often cited in support of the maturational disorder argument. For example, when compared with nonenuretics, enuretics have been reported to have slower physical growth (F. J. W. Miller, 1973), higher rates of motor and speech abnormalities (Douglas, 1973; Kaffman & Elizur, 1977; Lickorish, 1964) and, in older boys, a delay in the development of secondary sex characteristics (Douglas, 1973). Others have reported an increased risk of bedwetting among children with low birthweight resulting from short gestation (Kaffman & Elizur, 1977; Oppel et al., 1968), and children with low birthweight after normal gestation (Kolvin & Taunch, 1973; Neligan, Kolvin, Scott, & Garside, 1976), although Werner, Bierman, and French (1971) have cautioned against accepting low birthweight as evidence of developmental delay. Compared with the norms for the appropriate age group, electroencephalogram (EEG) records of persistent enuretics have been found to contain diffuse abnormalities, which have been interpreted as indicating immaturity of cortical development (Campbell & Young, 1966; Turton & Spear, 1953).

There is, however, contrary evidence in relation to such claims. For example, Oppel et al. (1968), found no relationship between a delay in the development of urinary continence and other development milestones. In respect of EEG studies, Salmon, Taylor and Douglas (1973) have pointed out that mechanisms governing the acquisition of urinary continence and the significance of statistically unusual features in the EEGs of children are insufficiently understood to support the notion of immaturity of cortical development. If, as has been suggested, the disrythmia in the EEGs of enuretics is a reflection of immaturity in cortical development, then a prospective study of patients with such EEGs is necessary to demonstrate the normalization of the recording over a given period of time coincident with the spontaneous establishment of bladder control. Shaffer (1980) has further noted that the development of sphincter control is often intermittent, which is different from the usual pattern of acquiring competence in other developmental disorders. This, together with the contradictory evidence noted previously, has led Shaffer (1980) to conclude that the available evidence does not indicate a clear relationship between delays in acquiring urinary continence and other forms of somatic immaturity.

A third source of evidence relevant to the issue of CNS immaturity as a cause of enuresis has been sought in studies that highlight the influence of genetic factors and gender differences in the incidence of enuresis. A greater prevalence of bedwetting among males than females has been noted in virtually all epidemiological surveys. A high incidence of enuresis occurring in the parents, siblings and other near relatives of bedwetters has also been reported in many studies (e.g., Bakwin, 1961; Kolvin, Taunch, Currah, Garside, Nolan, & Shaw, 1972; Turner, Young, & Rachman, 1970; Young & Turner, 1965). Furthermore, the frequency of occurrence of bedwetting in other members of the family may be directly related to the closeness of the genetic relationship. Bakwin (1973), for example, found concordance for enuresis between identical twins to be double that for fraternal twins.

Fourthly, various authors have reported that enuretics are "emotionally" immature compared with nonenuretics (Biering & Jespersen, 1959; Gunnarson & Melin, 1951; Hallgren, 1957; MacFarlane, Allen, & Honzick, 1954) and this is sometimes taken as additional evidence for a possible generalized maturational delay (De Jonge, 1969; Kolvin & Taunch, 1973). However, the evidence for such emotional immaturity is not clearcut. As has been pointed out earlier, the majority of enuretic children appear to differ little from the rest of the population in terms of emotional and social adjustment.

It seems likely that late maturation is an important factor in the nocturnal incontinence of some younger children. However, that slow maturation provides a sufficient explanation for the older enuretic's problem is difficult to maintain in the light of certain facts. For example, some children do not advance from incontinence in infancy to complete dryness in childhood, do nevertheless have occasional dry nights or even short sustained dry periods. One could argue that the more dry nights manifested, the more probable it is that maturation of the CNS mechanisms has already occurred. Miller et al. (1960) reported that among 5-year-old children who did not have complete nocturnal bladder control, 50 percent—while rarely dry—had had occasional dry nights; similarly, 20 percent had intermittent dryness and 29 percent experienced periods of dryness lasting from 3 to 9 months. Among the children studied by Oppel et al. (1968), one third of 5-year-olds nocturnally enuretic at the time of the study had been dry for at least 6 months at an earlier age.

Further evidence difficult to reconcile with the view that late maturation is predominantly responsible for enuresis is that alteration of the older enuretic child's environment may lead to temporary control. Stein and Susser (1967), for example, reported that students at boarding school were frequently dry on nights spent in sick bay, but reverted to regular bedwetting when returned to their usual quarters. Young (1965) suggested that the high rate of success achieved with conditioning treatment among nocturnally enuretic children aged 7 years or more provides evidence that in the majority of such children, maturation has already occurred.

Immaturity of the bladder. The suggestion that nocturnal enuresis is the result of failure to develop increased functional bladder capacity[2] originally gained impetus from the work of Hallman (1950) and Muellner (1960a, 1960b). It has subsequently received the support of Esperanca and Gerrard (1969), Starfield (1967), Troup and Hodgson (1971) and Zaleski, Gerrard, and Shokier (1973), all finding that enuretic children have smaller functional bladder capacities than non-enuretic children of the same age. Smaller capacity is held to not function as an adequate stimulus for the development of a micturition inhibitory response (Muellner, 1960a, 1960b), resulting in frequent diurnal voidings in response to small volumes of urine in the bladder.

It is difficult, however, to determine what degree of bladder capacity is adequate for nocturnal control. Diurnal frequency is an index of daytime functional bladder capacity but, since young children who pass urine hourly during the day can be dry at night, diurnal frequency is not a reliable index of an individual child's nocturnal status. In addition, attempts to increase functional bladder capacity as a means of improving bedwetting have met with mixed success. Thus, although increasing bladder capacity by retention control training has been found to decrease bedwetting (P. M. Miller, 1973; Paschalis, Kimmel, & Kimmel, 1972; Starfield & Mellits, 1968) more recent studies using similar bladder training programs have shown some increase in daytime bladder capacity but no significant reduction in bedwetting

[2]The term *functional bladder capacity* refers to the amount of urine a child will retain before voiding and not the actual structural size of the bladder.

(Doleys & Wells, 1975; Doleys, Ciminero, Tollison, Williams, & Wells, 1977; Harris & Purohit, 1977; Rocklin & Tilker, 1973). It is therefore difficult to establish the relative importance of bladder maturity to the development of nocturnal continence. Assessment of this view results in a similar conclusion to an evaluation of theories relating bedwetting to immaturity of the CNS; namely, that while inadequate functional bladder capacity may account for nocturnal incontinence in some cases, it is unlikely to be the only factor involved, especially when older enuretic children are considered.

Depth of sleep. The belief that bedwetting is associated with deep sleep is very common among the parents of enuretic children, and many authors have noted this anecdotal evidence (Baller, 1975; Bostock, 1962; Finley, Wansley, & Blenkarn, 1977; Hallgren, 1957). However, early studies of the relationship between sleep and enuresis based on clinical observations produced conflicting results. Bostock (1958) compared the "arousability from sleep" of 7 enuretic and 12 nonenuretic children using an auditory stimulus produced by a buzzer. The enuretic children took an average of 418 sec to awaken whereas the nonenuretics took 319 sec. Although statistical data were not provided, the author concluded that enuretics sleep more deeply than nonenuretics. However, Boyd (1960) has published results contrary to this conclusion. He examined 100 enuretic children aged between 5 and 15 years, comparing them with a control group matched for age and sex. The children were awakened by calling their names and, if they did not respond, by shaking them gently. The enuretic children took an average of 16 sec to awaken, compared to 20.5 sec among the nonenuretics, this difference not being significant.

A nonsignificant outcome was also obtained in a recent unpublished study by Bollard, Nettelbeck, and Saies (1984), comparing arousability of 8 enuretic 10-year-olds and 8 nonenuretic siblings or first cousins. The urine-alarm included an alarm clock preset to sound at 1, 4, and 7 hours after sleep onset on different nights. Enuretics were additionally awakened by a wetting accident. A stopwatch activated when the alarm sounded was switched off by the child, thereby measuring arousability directly. Enuretics were slower to arouse, taking an advantage of 56 sec compared to 37 sec among the nonenuretic controls, but the difference did not approach statistical significance. Notable features of the data were, firstly, the very wide between-individual differences in waking time, with light and heavy sleepers in both groups; secondly, within-individual differences were also very wide, the deepest sleepers nonetheless waking quickly on occasions.

Most empirical data relating to sleep and enuresis have come from studies employing EEG recordings of sleep patterns.[3] The issues of interest in relation to bedwetting are, firstly, whether the overall EEG sleep profiles of enuretics and nonenuretics differ in fundamental ways and, secondly, whether bedwetting episodes occur predominantly during stages 3 (i.e., slow-wave) and stage 4 (deep) sleep. In respect of the first issue, Graham (1973) reported that studies comparing the amount of time spent in the four sleep stages have generally not revealed any reliable differences between enuretic and nonenuretic children. A recent study by Gillin et al. (1982) found that enuretic boys had significantly more shallow sleep than nonenuretic controls but this is in the opposite direction to that predicted by proponents of the deep sleep hypothesis.

The evidence in respect of the second question is also equivocal. While bedwetting only very rarely occurs during the rapid-eye-movement (REM) phase when sleep is light (Broughton, 1968), several studies have observed that bedwetting can occur during all non-rapid-eye-movement (NREM) sleep stages, although enuretic episodes are more commonly associated with stages 3 and 4 (Broughton, 1968; Evans, 1971; Pierce, Whitman, Mass, & Gay, 1961; Ritvo et al., 1969). Arguner, Baybas, Gozukirmizi, and Zembilci (1980) also found that bedwetting tends to occur during the first sleep cycle of the night, when there is a predominance of slow-wave sleep However, more recent studies have reported that bedwetting events are not associated with any particular sleep stage (Kales, Kales, Jacobson, Humphrey, & Soldatos, 1977; Mikkelsen, Rapoport, Nee, Gruenau, Mendelson, & Gillin, 1980). Further Gillin et al. (1982) found that the percentage of time spent by enuretic boys in each sleep stage was essentially the same during nights when they wet the bed or remained dry.

The significant observation according to Broughton (1968) was not so much the particular sleep stage during which bedwetting occurred, but rather that bedwetting accompanied a marked "lightening" of deep

[3] Based largely on scoring the criteria for EEG patterns initially proposed by Dement and Kleitman (1957), human sleep is now typically classified into four stages, the number of these from 1 to 4 corresponding to the relative "depth of sleep," with stage 4 the deepest. In addition to these stages there is rapid-eye-movement (REM) sleep which has a number of separate behavioral and neurophysiological characteristics. After infancy, a night of normal sleep consists of a series of cycles, each containing non-rapid-eye-movement (NREM) sleep and REM sleep interspersed with occasional awakenings. The first cycle usually has more stage 3 and stae 4 sleep (slow-wave activity) and may lack a REM stage. As the cycles pass, the proportion of REM sleep increases and that of NREM sleep, especially slow-wave sleep, decreases.

NREM sleep, occurring during the transition from stage 4 to stage 1. Broughton considered that this result reconciles the different views on whether bedwetting episodes are synchronous with slow-wave sleep, light sleep, or even wakefulness. Thus, Broughton concluded that bedwetting is best thought of as a "disorder of the sleep-arousal system" and several others have confirmed that bedwetting occurs during arousal from deep sleep (Arguner, Baybas, Gozukirmizi, & Zembilci, 1978; Gastaut, Batini, Broughton, Fressy, & Tassinari, 1964; Pierce et al., 1961; Szabo & Popoviciu, 1969). Finley (1971) supported Broughton by demonstrating that the "arousal threshold" of enuretics is abnormally high compared with nonenuretics. (Finley defined arousal threshold in terms of progressive increments of stimulus intensity until the child is awake both behaviorally and according to the EEG record.)

De Perri and Meduri (1972) have demonstrated that, in addition to being unresponsive to external stimulation, enuretic children can also be relatively unresponsive to introceptive stimulation from a distended and rapidly contracting bladder. Simultaneous polygraphic and cystometric recordings were obtained during both spontaneous and pharmacologically induced sleep following artificial filling of the bladder, for 7 bedwetters (aged between 13 and 16 years) and 7 control subjects. Reflex micturition occurred without clinical signs of wakefulness in the enuretic group but with transient polygraphic evidence of arousal. The control group, on the other hand, showed definite electro-clinical arousal for cystometric pressure below threshold levels of reflex voiding. Thus, the weight of evidence is consistent with Broughton's (1968) suggestion, that the sleep-arousal system of bedwetters is impaired in some way.

Medical treatment. Medical therapists are likely to prescribe either of two treatments for bedwetting, the choice being determined by the child's age. On the assumption that bedwetting results from immaturity of physiological mechanisms governing bladder control, no formal treatment may be offered younger children, except for the advice that the child will eventually outgrow the problem. However, as demonstrated earlier this advice is difficult to reconcile with the evidence for children beyond the age of about 5 years. Surveys of prevalence do suggest that a certain proportion of children will spontaneously stop wetting the bed as they grow older but only about 1 in 6 become continent for each year between the ages of 5 to 15 years (De Jonge, 1973; Forsythe & Redman, 1974; Lovibond, 1964). At present one cannot predict those children who will become dry spontaneously, or the 2 percent or 3 percent who will remain enuretic into the latter teenage years.

The second and frequently practiced medical treatment, especially for older enuretic children, is to prescribe some form of medication. Although no major review of this area has appeared since Blackwell and Currah (1973), their findings from more than 100 studies were unequivocal and can be accepted as applying today. A wide range of medications have been used in attempts to control enuresis but effects have generally been disappointing. Only the tricyclic antidepressants have been shown consistently to be better than placebo, the most commonly used and extensively studied being imipramine (Tofranil).

The response of enuretics to tricyclic antidepressants is usually quite rapid, with a reduction in bedwetting frequency occurring in the first week of treatment. A plateau of reduced bedwetting (perhaps 2 or 3 wet nights less per week) subsequently results for most children still wetting (Stewart, 1975). However, while such reduction is typically statistically significant, it is nonetheless unsatisfactory for most families who hope for normal, total continence. Complete remission is usually obtained for less than 50 percent of those treated and is often in the range of only 10–20% at 6-months follow-up (Blackwell & Currah, 1973). In addition, relapse tends to occur immediately following the withdrawal of medication, an obvious shortcoming of treatment. Blackwell and Currah have reported that the lowest (i.e., most favorable) immediate relapse rate from among a number of well-controlled studies was 70 percent.

A further shortcoming of drug therapy often overlooked is the possibility of imipramine poisoning (Meadow, 1981), not only for the enuretic child but also for siblings having access to tablets. Imipramine poisoning is awkward to treat and may cause long-term heart damage (Goel & Shanks, 1974). Further, the long-term effects of such drugs on growth and development are yet to be established and are therefore of concern.

Blackwell and Currah (1973) suggested three possible mechanisms of action of tricyclic antidepressants: (a) the drug increases arousability during sleep in response to cues from a filling bladder; (b) the drug has certain biochemical (anticholinergic) properties which act at the level of the bladder and sphincter to prevent voiding; (c) in line with psychodynamic theory, the drug acts on the enuretic child's underlying depression for which bedwetting is a symptom. However, empirical evidence relevant to these explanations is inconclusive. Firstly, the capacity of tricyclics to make enuretics easier to arouse from sleep has not been demonstrated (Bennett-Johnson, 1980). In respect of the second explanation, anticholinergic drugs have not been found to produce a consistent effect, some reports indicating an increase in bladder capacity (Esperanca & Gerrard, 1969; Johnstone, 1972; Thompson & Lauvetz, 1976) but others not successful (Blackwell & Currah (1973). Thirdly, as discussed earlier, there is little evidence that enuresis is a symptom of underlying depression. Although Werry, Dowrick, Lampen, and Vamos (1975) demonstrated a reduction in wetting accompanied by positive behavioral changes following administration of imipramine, such changes may have occurred in response to decreased wetting rather than to any direct psychotrophic properties of the drug.

In summary then, the mechanism of action of tricyclic antidepressants in influencing enuresis remains unknown, although the anticholinergic property of these drugs (which seems to allow the storage of greater volume of urine in the bladder before voiding) appears the most promising. However, such treatment results in complete continence in only a minority of cases.

Behavioral Theories and Treatment

Standard conditioning. Like the physiological theories already discussed, behavioral theories of nocturnal enuresis conceive of the disorder as a failure to develop cortical control over subcortical effector mechanisms. However, whereas physiological theories attribute this failure to such processes as neural maturation, underdeveloped functional bladder capacity, and/or faulty sleep arousal, behavioral theories emphasize the role of conditioning in the development of processes necessary for continence.

The processes involved in achieving bladder control are complex and the importance of neural maturation is beyond question but it seems clear that conditioning is also involved. Various conceptualizations as to the nature of these conditioning processes have been suggested. Campbell (1934) and Mowrer and Mowrer (1938) were among the first to suggest that enuresis commonly reflects a deficiency in the inhibitory control of an essentially automatic function, because of faulty habit training. Morgan and Witmer (1939) believed that ordinary continence training teaches the child to respond to bladder stimulation by awakening and, ultimately, to substitute a toilet action for bedwetting. Smith (1948) extended the habit deficiency view by suggesting that bedwetting results from inefficient toilet training and becomes established because of the atmosphere of anxiety and frustration that it engenders. Crosby (1950) argued that bedwetting is not necessarily only a habit deficiency, but may represent the acquisition of the habit of urinating during sleep in response to specific environmental conditions.

Lovibond's (1964) summary of the behavioral viewpoint was that, for the majority of children, cause is related to the absence of environmental conditions ordinarily necessary for learning the response of sphincter inhibition and/or to low levels of conditionability. In a minority of cases, failure to develop control may be due to high levels of anxiety or nervous tension which produce inefficient learning, or the breakdown of previously established linkages.

Behavioral therapists have turned to the analysis of environmental conditions associated with learning bladder control, in attempting to elucidate the etiology of enuresis. Associated treatment has encompassed a collection of procedures based on the common theory that achievement of continence involves learning the discriminative cues that enable inhibition of urination until appropriate toileting is possible. The case for behavioral theories is supported by demonstration of the role of toilet training in establishing continence both diurnally and nocturnally.

Much of the earlier published information on this topic is of limited value, being sketchy and based on retrospective accounts given by mothers—evidence which is notoriously unreliable (Wenar & Coulter, 1962). However, in their prevalence survey of bedwetting Blomfield and Douglas (1956) found that where earlier toilet training had been given, a higher proportion of children developed earlier dryness. Then, in more recent years, researchers have clearly demonstrated the efficacy of daytime toilet training programs based on operant conditioning principles for bladder and bowel control (Azrin & Foxx, 1971, 1974; Bettison, 1978; Bettison, Davison, Taylor, & Fox, 1976; Foxx & Azrin, 1973a, 1973b). These programs have been used successfully with retarded persons, as well as with groups of normal children.

However, strongest support for the view that learning plays a facilitative role in the attainment of bladder control comes from the well-established high success rate associated with the bell-and-pad treatment of bedwetting, commonly referred to as the *standard conditioning* method. The first systematic rationale for the treatment of nocturnal enuresis based on conditioning principles was described by Mowrer and Mowrer (1938). They argued that enuresis results from failure to acquire the habit of responding to a filling bladder in the night by awakening and/or contracting the urethral sphincter muscles to prevent reflexive voiding. The bell-and-pad procedure was a logical outcome of the Mowrers' theoretical analysis, although the potential therapeutic effects of an apparatus of this type had earlier been recognized by Pfaundler (1904).

Treatment involves having the child sleep on a urine-sensitive pad connected to a loud bell or buzzer. When wetting occurs the alarm is triggered, causing the child to awaken and micturition to cease. The child is then required to complete micturition in the toilet before drying the detector pad, resetting the alarm and returning to bed. With younger children the alarm may also serve to waken an attendant, usually the parent, who helps the child through this procedure. Treatment is usually regarded as successful when 14 consecutive dry nights have been reached. Modern equipment follows the basic design of the Mowrers' apparatus, though incorporating more recent technological advances to eliminate hazards initially encountered, such as dangerous electrical currents and ulcers caused by contact with the pad electrodes, and to improve overall efficiency (Borrie & Fenton, 1966; Coote, 1965; Greaves, 1969; Neal & Coote, 1969; Pfeiffer & Lloyd, 1978).

Mowrer and Mowrer's (1938) explanation for the mechanisms of treatment was based on the principles of classical conditioning. They reasoned that increasing detrusor muscle tension acts as an unconditioned stimulus (US) to produce the unconditioned reflex voiding response (UR). With conditioning training, voiding in turn triggers the alarm (US2) which wakens the child (UR2) and results in the inhibition of urination (UR3) by producing reflexive sphincter contraction. However, Mowrer and Mowrer also argued that increasing detrusor muscle tension would act as a conditioned stimulus (CS), which, because it occurred in close contiguity with the alarm, would eventually come to wake the child (CR) and inhibit urination (CR2). Because increasing detrusor muscle tension involves a gradient of intensity, it was held that with training the process would move backwards in time and the child would wake without having urinated, before the alarm was triggered. Thus, as this CS became established by the conditioning procedure, the child would become dry.

Crosby (1950) introduced the "Dri-Nite" conditioning instrument, similar in concept to the Mowrers' apparatus except that the waking stimulus was an electric shock. Crosby was less explicit than Mowrer and Mowrer when describing the conditioning process by which the respective instruments were believed to have their effect but Crosby's comments suggest that he also had the classical conditioning model in mind.

Lovibond (1963a, 1963b, 1964) questioned the classical conditioning explanation on several grounds. Firstly, unlike the CS in the classical Pavlovian model, the presumed CS in the treatment of enuresis is not originally neutral with respect to micturition but the US for reflexive voiding. Secondly, the classical conditioning model would predict that, because of experimental extinction, dryness after treatment would not be sustained indefinitely. Thirdly, according to the Mowrers' model, awakening to urinate is essential to the conditioned linkage between bladder distention (CS) and the awakening response (CR), whereas some children respond to conditioning without waking to urinate. Furthermore the Mowerers' explanation does not account for the fact that children eventually sleep through the night without waking or wetting.

Lovibond (1963a) proposed an alternative explanation for the conditioning treatment based on passive avoidance learning (Church & Solomon, 1956; Mowrer, 1950, 1960), rather than on classical conditioning. Lovibond initially considered that escape from the alarm might facilitate the development of passive avoidance and, accordingly, he designed a "Twin-Signal" instrument that provided opportunity for escape. This apparatus emitted a brief, noxious signal at the onset of wetting and then, after one minute of silence, a second alarm (conventional buzzer) that operated continually until switched off. Appropriate sphincter contraction provided escape from the noxious signal and should become conditioned to stimuli associated with sphincter relaxation. Comparison of the Twin-Signal treatment with the continuous signal used in the Mowrers' procedure and Crosby's apparatus showed the Twin-Signal to be the most effective in initially arresting bedwetting. However, Lovibond (1964) recognized that the provision for escape and stimulus intensity were confounded in the Twin-Signal device and that stimulus aversiveness might account for its apparent superiority. Further, he commented that the case for adopting the Twin-Signal instrument for larger-scale services was not strong since the Mowrers' device is not only effective in arresting bedwetting but has the advantage of being relatively simple and cheap to construct and maintain. In a later study, Turner et al. (1970) found no difference in the effectiveness of the Twin-Signal and the Mowrers' devices. The Dri-Nite apparatus (Crosby, 1950) has not been shown to have significant therapeutic advantages over the Mowrers' device and has distinct drawbacks since most parents and enuretics find the delivery of electric shocks in response to bedwetting excessively frightening and distasteful. Thus, of the three types of conditioning apparatus developed, the case for the Mowrers' instrument for large-scale usage appears to be the strongest on practical grounds and this device has become the most extensively used and studied.

A review of 12 studies since 1965 by Doleys (1977) indicated that procedures utilizing conditioning instruments are very effective in arresting nocturnal enuresis. On average, bedwetting is arrested in about 75 percent of cases treated by the standard bell-and-pad procedure, with earlier reviews (Lovibond, 1964; Yates, 1970) suggesting that the rate of initial arrest can be as high as 80–90 percent. Among studies reviewed by Doleys (1977), the average duration of treatment with the standard procedure ranged from 5 to 12 weeks. This method has been shown to be more effective in arresting bedwetting than drug therapies (Blackwell & Currah, 1973; Meadow, 1974; Shaffer, Costello, & Hill, 1968), dynamic/supportive counselling psychotherapies (De Leon & Mandell, 1966; Novick, 1966; Werry & Cohrssen, 1965), advice and encouragement (Dische, 1971), and retention control training (Doleys et al., 1977; Fielding, 1980).

Despite this success, some problems associated with standard conditioning have been observed. Ulceration caused by contact with the electrode pads was common with early devices but this has virtually been eradicated by design improvements. However, the standard conditioning treatment can be inconvenient, resulting in failure to persist with treatment in about a third of cases (Young & Morgan, 1972). Frustrations can be particularly marked when the child wets several times in the night or when false alarms occur because of excessive sweating or machine malfunction. Treatment can be sabotaged by the child switching off the alarm before going to sleep, or by parents forgetting to switch it on. However, technological advances have reduced the incidence of malfunction in currently available devices (Coote, 1965; Pfeiffer & Lloyd, 1978) and problems of cooperation can largely be overcome by closer supervision from a clinician (Dische, 1973).

The influence of various subject variables on response to conditioning treatment has been investigated but few have been found to be significant; for example, bedwetting frequency, sex, and whether the enuresis was primary or secondary (Collins, 1973; Taylor & Turner, 1975; Turner et al., 1970). Sacks and De Leon (1978) reported no difference between disturbed and nondisturbed enuretic children in respect of the percentage cured and speed of cure, though their results suggested that disturbed children have a greater likelihood of relapse. Less favorable outcome has also been associated with high levels of maternal anxiety and disturbed family backgrounds (Young & Morgan, 1973) and unsatisfactory housing conditions (Dische et al., 1983).

The largest shortcoming of standard conditioning is the substantial number of children who resume wetting the bed after achieving a period of dryness. Doleys (1977) has noted relapse rates following standard conditioning ranging from 13 percent (Young & Turner,

1965) to 69 percent (Taylor & Turner, 1975), with an average relapse rate from 12 studies reviewed being approximately 40 percent.

Various attempts have been made to develop predictions of relapse following conditioning treatment. Lovibond (1964) and Young and Morgan (1973) between them examined such background factors as age, sex, general adjustment, and patterns of bedwetting, but found none to be significantly associated with probability of relapse. However, other evidence has suggested an association between proneness to relapse and diurnal urinary symptoms (Bollard, 1982; Fielding, 1980; Lovibond & Coote, 1970), deviant scores on a teacher's behavior rating scale and the presence of family difficulties (Dische et al., 1983), and bedwetting frequency at the commencement of treatment (Finley, Rainwater, & Johnson, 1982).

Countermeasures to relapse have generally followed two strategies; an intermittent schedule with the alarm following some variable proportion of wets; and overlearning training in combination with standard conditioning (i.e., increasing the child's fluid intake towards the end of treatment). Morgan (1978) reviewed eight studies involving either intermittent schedules and/or overlearning. He concluded that both procedures are superior to standard conditioning with respect to reducing subsequent relapse and that, as a single procedure, overlearning is superior to intermittent reinforcement. However, Morgan concluded that both alternatives increase the time required to attain dryness. The only study to compare standard conditioning directly with intermittent reinforcement and overlearning (Taylor & Turner, 1975) showed a clear difference in acquisition time, durations of treatment being 68, 113, and 86 days respectively for each of these procedures.

Finley et al. (1982) examined relapse rates for 168 enuretic children given conditioning treatment involving varying intermittent alarm schedules, claiming that intermittent schedules resulted in significantly lower relapse rates without prolonging treatment, compared with continuous reinforcement. However, these claims are severely weakened by the study's design, 22 "rapid responders" (i.e., 13 percent of the sample) who attained the dryness criterion during the initial, continuous reinforcement phase of treatment not being included in the subsequent comparisons of acquisition and relapse rates. Thus the effect of excluding these children from analysis was to increase the average treatment time and relapse rate for children undergoing continuous reinforcement.

In summary, intermittent reinforcement and overlearning have been shown to reduce relapse rates but at the expense of increasing the duration of treatment (Taylor & Turner, 1975). Thus, relapse remains a problem with the standard conditioning procedure, an issue that is discussed further in a later section.

Dry-bed training. Azrin, Sneed, and Foxx (1973, 1974) view nocturnal continence as an operant learning process in which social and motivational factors are as important as sensitivity to bladder sensation. Enuresis is held to result from insufficient social reinforcement and inhibitory influences. In line with this model, Azrin et al. have incorporated a variety of operant training procedures shown in other studies to curb bedwetting into one comprehensive program termed Dry-Bed Training (DBT) that emphasizes positive reinforcement for nocturnal bladder control and aversive consequences immediately following bedwetting accidents. DBT employs the standard urine-alarm apparatus but regards this as a convenient tool for contiguously applying social reinforcement to a bedwetting accident, rather than providing direct conditioning of the bladder sphincter. Additional major features include regular nighttime awakenings, increased fluid intake, and practice in withholding urine before voiding, practice in correct nighttime toileting behavior, positive reinforcement for nocturnal control, and punishment for bedwetting accidents. Punishment consists of verbal admonishment following an accident, "cleanliness training" (the requirement that the child change wet sheets, deposit them in the laundry, and remake the bed), and "positive practice" (the child must count to 50, then go to the toilet, this practice being repeated 20 times once cleanliness training has been performed). Initial all-night intensive training is done by a professional trainer in the child's home. Posttraining supervision by the child's parents then continues until the child becomes continent.

Azrin et al. (1974) conducted an experiment involving 24 enuretic children (average age = 8 years). The experimental design provided a within-subject as well as a between-subjects comparison of standard conditioning with DBT. In one condition the urine-alarm sounded in the parents' bedroom and in the child's room. In another condition the alarm sounded only in the parents' room. The within-subject comparison was provided by instituting DBT after two weeks for those children who began with standard conditioning.

Results indicated that DBT was more effective than standard conditioning in arresting bedwetting. Before treatment, all subjects were reported to be wetting the bed every night. Standard conditioning reduced accidents to an average of 6 during the first week of treatment and to 5 during the second week. However, after one night of DBT, the average number of accidents was only 1 during both the first week and second week and none after the third week. Ultimately, all 24 subjects treated by DBT reached the criterion of 14 consecutive dry nights, in an average time of 4 weeks. None relapsed to pretraining level of bedwetting during a 6-month follow-up. In seven instances during follow-up two or more such accidents occurred within seven days but in each instance bedwetting was arrested within a week following reinstatement of DBT. A second finding was that bedwetting was eliminated as effectively when the alarm sounded only in the parents' bedroom as when the alarm sounded in both the child's and the parents' bedroom. Azrin et al. (1974) therefore concluded that Pavlovian conditioning did not contribute to the success of DBT, since omission of the alarm from the child's room precluded direct conditioning of the bladder, but that the alarm was a means of producing operant reinforcement.

Despite these promising results, however, closer scrutiny of the Azrin et al. study reveals significant deficiencies in the control procedures. Firstly, the DBT group included 11 subjects treated by the standard procedure for 2 weeks prior to the introduction of DBT. The alarm-only phase of treatment reduced bedwetting frequency, albeit slightly, and this initial gain, together with general experience of the urine-alarm, could have affected subjects' progress during subsequent treatment by DBT. Secondly, alarm-only treatment was very brief, and it has been shown that significant treatment effects are not usually seen for standard conditioning until after the first few weeks (Baker, 1969; Turner et al., 1970). Thirdly, the relative success of DBT might be attributable to a higher degree of patient/therapist contact within DBT's initial all-night training session, resulting in higher motivation directed towards correct alarm usage on the part of parents and children. Doleys et al. (1977) have supported the general effectiveness of DBT, while noting that success rate among their 13 subjects (average age = 6.6 years) was less remarkable than that reported by Azrin et al. (1974).

Bollard and Woodroffe (1977) examined the effectiveness of DBT with two important modifications to the original procedure. Firstly, parents participating were instructed to administer the intensive all-night training, rather than introducing an outside trainer into the child's home. Secondly, the Dry-Bed procedure was administered to some subjects without the adjunct of a urine-alarm. Fourteen children (ages ranged from 4 to 14 years) were assigned to DBT with an alarm and 10 to the same procedure but without an alarm. A control group of 10 children received no treatment at all. All children in the DBT-with-alarm condition reached the success criterion of 14 consecutive dry nights, the median time being just less than 4 weeks. Two of the 14 children relapsed during a 6- month follow-up although, as it was left to parents to indicate if bedwetting recurred, this may be an underestimate. None of the children undergoing DBT without the alarm reached the dryness criterion within a 13-week treatment period, although there was a substantial drop in mean wetting frequency for this group during the first week of training, followed by a plateau of reduced bedwetting. Parents of control children reported that bedwetting frequency was unchanged throughout the 13-week experimental period.

Nettelbeck and Langeluddecke (1979) criticized Bollard and Woodroffe's claim of reduced bedwetting frequency in the DBT without an alarm condition, on the grounds that baseline measures and control data had not been collected but assumed on the basis of parents' reports to be seven wet nights per week throughout. Nettelbeck and Langeluddecke treated 8 children (mean age = 8 years) by DBT with an alarm and 7 by DBT but without an alarm, confirming the effectiveness of DBT with an alarm but finding it to be ineffective without an alarm when compared with a no-treatment control group over a 10-week period.

Bollard and Nettelbeck (1981) compared standard conditioning with DBT administered under four different conditions; by the child's parents at home with and without an alarm, by a professional trainer at home with an alarm, or by a professional trainer in hospital with an alarm. One hundred and twenty children (mean age = 9 years) took part and treatment continued for 20 weeks. DBT with an alarm was equally effective under all conditions and significantly though marginally more effective than standard conditioning, both for the proportion of children successfully treated and the overall speed of treatment. The superiority of DBT was not simply attributable to greater therapist contact. Although DBT without an alarm resulted in significantly fewer bedwettings than a no-treatment control, it was markedly less effective in arresting bedwetting than any of the alarm-based treatments. Further support for the general effectiveness of DBT with an alarm has been provided by Barrett (1983), Bollard, Nettelbeck, and Roxbee (1982), and Griffiths, Meldrum, and McWilliam (1982).

In spite of the impressive results of DBT in terms of the proportion who achieve initial arrest of bedwetting and the speed of treatment, there are important limitations to its large-scale use in clinical practice that do not apply to the same degree to the standard conditioning method. The program involves a complicated schedule of tasks that is time-consuming and that can undermine the child's and the parents' motivation to persist. Although it has been shown that parents can replace the professional trainer in the home for the initial all-night session without reducing the program's effectiveness (Bollard & Nettelbeck, 1981; Bollard & Woodroffe, 1977), such training is time consuming. In our experience, instructing parents in DBT requires about 90 mins, which is considerably longer than is required for instruction of standard conditioning.

Bollard and Nettelbeck (1982) addressed this limitation by instructing the parents of enuretic children within small groups settings to administer DBT with and without an alarm. Results were virtually the same as those from Bollard and Nettelbeck (1981), suggesting that instructing parents in a group to administer DBT with an alarm is a viable large-scale method of treating nocturnal enuresis that should save therapist and administrative time.

Even with the advantages of small-group instruction, however, DBT still places heavy demands on parents and children, especially in its initial phase. Considerable effort is required to maintain compliance from children, especially during the positive practice components. Similar difficulties have been noted by Barrett (1983) and by Griffiths et al. (1982). For these reasons, Bollard and Nettelbeck (1982) attempted to delineate which aspects of DBT, in addition to the alarm, contribute most to the procedure's overall effectiveness, with the intention of subsequently simplifying the procedure. Main components were first identified as (a) the waking schedule, (b) retention control training, and (c) positive practice. Combinations of these yielded six treatment groups each comprising 12 subjects. These groups were compared for effectiveness, together with a standard alarm-only group and a DBT group from the Bollard and Nettelbeck (1981) study. None of the effects of the single components was statistically significant although bedwetting was reduced to levels slightly below the level achieved with the alarm-only treatment by the addition of either retention control training, or positive practice, with a more substantial decrease in bedwetting resulting from the waking schedule. The effects of the three components were cumulative, so that the more components added to the alarm-only procedure, the better the therapeutic response but retention control training and positive practice could be eliminated from the DBT schedule without sacrificing its overall effectiveness since a combination of the waking schedule with the urine alarm was almost as effective as the complete DBT program. For practical purposes, this finding is of considerable advantage because of the demands of the full DBT program. Although the waking schedule does present additional demands to standard conditioning, this is only substantial on the initial night when the child is awakened hourly for toileting. Following the intensive all-night session, the child is awakened once only during the night and most parents and children appear to cope with this requirement. Indeed, prior to treatment most parents reported that they had previously employed the practice of regular lifting during the night in an attempt to manage the child's bedwetting.

Adequate data on relapse following DBT are as yet limited. Williams, Doleys, and Ciminero (1978) have provided a 2-year follow-up of eight enuretic children successfully treated by DBT, finding that five averaged less than one wet a month but that the other three were wetting four or more times a month. Bollard (1982) followed up 60 enuretic children treated by DBT and 35 treated by standard conditioning over a 2-year period. Relapse was defined as renewed bedwetting at a frequency of more than one wet bed per week over a 4-week period. Results showed that after achieving the initial success criterion of 14 consecutive dry nights, 39 percent of the DBT and 41 percent of the standard conditioning group relapsed. Thus it seems at present that DBT, in common with standard conditioning, is associated with a high relapse rate.

The use of DBT without an alarm by Bollard and Woodroffe (1977), Bollard and Nettelbeck (1981), Bollard and Nettelbeck (1982), and Nettelbeck and Langeluddecke (1979) has been only moderately successful and these findings differ substantially from reports by Azrin and his colleagues that bedwetting can be eliminated effectively by a training program similar to the original DBT schedule but without an alarm and with some modifications to the intensive training session and the way parents were instructed. (Azrin & Thienes, 1978; Azrin, Thienes-Hontos, & Besalel-Azrin, 1979; Besalel-Azrin, Azrin, Thienes-Hontos, & McMorrow, 1980). One possible explanation for this difference is that the various modifications to the original DBT schedule made by Azrin and his colleagues have increased the effectiveness of treatment, although the basic training features of both versions are much the same. Another reason could be that Azrin's subjects were generally younger than subjects treated by us. It is apparent, for example that Azrin and Thienes (1978) included a high proportion of 3-year-olds treated in the modified operant procedure and these children were likely to have been more responsive to most forms of therapy.

Caceres (1982) has found standard conditioning to be more effective than the no-alarm procedure described by Azrin and Thienes (1978), both in terms of the number of children reaching dryness and the speed of treatment. Caceres also found that parents experienced less difficulty administering standard conditioning. However, a recent report by Keating, Butz, Burke, and Heimberg (1983) supports the effectiveness of the no-alarm program. Three variations in the mode of delivery of DBT were investigated. Twenty-three children ranging in age from 4 to 14 years received DBT without the use of a urine-alarm. Treatment variations included: (a) in-home training of parents and child, (b) office-based training of parents and child, and (c) office-based training of parents only. An additional seven children served as a waiting list control group during the first eight weeks of the study. A variety of outcome measures showed improvement for the entire treatment sample regardless of specific mode of delivery. Eighteen of 23 subjects reached the dryness criterion (14 consecutive dry nights) within a mean of 74 days. However, Keating et al. (1983) concede that this procedure appears less effective than DBT with an alarm in terms of the success rate and speed of response, the latter result also raising the likelihood of a higher dropout rate.

Even though further research might substantiate the effectiveness of the modified operant program, this procedure still has significant practical limitations since it involves further additions to an already complicated and demanding training regimen. However, setting aside the practical considerations, the results of the no-alarm treatment do raise interesting theoretical issues in respect of the role of operant variables in reducing bedwetting. Procedures such as training in rapid awakening, practice in withholding urination, massed practice in correct nighttime toileting behavior, and differential social reinforcement for wet or dry nights, appear to contribute to the overall effectiveness of the DBT program, in addition to the specific stimulus effects of the urine-alarm.

Summary of conditioning treatments. There is now a substantial body of literature attesting to the greater superiority of conditioning treatments of enuresis, compared with psychotherapy and medication. In deciding whether to provide DBT or standard conditioning the therapist is faced with considerations of the speed and endurance of treatment and the comparative ease of implementation of each method. Taking these into account, we believe that standard conditioning combined with a nighttime waking schedule provides the most cost-effective treatment for large scale clinical practice. A more detailed protocol for the management of bedwetting in this way is presented in the next section.

MANAGEMENT OF THE ENURETIC PATIENT

Initial Investigations

Medical. Although underlying organic causes for enuresis are rare, every child with this condition should nonetheless be investigated by a medical practitioner before proceeding with treatment. A detailed history should be taken and, on physical examination, the child's growth percentiles and blood pressure measured. Urine analysis is also mandatory. Additional radiologic and/or urologic investigation generally would not be required unless an underlying physical defect was apparent or the child failed to respond to treatment. More detailed accounts of the initial medical workup are provided by McKendry and Stewart (1974) and Jureidini (1982).

Psychological

Assessment interview. Before embarking on treatment, it is essential that the child and parents are interviewed. Areas covered should include: the child's history, pattern of bedwetting, previous attempts to manage the problem and a check on the outcome of the medical investigation; the presence of other continence problems (e.g., excessive frequency and/or urgency of micturition, diurnal enuresis, encopresis); family history of enuresis; the parents' perception of the nature and etiology of enuresis; assessment of the child's social and emotional adjustment; accommodation arrangements; the child and parents' motivation for treatment; and parental ability to conduct treatment. Evidence of fear of the dark or toilet phobia that may be related functionally to bedwetting should be explored and such behaviors eliminated prior to commencing treatment of the bedwetting itself.

Psychological preparation for treatment. The therapist should explain the nature of enuresis and the rationale for treatment, and dispel any misunderstanding held about the problem. It is worthwhile emphasizing that enuresis is common in childhood, that in the vast majority of cases it does not represent underlying emotional or organic pathology, and that with appropriate treatment the prospects of a cure are high. We favor an explanation based on the notion that bedwetting results from failure to learn to perceive the signals from a filling bladder during sleep and to respond by contracting the bladder sphincter and/or by awakening to go to the toilet. The explanation should be tailored to fit the parents' level of comprehension and in many instances a separate, less sophisticated explanation will be required for the child. As a general guide, the reader is directed to Bollard and Nettelbeck (1989) for more detail of such explanations and in addition, comprehensive comments about psychological preparation in conditioning treatment.

Establishment of baseline. For at least two weeks following the initial assessment and prior to treatment, bedwetting incidents should be recorded in order to establish baseline wetting frequency. It is advantageous to provide parents with a simple calendar or chart for recording. During this baseline period, all preexisting management procedures (including lifting and fluid restriction) must cease.

Demonstration of the conditioning procedure and waking schedule. The urine-alarm equipment is demonstrated by pouring a small amount of sterile saline on to the detector pad, thereby triggering the alarm. The child is then encouraged to repeat this with one hand placed on the pad, thus being reassured that there is no electric shock and nothing to fear. The conditioning procedure is described in detail and the child required to role-play the various steps, using a demonstration bed, to ensure that the method is understood. Written instructions for the procedure and for recording are issued. The conditioning procedure involves placing the pad in the child's bed such that when the alarm is triggered by a wetting accident the child is awakened. The alarm unit is placed at a sufficient distance from the bed so that the child cannot switch it off while still in bed, but not too far away to reduce the intensity of the signal.

Next, the waking schedule is described. A comprehensive description is provided by Azrin et al. (1974) but, briefly, it involves the child being woken hourly during the first night of training and sent to the toilet each time. Thereafter the child is woken for toileting once only each night, according to a predetermined schedule of times. This schedule is systematically phased out as the child acquires bladder control.

The child is encouraged to sleep without pajama pants in order to minimize delay between voiding and triggering the alarm. Following an accident, the child is required after awakening to go quickly to the toilet in order to finish voiding. After returning to the bedside, the wet sheet is removed, the detector pad dried thoroughly and the alarm reset. Then the child gets back into bed and returns to sleep. The child is encouraged to take full responsibility for this process but the parents are required to assist if the child is unable to manage alone.

The parent (or child if mature enough) must contact the therapist weekly by telephone and report on progress and a specific time for reporting is arranged. Parents are encouraged to make contact immediately if difficulties arise before the weekly designated time. Any cases not reporting at the designated time are contacted by the therapist. If resources permit, it is advantageous to supplement telephone contacts by visits to the therapist, at monthly intervals. Close supervision maintains progress, increasing the likelihood that the procedure is followed correctly and providing support to persist with the program.

Treatment continues until the child achieves 14 consecutive dry nights. If little progress is achieved after a 4-month period the child is reviewed by the therapist. In such cases, a break from the procedure might be indicated before resuming later. A further medical review should also be considered in the case of slow responders.

Follow-up after the dryness criterion has been reached is essential. Parents are encouraged to contact the therapist if the child relapses, this being defined as a resumption of bedwetting more than once per week over a 4-week period. In light of the high relapse rate associated with conditioning treatment, it is best to warn parents from the outset that success may require more than one course of treatment with the alarm.

DIRECTIONS FOR FUTURE RESEARCH

The Sleep-Arousal System and Enuresis

It has been noted that there are frequent anecdotal reports of bedwetters sleeping more deeply than nonenuretics and that there is empirical evidence for an association between enuresis and an impairment of the sleep-arousal system, although the precise nature of this remains unclear. In order to explore the sleep-arousal issue further, sleep patterns might be monitored by EEG under the following conditions: (a) just prior to and during the act of bedwetting; (b) throughout the course of treatment, comparing various adjuvant therapies to standard conditioning aimed at facilitating arousal from sleep; (c) following achievement of nocturnal continence; and (d) at the time of relapse, should this occur. EEG monitoring of sleep patterns could be supplemented by other measures of arousability, such as the degree of auditory stimulus required to achieve wakefulness, a procedure suggested by Finley (1971). In this way it would be possible to observe whether the development of bladder control is related to changes within the sleep-arousal system and, if so, whether such changes need be permanent for sustained continence to be achieved. Such observations would also permit determination of the degree of cortical arousal caused by the alarm or other stimulus which was necessary for effective conditioning treatment.

Related issues are whether adjuvant therapies to the urine alarm would facilitate necessary cortical arousal and the relative effectiveness of such additional procedures. One of the more obvious possible adjuvant therapies would seem to be the use of drugs to facilitate waking. Lovibond (1964) noted that stimulant drugs such as amphetamine sulphate have been used in clinical practice as an adjunct to conditioning treatment in difficult cases. Young and Turner (1965) found that CNS stimulants Methedrine and Dexedrine administered during conditioning treatment resulted in more rapid initial arrest of bedwetting, although relapse was high for subjects taking Dexedrine.

Further research into the use of waking schedules as an adjuvant therapy is also necessary. It seems likely that the facilitatory effect of the DBT waking schedule is due to this procedure enhancing the enuretic child's ease of arousability from sleep but this has not yet been directly tested. It may also be possible to improve the effectiveness of the DBT waking schedule by staggering the time of the awakenings throughout the night as was done by Creer and Davis (1975) and Young (1964) and/or by the use of an intermittent schedule of awakenings.

Oswald, Taylor, and Treisman (1960) found that sleeping subjects can make discriminations between incoming stimuli on the basis of their meaningfulness (e.g., the subject's own name) compared with less meaningful material. Furthermore, the probability of such a discriminative response can be raised by contingent reinforcement, like monetary reward (Zung & Wilson, 1961). It might therefore be possible to enhance the effectiveness of conditioning when the child is difficult to arouse by using a signal more meaningful than the alarm, such as the child's name, and to reward arousal to the signal as well as rewarding a dry night.

Matching Treatment with Individual Differences in Etiology

The tendency of research into the treatment of bedwetting has been to develop procedures and to apply these routinely to all enuretic children. However, in any large group of such children one finds considerable heterogeneity in terms of frequency of bedwetting, functional bladder capacity, the presence of diurnal symptoms, ease of arousability from sleep, and motivation to become dry (Bennett-Johnson, 1980). Thus, if a single treatment program is to accommodate these individual differences, it must combine a variety of training strategies. Essentially this is what has been attempted by Azrin et al. (1973, 1974) when developing DBT and, as discussed earlier, research has shown that this composite treatment approach is highly successful. A problem with such a comprehensive program, however, is that the treatment becomes excessively burdensome. Furthermore, if the full program is used for all children treated, some training for some individuals will be unnecessary.

A more efficient approach would be to assess the enuretic child beforehand and to match particular procedures with training needs. Although research reviewed here suggests that the standard urine-alarm procedure provides the most suitable "core" treatment for bedwetting, assessment prior to treatment could in some cases indicate additional forms of therapy likely to be beneficial. For example, functional bladder capacity could be measured by the water load technique described by Harris and Purohit (1977)[4] and, if significantly low, conditioning could be supplemented by daily retention control training. Arousability from sleep could be assessed beforehand or during the first few days of treatment, by measuring the degree of auditory stimulation necessary to wake the child, or by timing the interval between presentation of an auditory stimulus and the child awakening. Where the child was difficult to wake, standard conditioning could be supplemented by a nightly waking schedule, or even an appropriate drug. If poor motivation was a feature before treatment, then the urine-alarm program could be supplemented by more intensive differential reinforcement for wet or dry nights.

The problem of relapse. It has been noted earlier that attempts to overcome the problem of relapse following treatment by standard conditioning or DBT have met with only limited success. In view of these findings, one could adopt the view that the major goal of treatment should be to achieve initial dryness as quickly as possible, warn parents beforehand that a subsequent period of alarm-based treatment may be necessary, and deal with any relapses as they occur (Sacks & De Leon, 1983). However, in a clinical setting there are at least two issues of concern relating to relapse. One is the additional time required for alarm usage, a logistical problem when available urine alarms are under heavy demand. The other problem concerns the possibility that parents and child will become disillusioned with the training program following relapse and therefore be less motivated to continue treatment. Thus, there is still a need to develop a treatment that arrests bedwetting quickly and has a lower relapse rate. A starting point could be the combination of retention control training with the urine alarm. The only factor yet found to predict proneness to relapse reliably is the child's history of diurnal micturitional difficulty (Fielding, 1982). Problems of diurnal urgency, frequency, and wetting accidents are most likely explained by severely low levels of functional bladder capacity. Findings from studies employing retention control training suggest that while this procedure is of limited value in

[4] This procedure involves the child refraining from drinking any fluid for two hours. At the end of this period the child is required to void and then to drink water according to the following specifications: (a) A child weighting 55 lbs receives 1 oz of water per 2 lbs of body weight to a maximum of 1 liquid pint; one weighing more than 55 lbs receives 1 oz of water per 3 lbs of body weight to a maximum of 2 liquid pints. The child is urged to refrain from voiding as long as possible. The resulting voided specimen serves as the index of bladder capacity.

arresting bedwetting, it can be quite effective in increasing functional bladder capacity. Thus retention control training in conjunction with the urine-alarm device may lead in some cases to a more permanent dryness response.

SUMMARY

Functional nocturnal enuresis persists beyond an age by which most children have acquired normal bladder control in the absence of neurologic or urologic pathology for approximately 15 percent of 5-year-olds and 2 percent of teenagers. Theoretical explanations and associated treatments of enuresis fall into three main categories. Psychodynamic formulations view enuresis as a surface indicator of underlying emotional disturbance and some form of psychotherapy as the treatment of choice. Physiological theories attribute a failure to develop control of micturition to either immaturity of CNS connections governing bladder control, immaturity of the bladder itself, or faulty sleep-arousal-mechanisms. Forms of therapy advocated by physiological theorists include exercises to increase functional bladder capacity, the use of drugs (usually tricyclic antidepressants), or no active treatment at all except for the advice that the child will eventually outgrow the problem. Behavioral theorists emphasize the role of conditioning in the development of bladder control and view enuresis as resulting from incomplete or faulty learning. The two major forms of behavior therapy for enuresis are the *standard conditioning* urine-alarm procedure and *Dry-Bed training* (DBT), which incorporates a variety of operant procedures together with a urine alarm. Research has shown that such conditioning treatments are much more effective in arresting bedwetting than psychotherapy or drug therapy. In spite of this finding, however, conditioning treatments are associated with a high subsequent relapse rate and, to date, attempts to overcome this problem have met with only limited success.

A detailed protocol for the management of the enuretic patient is presented. This includes an initial medical and psychological assessment of the child, psychological preparation for treatment, demonstration of the conditioning procedure, and close supervision and follow-up. On a cost-effectiveness basis, the standard conditioning procedure, combined with a nighttime waking schedule, is recommended for the vast majority of bedwetters.

Suggestions for future research include further investigation into: (a) the sleep-arousal system using EEG monitoring of sleep patterns during various stages in the acquisition of nocturnal bladder control;

(b) individual differences in etiology with a view to matching particular treatment procedures with the enuretic child's individual needs; and (c) the possible use of retention control training as an adjunct to conditioning treatment in order to reduce relapse.

REFERENCES

Arguner, A., Baybas, S., Gozükirmizi, E., & Zembilci, N. (1980). Focal and generalized abnormalities during sleep in cases of enuresis nocturna. In L. Popoviciu, B. Asgia, & G. Badiu (Eds.), *Sleep, 1978. Fourth European Congress on Sleep Research* (pp. 717–720). Munchen: S. Karger, Basel.

Azrin, N. H., & Foxx, R. M. (1971). A rapid method of toilet training the institutionalzied retarded. *Journal of Applied Behavior Analysis, 4*, 89–99.

Azrin, N. H., & Foxx, R. M. (1974). *Toilet training in less than a day*. New York: Simon and Schuster.

Azrin, N. H., Sneed, T. J., & Foxx, R. M. (1973). Dry bed: A rapid method of eliminating bedwetting (enuresis) of the retarded. *Behaviour Research and Therapy, 11*, 427–434.

Azrin, N. H., Sneed, T. J., & Foxx, R. M. (1974). Dry-bed training: Rapid elimination of childhood enuresis. *Behaviour Research and Therapy, 12*, 147–156.

Azrin, N. H., & Thienes, P. M. (1978). Rapid elimination of enuresis by intensive learning without a conditioning apparatus. *Behavior Therapy, 9*, 342–354.

Azrin, N. H., Thienes-Hontos, P., & Besalel-Azrin, V. (1979). Elimination of enuresis without a conditioning apparatus—an extension by office instruction of the child and parents. *Behavior Therapy, 10*, 14–19.

Baker, B. L. (1969). Symptom treatment and symptom substitution in enuresis. *Journal of Abnormal Psychology, 74*, 42–49.

Bakwin, H. (1961). Enuresis in children. *Journal of Pediatrics, 58*, 806–819.

Bakwin, H. (1973). The genetics of enuresis. In I. Kolvin, R. C. MacKeith, & S. R. Meadow (Eds.), *Bladder control and enuresis* (pp. 73–77). Philadelphia: Lippincott.

Bakwin, H., & Bakwin, R. M. (1972). *Clinical management of behavioral disorder in children* (4th ed.). Philadelphia: Saunders.

Baller, W. R. (1975). *Bed-wetting: Origins and treatment*. New York: Pergamon.

Barbour, R. F., Borland, E. M., Boyd, M. M., Oppe, T. E., & Miller, A. (1963). Enuresis as a disorder of development. *British Medical Journal, 2*, 787.

Barrett, D. W. (1983). Modified dry bed training: A review, critique and case study. *Journal of Clinical Child Psychology, 12*, 187–191.

Behrle, F. C., Elkin, M. T., & Laybourne, P. C. (1956). Evaluation of a conditioning device in the treatment of nocturnal enuresis. *Pediatrics, 17*, 849–855.

Bennett-Johnson, S. (1980). Enuresis. In R. J. Daitzman (Ed.), *Clinical behav-*

ior therapy and behavior modification (Vol. 1, pp. 81–142). New York: Garland STPM Press.

Besalel-Azrin, V. A., Azrin, N. H., Thienes-Hontos, P., & McMorrow, M. (1980). Evaluation of a parent's manual for training enuretic children. *Behaviour Research and Therapy, 18*, 358–360.

Bettison, S. (1978). Toilet training the retarded: Analysis of the stages of development and procedures for designing programmes. *Australian Journal of Mental Retardation, 5*, 95–100.

Bettison, S. (1979). Toilet training. In M. Griffin & A. Hudson (Eds.), *Children's problems*. Melbourne: Circus Books.

Bettison, S. (in press). Research into behavioral approaches to toilet training and the acquisition of daytime bladder and bowel control by retarded persons. *International Review of Research in Mental Retardation*.

Bettison, S., Davison, D., Taylor, P., & Fox, B. (1976). The long-term effects of a toilet training programme for the retarded: A pilot study. *Australian Journal of Mental Regardation, 4*, 28–35.

Bieger, P. P. (1954). Enuresis nocturna is het lager. *Nederlandsch Tijdschriht voor Geneeskunde, 98*, 1839.

Biering, A., & Jespersen, T. (1959). The treatment of enuresis nocturna with conditioning devices. *Acta Paediatrica, 48* (Suppl. 118), 152–153.

Blackwell, B., & Currah, J. (1973). The pharmacology of enuresis. In I. Kolvin, R. C. MacKeither, & S. R. Meadow (Eds.), *Bladder control and enuresis* (pp. 231–257). Philadelphia: Lippincott.

Blomfield, J. M., & Douglas, J. W. B. (1956). Bedwetting: Prevalence among children aged 4–7 years. *Lancet, 1*, 850–852.

Bollard, J. (1982). A two-year follow-up of bedwetters treated by Dry-Bed Training and standard conditioning. *Behaviour Research and Therapy, 20*, 571–580.

Bollard, J., & Nettelbeck, T. (1989). *Bedwetting: A treatment manual for professional staff.* London: Chapman & Hall.

Bollard, J., & Nettelbeck, T. (1981). A comparison of Dry-Bed Training and standard unine-alarm conditioning treatment of childhood bedwetting. *Behaviour Research and Therapy, 19*, 215–226.

Bollard, J., & Nettelbeck, T. (1982). A component analysis of Dry-Bed Training for treatment of bedwetting. *Behaviour Research and therapy, 20*, 383–390.

Bollard, J., Nettelbeck, T., & Roxbee, L. (1982). Dry-Bed Training for childhood bedwetting: A comparison of group with individually administered parent instruction. *Behaviour Research and Therapy, 20*, 209–217.

Bollard, J., Nettelbeck, T., & Saies, J. M. (1984). *An analysis of the association between arousal from sleep and nocturnal enuresis.* Unpublished raw data.

Bollard, J., & Woodroffe, P. (1977). The effect of parent-administered Dry-Bed Training on nocturnal enuresis in children. *Behaviour Research and Therapy, 15*, 159–165.

Borrie, P., & Fenton, J. C. B. (1966). Buzzer ulcers. *British Medical Journal, 2*, 151–152.

Bostock, J. (1958). Exterior gestation, primitive sleep, enuresis and asthma: A study in aetiology. *Medical Journal of Australia, 149*, 185.
Bostock, J. (1962). The deep sleep-enuresis syndrome. *Medical Journal of Australia, 49*, 240–243.
Boyd, M. M. (1960). The depth of sleep in enuretic school children and in nonenuretic controls. *Journal of Psychosomatic Research, 4*, 274.
Broughton, R. F. (1968). Sleep disorders: Disorders of arousal? *Science, 159*, 1070–1078.
Caceres, J. (1982). Corticol control or social reinforcmeent? *The Behaviour Therapist, 5*, 65–67.
Campbell, E. W., & Young, J. D. (1966). Enuresis and its relation to electroencephalographic disturbances. *Journal of Urology, 96*, 947.
Campbell, M. F. (1934). A clinical study of persistent enursis. *New York State Journal of Medicine, 34*, 190.
Campbell, M. F. (1970). Neuromuscular uropathy. In M. F. Campbell & J. H. Harrison (Eds.), *Urology* (Vol. 2, pp. 1935–1948). Philadelphia: Saunders.
Church, R. M., & Solomon, R. L. (1956). Traumatic avoidance learning: The effects of delay and shock termination. *Psychological Reports, 2*, 317–326.
Collins, R. W. (1973). Importance of the bladder—cue buzzer contingency in the conditioning treatment of enuresis. *Journal of Abnormal Psychology, 82*, 299–308.
Coote, M.A. (1965). Apparatus for conditioning treatment of enuresis. *Behaviour Research and Therapy, 2*, 233–238,
Creer, T. L., & Davis, M. H. (1975). Using a staggered waking procedure with enuretic children in an institutional setting. *Journal of Behavior Therapy and Experimental Psychiatry, 6*, 23–25.
Crosby, N. D. (1950). Essential enuresis: Successful treatment based on psychological concepts. *Medical Journal of Australia, 2*, 533–543.
De Jonge, G. A. (1969). *Kinderen met enuresis een epidemiologische klinisch onderzoek*. Assen: Van Gorcum.
De Jonge, G. A. (1973). Epidemiology of enuresis: A survey of the literature. In I. Kolvin, R. C. MacKeither, & S. R. Meadow (Eds.), *Bladder control and enuresis* (pp. 39–46). Philadelphia: Lippincott.
De Leon, G., & Mandell, W. (1966). A comparison of conditioning and psychotherapy in the treatment of functional enuresis. *Journal of Clinical Psychology, 22*, 326–330.
Dement, W., & Kleitman, N. (1957). Cyclic variations in EEG during sleep and their relation to eye movements, body mobility and dreaming. *Electroencephalography and Clinical Neurophysiology, 9*, 673.
De Perri, R., & Meduri, M. (1972). L'enuresi notturna: Ulteriori elementi in tema di diagnostica strumentale. *Acta Neuroligica Napoli, 27*, 22–27.
Dische, S. (1971). Management of enuresis. *British Medical Journal, 2*, 33–36.
Dische, S. (1973). Treatment of enuresis with an enuresis alarm. In I. Kolvin, R. C. MacKeith, & S. R. Meadow (Eds.), *Bladder control and enuresis* (pp. 211–230). Philadelphia: Lippincott.

Dische, S., Yule, W., Corbett, J., & Hand, D. (1983). Childhood nocturnal enuresis: Factors associated with outcome of treatment with an enuresis alarm. *Developmental Medicine and Child Neurology, 25*, 67–80.

Doleys, D. M. (1977). Behavioral treatments for nocturnal enuresis in children: A review of the recent literature. *Psychological Bulletin, 84*, 30–54.

Doleys, D. M., Ciminero, A. R., Tollison, J. W., Williams, C. L., & Wells, K. C. (1977). Dry-Bed training and retention control training—a comparison. *Behavior Therapy, 8*, 541–548.

Doleys, D. M., & Wells, K. C. (1975). Changes in functional bladder capacity and bedwetting during and after retention control training: A case study. *Behavior Therapy, 6*, 685–688.

Douglas, J. W. B. (1973). Early disturbing events and later enuresis. In I. Kolvin, R. C. MacKeith, & S. R. Meadow (Eds.), *Bladder control and enuresis* (pp. 109–117). Philadelphia: Lippincott.

Douglas, J. W. B., & Blomfield, J. M. (1958). *Children under five*. London: Allen & Unwin.

Esperanca, M. D., & Gerrard, J. W. (1969). Nocturnal enuresis: Studies in bladder function in normal children and enuretics. *Canadian Medical Association Journal, 101*, 324–327.

Essen, J., & Peckham, C. (1976). Nocturnal enuresis in childhood. *Developmental Medicine and Child Neurology, 18*, 577–589.

Evans, J. I. (1971). Sleep of enuretics. *British Medical Journal, 3*, 110.

Fielding, D. (1980). The response of day and night wetting children and children who wet only at night to retention control training and the enuresis alarm. *Behaviour Research and Therapy, 18*, 305–317.

Fielding D. (1982). An analysis of the behaviour of day and night wetting children: Towards a model of micturition control. *Behaviour Research and Therapy, 20*, 49–60.

Finley, W. W. (1971). An EEG study of the sleep of enuretics at three age levels. *Clinical Electroencephalography, 2*, 35–39.

Finley, W. W., Rainwater, A. J., & Johnson, G. (1982). Effect of varying alarm schedules on acquisition and relapse parameters in the conditioning treatment of enuresis. *Behaviour Research and Therapy, 20*, 69–80.

Finley, W.W., Wansley, R. A., & Blenkarn, M. M. (1977). Conditioning treatment of enuresis using a 70% intermittent reinforcement schedule. *Behaviour Research and Therapy, 15*, 419–427.

Forsythe, W. I., & Redman, A. (1974). Enuresis and spontaneous cure rate. *Archives of Disease in childhood, 49*, 259–263.

Foxx, R. M., & Azrin, N. H. (1973a). *Toilet training the retarded: A rapid program for day and nighttime independent toileting*. Champaign, IL: Research Press.

Foxx, R. M., & Azrin, N. H. (1973b). Dry pants: A rapid method of toilet training children. *Behaviour Research and Therapy, 11*, 435–442.

Gastaut, H., Batini, C., Broughton, R., Fressey, J., & Tassinari, C. A. (1964). Etude electrographique des manifestations paroxystiques, non-épileptiques, au cours du sommeil nocturne. *Review Neurologique, 110*, 309–310.

Gillin, J. C., Rapoport, J. L., Mikkelsen, E. J., Langer, D., Vanskiver, C., & Medelson, W. (1982). EEG sleep patterns in enuresis: A further analysis and comparison with normal controls. *Biological Psychiatry, 17*, 947–953.

Goel, K. M., & Shanks, R. A. (1974). Amitriptyline and imipramine poisoning in children. *British Medical Journal, 1*, 261–263.

Graham, P. (1973). Depth of sleep and enuresis: A critical review. In I. Kolvin, R. C. MacKeith, & S. R. Meadow (Eds.), *Bladder control and enuresis* (pp. 78–83). Philadelphia: Lippincott.

Greaves, M. W. (1969). Hazards of enuresis alarm. *Archives of Disease in Children, 44*, 285–286.

Griffiths, P., Meldrum, C., & McWilliam, R. (1982). Dry-Bed training in the treatment of nocturnalenuresis in childhood: A research report. *Journal of Child Psychology and Psychiatry, 23*, 485–495.

Gunnarson, S., & Melin, K. A. (1951). The electro-encephalgram in enuresis. *Acta Paediatrica, 40*, 496–501.

Guyton, A. C. (1966). *Textbook of medical physiology*. Philadelphia: Saunders.

Hallgren, B. (1956). Enuresis: 1. A study with reference to the morbidity and symptomatology. *Acta Psychiatrica et Neurologica Scandinavica, 31*, 379–436.

Hallgren, B. (1957). Enuresis: A clinical and genetic study. *Acta Psychiatrica et Neurologica Scandanavica, 32* (Suppl. 114), 1–159.

Hallman, N. (1950). On the ability of enuretic children to hold urine. *Acta Paediatrica, 39*, 87–93.

Harris, L. S., & Purohit, A. P. (1977). Bladder training and enuresis: A controlled trial. *Behaviour Research and Therapy, 15*, 485–490.

Hawkins, D. N. (1962). Enuresis: A survey. *The Medical Journal of Australia, 1*, 979–980.

Illingworth, R. S. (1968). *The normal child* (4th ed.). London: Churchill.

Johnstone, J. (1972). Cystometry and evaluation of anticholinergic drugs in enuretic children. *Journal of Pediatric Surgery, 7*, 18–20.

Jureidini, K. (1982, December). Enuresis: Helping the patients and parents. *Patient Management*, pp. 25–28.

Kaffman, M., & Elizur, E. (1977). Infants who become enuretics. A longitudinal study of 161 Kubbutz children. *Monographs of the Society for Research in Childhood Development, 42* (2, Serial No. 170).

Kales, A., Kales, J. D., Jacobson, A., Humphrey II, F. J., & Soldatos, C. R. (1977). Effects of imipramine on enuretic frequency and sleep stages. *Pediatrics, 60*, 431–436.

Keating, J. C., Butz, R. A., Burke, E., & Heimberg, R. G. (1983). Dry Bed training without a urine alarm: Lack of effect of setting and therapist contact with child. *Journal of Behavior Therapy and Experimental Psychiatry, 14*, 109–115.

Kolvin, I., & Taunch, J. (1973). A dual theory of nocturnal enuresis. In I. Kolvin, R. C. MacKeith, & S. R. Meadow (Eds.), *Bladder control and enuresis* (pp. 156–172). Philadelphia: Lippincott.

Kolvin, I., Taunch, J., Currah, J., Garside, R. F., Nolan J., & Shaw, W. B. (1972). Enuresis: A descriptive analysis and a controlled trial. *Developmental Medicine and Child Neurology, 14.* 715.

Levine, A. (1943). Enuresis in the navy. *American Journal of Psychiatry, 100,* 320.

Lickorish, J. R. (1964). One hundred enuretics. *Journal of Psychosomatic Research, 7,* 263.

Lovibond, S. H. (1963a). The mechanism of conditioning treatment of enuresis. *Behaviour Research and Therapy, 1,* 17–24.

Lovibond, S. H. (1963b). Intermittent reinforcement in behaviour therapy. *Behaviour Research and Therapy, 1,* 127–132.

Lovibond, S. H. (1964). *Conditioning and enuresis.* Oxford: Pergamon Press.

Lovibond, S. H., & Coote, M. A. (1970). Enuresis. In C. G. Costello (Ed.), *Symptoms of psychopathology* (pp. 373–396). New York: Wiley.

MacFarlane, J. W., Allen, L., & Honzik, M. P. (1954). *A developmental study of the behavior problems of normal children between 21 months and 14 years.* Berkeley: University of California Press.

Martin, C. R. A. (1966). *A new approach to nocturnal enuresis.* London: H. K. Lewis.

McGee, R., Mackinson, T., Williams, S., Simpson, A., & Silva, P. A. (1984). A longitudinal study of enuresis from five to nine years. *Australian Paediatric Journal, 20,* 39–42.

McKendry, J. B. J., & Stewart, D. A. (1974). Enuresis. *Pediatric Clinics of North America, 21,* 1019–1028.

Meadow, S. R. (1970). Childhood enuresis. *British Medical Journal, 4,* 787–789.

Meadow, S. R. (1974). Drugs for bedwetting. *Archives of Disease in Childhood, 49,* 257–258.

Meadow, S. R. (1981). *Help for bed wetting.* Edinburgh: Churchill Livingstone.

Mikkelsen, E. J., Rapoport, J. L., Neel, L., Gruenau, C., Mendelson, W., & Gillin, J. C. (1980). Childhood Enuresis 1. Sleep patterns and psychopathology. *Archives of General Psychiatry, 37,* 1139–1144.

Miller, F. J. W. (1973). Children who wet the bed. In I. Kolvin, R. C. MacKeith, & S. R. Meadow (Eds.), *Bladder control and enuresis* (pp. 47–52). Philadelphia: Lippincott.

Miller, F. J. W., Court, S. D. M., Walton, W. S., & Knox, G. G. (1960). *Growing up in Newcastle-upon-Tyne.* Oxford: Oxford University Press.

Miller, P. M. (1973). An experimental analysis of retention control training in the treatment of nocturnal enuresis in two institutionalized adolescents. *Behavior Therapy, 4,* 288–294.

Morgan, J. J. B., & Witmer, F. J. (1939). The treatment of enuresis by the conditioned reaction technique. *Journal of Genetic Psychology, 55,* 59–65.

Morgan, R. T. T. (1978). Relapse and therapeutic response in the conditioning treatment of enuresis: A review of recent findings on intermittent reinforcement, overlearning and stimulus intensity. *Behaviour Research and Therapy, 16,* 273–279.

Mowrer, O. H. (1950). *Learning theory and behaviour.* New York: Wiley.

Mowrer, O. H., & Mowrer, W. M. (1938). Enuresis: A method for its study and treatment. *American Journal of Orthopsychiatry, 8*, 436–459.

Muellner, S. R (1960a). Development of urinary control in children. *Journal of the American Medical Association, 172*, 1256–1261.

Muellner, S. R. (1960b). Development of urinary control in children. A new concept in cause, prevention and treatment of primary enuresis. *Journal of Urology, 84*, 714–716.

Neal, B. W., & Coote, M. A. (1969). Hazards of enuresis alarm. *Archives of Disease of Children, 44*, 651.

Neligan, G. A., Kolvin, I., Scott, D. Mc., & Garside, R. F. (1976). *Born too soon or born too small* (Clinics in Developmental Medicine No. 61). London: Heinemann/S.I.M.P.

Nettelbeck, T., & Langeluddecke, P. (1979). Dry-Bed training without an enuresis machine. *Behaviour Research and Therapy, 17*, 403–404.

Notschaele, L.A. (1964). Bedwaterne by kinderen van de kleuter—en lagere school. *Tijdschrift voor Sociale Geneeskunde, 42*, 226.

Novick, J. (1966). Symptomatic treatment of acquired and persistent enuresis. *Journal of Abnormal Psychology 77*, 363–368.

Oppel, W. C., Harper, P. A., & Rider, R. V. (1968). The age of attaining bladder control. *Pediatrics, 42*, 614.

Oswald, I., Taylor, A. M., & Treisman, M. (1960). Discriminative responses to stimulation during human sleep. *Brain, 83*, 440–453.

Paschalis, A. P., Kimmel, H. D., & Kimmel, E. (1972). Further study of diurnal instrumental conditioning in the treatment of enuresis nocturna. *Journal of Behavior Therapy and Experimental Psychiatry, 3*, 253–256.

Pfaundler, M. (1904). Demonstration eines apparatus zur selstätigen stattgehabter Bettnäsung. *Verhandlungen der Gesellschaft für Kinderheilkunde, 21*, 219.

Pfeiffer, D. G., & Lloyd, D. T. (1978, September/October). Enuresis alarm innovations. *Monitor-Proceedings of the I.R.E.E., Australia*, pp. 148–150.

Pierce, C. M., Whitman, R. M., Mass, J. W., & Gay, M. L. (1961). Enuresis and dreaming. *Archives of General psychiatry, 4*, 166.

Rentfrow, R. K., & Rentfrow, D. K. (1969). Studies related to toilet training of the mentally retarded. *American Journal of Occupational Therapy, 23*, 425–430.

Ritvo, E. R., Ornitz, E. M., Gottlieb, F., Poussaint, H. F., Maron, B. J., Ditmon, K. S., & Blinn, K. A. (1969). Arousal and non-arousal enuretic events. *American Journal of Psychiatry, 126*, 77–84.

Rocklin, N., & Tilker, H. (1973). Instrumental conditioning of nocturnal enuresis: A reappraisal of some previous findings. *Proceedings of the 81st Annual Convention of the American Psychological Association, 8*, 915–916.

Rutter, M., Yule, W., & Graham, P. (1973). Enuresis and behavioral deviance: Some epidemilogical considerations. In I. Kolvin, R. C. MacKeith, & S. R. Meadow (Eds.), *Bladder control and enuresis* (pp. 137–150). Philadelphia: Lippincott.

Sacks, S., & De Leon, G. (1973). Conditioning two types of enuretics. *Behaviour Research and Therapy, 11*, 653–654.
Sacks, S., & De Leon, G. (1978). Training the disturbed enuretic. *Behaviour Research and Therapy, 16*, 296–299.
Sacks, S., & De Leon, G. (1983). Conditioning functional enuresis: Follow-up after retraining. *Behaviour Research and Therapy, 21*, 693–694.
Sacks, S., De Leon, G., & Blackman, S. (1974). psychological changes associated with conditioning functional enuresis. *Journal of Clinical Psychology, 30*, 271–276.
Salmon, M. A., Taylor, D. C., & Douglas, L. (1973). On the EEG and enuresis. In I. Kolvin, R. C. MacKeith, & S. R. Meadow (Eds.), *Bladder control and enuresis* (pp. 189–194). Philadelphia: Lippincott.
Shaffer, D. (1973). The association between enuresis and emotional disorder: A review of the literature. In I. Kolvin, R. C. MacKeith, & S. R. Meadow (Eds.), *Bladder control and enuresis* (pp. 118–136). Philadelphia: Lippincott.
Shaffer, D. (1980). The development of bladder control. In M. Rutter (Ed.), *Scientific foundations of developmental psychiatry* (pp. 129–137). London: William Heinemann.
Shaffer, D., Costello, A. J., & Hill, I. D. (1968). Control of enuresis with imipramine. *Archives of Disease in Childhood, 43*, 665–671.
Smith, L. J. (1981). Training severely and profoundly mentally handicapped nocturnal enuretics. *Behaviour Research and Therapy, 19*, 67–74.
Smith, S. (1948). *The psychological origin and treatment of enuresis*. Seattle: University of Washington Press.
Starfield, B. (1967). Functional bladder capacity in enuretic and non-enuretic children. *Journal of Pediatrics, 70*, 777–781.
Starfield, B., & Mellits, E. D. (1968). Increase in functional bladder capacity and improvement in enuresis. *Journal of Pediatrics. 74*, 483–487.
Stein, Z. A., & Susser, M. (1967). the social dimensions of a symptom: A sociomedical study of enuresis. *Social Science and Medicine. 1*, 183.
Stewart, M. A. (1975). Treatment of bedwetting. *Journal of the American Medical Association, 232*, 281.
Szabo, L., & Popoviciu, L. (1969). Clinical EEG and polygraphic investigations of sleep in children with simple enuresis or associated with other nonconvulsive nocturnal episodic manifestations. *Electroencephalography and Clinical Neurophysiology, 27*, 635–636.
Taylor, P. D., & Turner, R. K. (1975). A clinical trial of continuous, intermittent and overlearning "bell-and-pad" treatments for nocturnal enuresis. *Behaviour Research and Therapy, 2*, 567–574.
Thompson, I., & Lauvetz, R. (1976). Oxybutynin in bladder spasm, neurogenic bladder, and enuresis. *Urology, 8*, 452–454.
Thorne, F. C. (1944). The incidence of nocturnal enuresis after the age of five years. *American Journal of Psychiatry, 100*, 686.
Troup, C. W., & Hodgson, N. B. (1971). Nocturnal functional bladder capacity in enuretic children. *Pediatric Urology, 105*, 129–132.
Turner, R. K., Young, G. C., & Rachman, S. (1970). Treatment of nocturnal

enuresis by conditioning techniques. *Behaviour Research and Therapy, 8*, 367–381.
Turton, E. C., & Spear, A. R. (1953). EEG findings in 100 cases of severe enuresis. *Archives of Disease in Children, 28*, 316–320.
Wenar, C., & Coulter, J. B. (1962). A reliability study of developmental histories. *Child Development, 33*, 453.
Werner, E., Bierman, J. M., & French, F. (1971). *The children of Kanai. A longitudinal study from the prenatal period to age ten.* Honolulu: University of Hawaii Press.
Werry, J., Dowrick, P., Lampen, E., & Vamos, M. (1975). Imipramine in enuresis - psychological and physiological effects. *Journal of Child Psychology and Psychiatry, 16*, 289–299.
Werry, J. S., & Cohrssen, J. (1965). Enuresis: An etiologic and therapeutic study. *Journal of Pediatrics, 67*, 423–431.
White, M. A. (1968). A thousand consecutive cases of enuresis: Results of treatment. *Medical Officer, 120*, 151–155.
Williams, C. L., Doleys, D. M., & Ciminero, A. R. (1978). A two-year follow-up of enuretic children treated with dry-bed training. *Journal of Behavior Therapy and Experimental Psychiatry, 9*, 285–286.
Yates, A. J. (1970). *Behavior therapy.* New York: Wiley.
Young G. C. (1964). A "staggered-awakening" procedure in the treatment of enureis. *Medical Officer, 111*, 142–143.
Young, G. C. (1965). The aetiology of enuresis in terms of learning theory. *Medical Officer, 113*, 19–22.
Young, G. C., & Morgan, R. T. T. (1972). Childhood enuresis: termination of treatment by parents. *Community Medicine, 129*, 247–250.
Young, G. C., & Morgan, R. T. T. (1973). Analysis of factors associated with the extinction of a conditioned response. *Behaviour Research and Therapy, 11*, 219–222.
Young, G. C., & Turner, R. K. (1965). CNS stimulant drugs and conditioning of nocturnal enuresis. *Behaviour Research and Therapy, 3*, 93–101.
Zaleski, A., Gerrard, J. W., & Shokeier, M. H. K. (1973). Nocturnal enuresis: The importance of a small bladder capacity. In I. Kolvin, R. C. MacKeith, & S. R. Meadows (Eds.), *Bladder control and enuresis* (pp. 95–101). Philadelphia: Lippincott.
Zung, W. W. K., & Wilson, W. P. (1961). Response to auditory stimulation during sleep. *Archives of General Psychiatry, 4*, 548–552.

IV

BEHAVIORAL PEDIATRICS

8

Psychological Contributions to Primary Pediatric Health Care

Mary L. Kelley
Louisiana State University Medical Center

Ronald S. Drabman
University of Mississippi Medical Center

The interfacing of psychological and pediatric health care providers has increased dramatically during the past 20 years. In part, this growth in collaborative management of children has occurred as a result of changes in pediatric practices. the development of vaccinations and antibiotics, which virtually eliminated or quickly treated many childhood illnesses, allowed pediatricians to redirect their efforts toward the early detection, treatment, and prevention of developmental and behavioral problems (Richmond, 1985; Russo & Varni, 1982).

Pediatricians and other child health care providers are called upon very frequently to address parental concerns about children's behavior and development and to offer advice for the treatment or prevention of minor behavior problems such as sleeping or feeding difficulties (Christophersen, 1983a). In fact, approximately 50 percent of pediatricians' time is spent providing well child care (Reisinger & Bires, 1980). Likewise, in a study authorized by the American Academy of Pediatrics (1978), pediatricians indicated that parents' requests for assistance with school problems and behavioral counseling were two of the greatest areas of change in pediatric practice during the previous five years. An additional point of emphasis in current pediatric practices is the early detection and treatment of development delays (Richmond, 1985).

The American Academy of Pediatrics has placed increasing emphasis on pediatricians' responsibility to promote children's optimal social and cognitive development (MacPhee, 1984). Survey results, however, indicate that a clear majority of pediatricians view their training in child development and behavioral problems as inadequate (Task Force on Pediatric Education, 1978; as cited in Christophersen, Barrish, Barrish, & Christophersen, 1984). In fact, another study found that although pediatricians detected 78 percent of mothers' concerns about their children's physical functioning, they recognized only 41 percent of parental concerns about behavior (Starfield & Barkowf, 1969). Pediatricians' failure to recognize children's behavior problems may be explained, in part, by deficiencies in their training. For example, they may avoid inquiring about children's developmental and behavioral status because they lack answers to many parental concerns (Christophersen, 1983a).

One outgrowth of the changing demands of pediatric care has been the collaboration of psychologists and pediatricians in promoting children's optimal functioning. Numerous authors have discussed the role of psychologists working with pediatricians in both inpatient and outpatient settings and have attested to the benefits of these collaborative efforts (Drotar, 1982, 1985; Freidman, 1985). During the past 20 years (as illustrated in other chapters in this book) researchers have documented with increasing frequency the influence of psychological and environmental variables on the development, maintenance, and treatment of many physical disorders. Although the emphasis has been on the assessment, treatment, and prevention of chronic illnesses and other physical disorders, a growing number of psychologists have become involved in improving primary pediatric care. In fact, Christophersen (1983a) has suggested that if pediatricians are to incorporate much of behavioral psychology into their practices, efforts should be directed toward problems encountered in well child care or primary pediatric settings.

DEFINITION AND SCOPE OF BEHAVIORAL PEDIATRICS

Numerous labels have been applied to psychologists working in non-psychiatric, pediatric settings. The first such term, pediatric psychologist, was coined by Wright in 1967 (as cited in Mesibov, 1983). Since that time, the field of pediatric psychology has been referred to as behavioral pediatrics, pediatric behavioral medicine, and child health care psychology (La Greca & Stone, 1985; Hobbs, Beck, & Wansley, 1984; Russo & Varni, 1982). Each term connotes a different point of emphasis. The more commonly used term, behavioral pediatrics, has its root in pediatric medicine and now is used to describe an array of activities performed by individuals from many disciplines (Russo & Varni, 1982; Varni & Dietrich, 1981). These authors suggest that the field of behavioral pediatrics is interdisciplinary, empirically based, concerned with illness *and* child management, and oriented to treatment and prevention. Based on these considerations, Varni and Dietrich (1981) defined behavioral pediatrics as:

> Represent[ing] the interdisciplinary integration between biobehavioral science and pediatric medicine with emphasis on multidimensional and comprehensive diagnosis, prevention, treatment, and rehabilitation of physical disease and disabilities in children and adolescents. (p. 5)

The definition and conceptualization of behavioral pediatrics put forth by Varni and his colleagues is, in our opinion, preferred over other definitions. The definition does not limit the scope of the field to those activities performed by only a single specialty or orientation as does the term pediatric psychology (Varni, 1983). A multidisciplinary approach will increase the likelihood that assessment and treatment are comprehensive and accurate. Furthermore, the definition is adequately broad to include activities that deal with well child care and prevention.

Although the scope of behavioral pediatrics is broad, the psychological research in the area has focused on the assessment and treatment of illness and health-related behavior. With the exception of Christophersen and his colleagues, relatively few contributions have been designed to improve well child care. Given the extent to which pediatricians and other health care providers are engaged in well child care (e.g., Christophersen, 1982, 1983b; Christophersen & Rapoff, 1980), the paucity of research is perplexing. Furthermore, psychological contributions to primary pediatric care might facilitate the prevention of behavior disorders in children in a cost-effective manner. For example, pediatricians properly trained in the use of behavior management procedures could provide parents with information on effective methods of disciplining their children.

The remainder of this chapter focuses on the potential benefits that behavioral pediatrics could have (and to a certain extent has had) on primary pediatric care. Specifically, the emphasis is on discussing psychological contributions to the prevention, early detection, and treatment of behavior and developmental problems by pediatricians. Each section emphasizes the psychologist's role in training and collaborating with pediatricians. The role of behavioral pediatrics in the treatment of chronic illnesses, pain, or terminal illnesses is not emphasized as this topic is discussed elsewhere in this book. Prior to discussing well child care, however, the relevance of behavior analysis to pediatrics will be discussed. This conceptual framework is considered fundamental to behavioral pediatrics in general and well child care in particular and, thus, worthy of separate emphasis and discussion.

RELEVANCE OF BEHAVIOR ANALYSIS TO PEDIATRICS

Several authors have discussed the use of behavioral assessment strategies in understanding the complex interplay of biological and psychological variables (Redd & Rusch, 1985; Schwartz, Tapp, & Brucker, 1985). In doing so, however, some authors have presented behavioral assessment as a separate, albeit interactive, diagnostic tool that accompanies traditional, medical approaches (e.g., Williams, Foreyt, & Goodrick, 1981). Models that emphasize the relatively independent and different approaches to assessment used by physicians and psychologists are useful to understanding the medical field. However, such models often do not emphasize an overall theoretical approach that serves to integrate data from multiple sources.

An alternative approach is to view behavior analysis as a theoretical perspective that can incorporate both biological and psychological variables (Redd & Rusch, 1985). It is our bias that the behavior analytic model of assessment is a useful heuristic which can guide the assessment of psychological and biological variables relevant to the maintenance of illness and related behavior problems. Figure 8.1 illustrates our conceptualization of this model taking into account biological variables. The underlying assumption of the model is that the purpose of assessment is to understand and predict behavior in ways that lead to behavior change (Witt & Cavell, 1986). Similar models

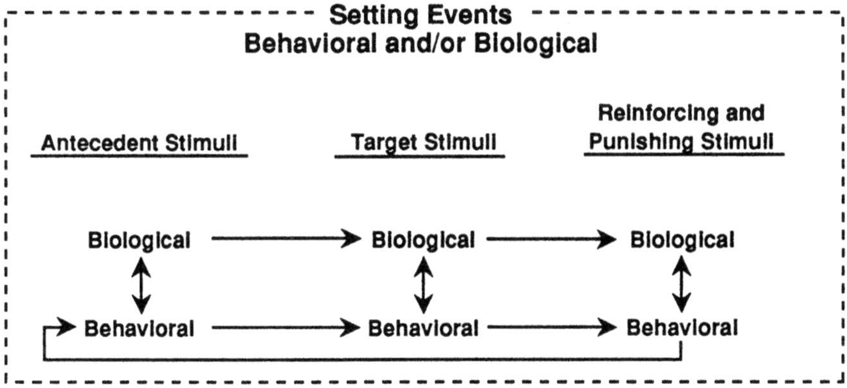

FIGURE 8.1. Behavioral Analytic Model.

have been proposed elsewhere (Bijou & Baer, 1978; Redd & Rusch, 1985; Schwartz et al., 1985)

As shown in Figure 8.1., biological, behavioral (covert and overt), and environmental variables may serve as antecedents to disease, illness, or behavior problems associated with illness. Antecedent variables can be immediate or temporally distant, in which case they are termed setting events (Bijou & Baer, 1978). In many instances, the presence of disease, infection, or trauma might be considered a setting event which is functionally related to subsequent stimulus-response interactions. Figure 8.1 indicates that biological, behavioral, and environmental variables may all function to maintain illness or behavior disturbance. Such a model is idiographic; the degree to which biological and behavioral variables occasion or maintain illness related behavior may vary substantially across individuals with similar illnesses or across illnesses. Of course, this model is familiar to most readers. The utility of the model, however, often does not receive appropriate emphasis when dealing with medical problems.

The application of behavior analysis to pediatric problems might best be understood and appreciated through an illustration. For example, a relatively serious pediatric problem during infancy is failure to thrive (Bithony & Rathbun, 1983). The condition is defined in terms of the infant's failure to gain weight in an appropriate manner. Traditionally, the literature has distinguished organic from nonorganic failure to thrive with the former being diagnosed when failure to gain weight can be attributed to a physical disorder (Roberts & Maddux, 1982). Recently, however, researchers have suggested that a simple dichotomy of failure to thrive is inadequate and have added a third category referred to as "mixed" which represents cases of failure to thrive in which both organic and nonorganic factors appear to influence weight gain (Homer & Ludwig, 1981).

Applying the behavior analytic model to the assessment of failure to thrive makes categorizing these infants unnecessary. Instead, the model suggests any number of variables may be affecting lack of weight gain and that specification of these variables will lead directly to treatment. For example when a biological condition exists which interferes with feeding, aversive parent–child interactions are commonly seen. Thus, one could conceptualize the physical problems as setting events that effect subsequent parent–child interactions. The functional analysis of dyadic interactions may reveal a coercive process characterized by forced and ineffective feeding behavior by the mother as well as aversive child behavior which function to terminate the interaction. Correction of physical problems may or may not be adequate to produce more positive, effective feeding interactions between parent and child. Of course, many other variables also may be associated with the child's failure to gain weight. (See Redd & Rusch 1985, for a more detailed case example of the application of behavior analysis to behavioral-biological problems.)

Many disadvantages exist for conceptualizing pediatric problems from a behavior analytic perspective. The model is idiographic and emphasizes functional relationships and therefore facilitates individualization of treatment regimens. The approach also provides an overall theoretical perspective that better approximates the complex interactions between biological, behavioral, and environmental variables (Schwartz et al., 1985). Finally, use of behavior analysis to conceptualize patients' problems represents a dynamic rather than static approach to problem solving. This is in contrast to the more rule-governed approaches to assessment and treatment that typify traditional medicine. For example, on more than one occasion pediatric residents or faculty have pressed us to determine whether a patient's symptoms were due to psychological or physical factors. Their inquiries, sometimes born out of frustration in managing difficult cases, appeared to reflect a dualistic, mind–body perspective of health. Occasionally, their inquiries involved the hidden agenda of finding *the* specialist responsible for treatment. On one such occasion, a 9-year-old asthmatic displayed symptoms that appeared resistant to medical intervention. Psychology was asked to determine whether his symptoms were induced by psychological factors. In discussing the case, it was emphasized that the question could not be answered in a categorical fashion. It also was stressed that the variables maintaining disease or illness behavior often change over time and that many factors could be maintaining the child's symptoms. Thus, assessment and treatment should take place in a collaborative, systematic fashion.

The utility of behavioral analytic strategies to improving well child care is unquestionable (Christophersen & Rapoff, 1979; Christophersen, 1983a). Given the frequency with which pediatricians encounter problems related to such behaviors as toileting and eating, their ability to functionally analyze the contingencies maintaining problem behavior could facilitate their delivery of appropriate recommendations.

Unfortunately, training in applied behavior analysis typically is provided in only a cursory fashion in many residency programs (Mastria & Drabman, 1979). Furthermore, with the availability of psychologists and other health-related personnel in training hospitals, pediatric residents may rely heavily on individuals other than themselves to deal with parents' concerns about children's behavior. A common complaint of pediatric residents has been that outpatient caseloads are so heavy they do not have time to address patients' behavioral concerns. Although this may be true, until pediatricians are trained and required to recognize behavior and developmental problems and to provide behavioral counseling when appropriate, they are unlikely to fully appreciate the importance of their responsibility to promoting children's social and cognitive development. The availability of behavior therapists to pediatric residents in training hospitals may, in some instances, actually diminish the likelihood they will acquire and use skills for preventing, detecting, or treating minor behavior problems once they finish their residency. For example, some cases may be referred to psychologists that could be treated by a pediatrician. However, as the following sections indicate, these problems may represent exceptions rather than normative behavior.

HEALTH EDUCATION AND PREVENTION

Finney and Christophersen (1984) argue that pediatric health education entails "strategies designed to inform parents about ways in which they can improve and protect their children's health and to motivate them to change to healthier practices." Moreover, it was recommended that children become involved in the educational process at the earliest appropriate age (Finney & Christophersen, 1984). Pediatricians and other health care professionals (including psychologists) are in a unique position to educate parents and thereby reduce health risks. In Finney and Christophersen's review of educational efforts within pediatrics, the authors target five areas for education relevant to behavioral pediatrics: accident prevention, behavior problems, child development, nutrition, and medical adherence. The following sections discuss several topics relevant to parent, child, and adolescent health education that have been emphasized in the pediatric literature as important to optimal well child care.

Accident and trauma prevention. Accidents are the most frequent cause of death in children and adolescents. Frequent causes of accidental deaths in preschoolers and young children have included automobile accidents, poisoning, burns, and drowning (Finney & Christophersen, 1984). With regard to automobile accidents, use of car seat restraints is considered an important method of reducing injury to children. However, pediatricians' attempts to increase parents' use of car seats via educational efforts have only been moderately effective (Bergman, 1982). Christophersen and Gyulay (1981) recommend shifting the focus of educational efforts away from the dangers of *not* using a car seat to a positive approach which emphasizes that improved child behavior through car seat use may produce more effective outcomes. This positive educational approach was effective in increasing car seat use over a 12-month period which, in turn, resulted in marked decreases in children's inappropriate behavior while traveling (Christophersen & Gyulay, 1981). The prevention of burns in children is another important target for health education. Efforts in this area have included educating parents during well child care visits regarding the importance of smoke detectors, outlet covers, and the necessity of removing fire hazards such as matches (Bergman, 1982; Finney & Christophersen, 1984). Other researchers have developed programs for teaching children appropriate behavior in the event of a fire (Jones, Kazdin, & Haney, 1981; Rosenbaum, Creedon, & Drabman, 1981).

Child development. A great many interventions have been conducted to provide parents with information on child development and methods of facilitating cognitive and language development (Casey, Bradley, Caldwell, & Edwards, 1986; Finney & Christophersen, 1984). Whether pediatricians routinely provide parents with sufficient information on normal child development is questionable (MacPhee, 1984). Some authors believe that pediatricians' training in child development is inadequate and therefore their ability to provide accurate information to parents is limited (Richmond, 1967). The results of one study contradicted this belief as the authors found that pediatricians did not differ from child developmentalists in their knowledge of normal behavior (MacPhee, 1984). It may be that pediatricians do not routinely provide information on normal development because they believe such discussion is unnecessary, impractical given time constraints, or not their responsibility (MacPhee, 1984; Green, 1985).

There are many potential benefits to informing parents about normal development during well child visits. Information on such topics as the appropriate age to begin toilet training or the course of language development might reduce parents' age-inappropriate demands and stress. Discussing ways to provide stimulating environments, such as methods for enhancing language, may function to facilitate normal development and prevent developmental delays (Finney & Christophersen, 1984; MacPhee, 1984).

A related, yet rarely mentioned, topic to discuss during well child care visits is the impact child rearing can have on marriage, career, and family life. The effect of children's behavior on their parents is often underestimated. For example, marital satisfaction is lowest when couples have very young children (Glenn & Weaver, 1978). As anyone with children can attest, the impact of having children on job performance, leisure time, and finances can be great. It seems that pediatricians are in a unique position to prepare new or expectant parents for the many lifestyle changes that are about to take place. For example, discussing such topics as methods for finding good babysitters or the importance of scheduling parent activities that do not include the child can be helpful in alleviating some of the stresses associated with parenthood.

Parent educational strategies. One approach to providing parents with information on normal child behavior and other health education topics is to provide handouts (Christophersen, 1982, 1983a; Christophersen & Rapoff, 1980). The use of parent handouts that discuss health concerns of children of varying ages can be time-efficient and provide parents with an opportunity to review information presented orally. For example, pediatricians with whom we work routinely distribute educational handouts to parents that are age-specific. These handouts provide parents with nutritional, safety and developmental information specific to their child's age group.

Although bibliotherapy may be a good first step towards improving health education efforts above and beyond oral presentation during well child visits, they are not adequate to ensure compliance (Bergman, 1982). It is quite likely that efforts to improve compliance must be tailored to individual families. It may be beneficial to discuss only those topics that are relevant to the age of the child being seen (Christophersen, 1983a). For example, discussion of poison prevention might best be reserved for parents of children who are about to begin walking. Low-income families are likely to present many obstacles to compliance. For example, simply instructing these parents to place safety locks on their cabinet doors may be insufficient to produce compliance. With these families, it may be necessary to assist the parent in planning how the items will be purchased and installed as well as making purchase of the items available at the facility.

The education of parents can suffer if physicians do not follow through with routine, systematic review of important topics in their well child visits. To help address this problem, Christophersen (1983b) recommends use of flow charts which remind pediatricians of topics to be discussed and activities to be performed during well child visits. The chart is kept in each patient's medical folder and items are checked off when completed. Thus, the physician can quickly see what well care activities have been performed for a given child (Christophersen, 1983b).

Use of a flow chart is likely to remind physicians to discuss important health education topics during their patient visits. As mentioned earlier, however, discussion alone may be insufficient to promote compliance. It may be that physicians' interpersonal skills are directly related to whether parents follow suggestions.

Parent education regarding the health, safety, and development of children is clearly important to prevention of injury, developmental delay, and death (Finney & Christophersen, 1984). It also may serve to facilitate parents' acquisition of appropriate expectations for their children and to reduce family stress (Christophersen, 1986). However, many questions regarding optimal educational strategies are unanswered. For example, it is unclear in what ways socioeconomic and cultural variables mediate parents' responsivity to traditional educational efforts. Although the importance of educating parents about certain topics such as safety is obvious, the outcomes of including other topics such as methods of promoting child development and family satisfaction are less clear. One problems lies in the fact that the topics may be more relevant to certain families than others. It also is unknown what additional topics not mentioned in the literature may be important in promoting family health and adjustment.

Because so many research questions remain unanswered, the incorporation of applied behavior analysis in the practice of health education takes on added significance. The functional analysis of variables that facilitate or impede an individual's compliance with educative suggestions seems essential. For example, imagine a pediatrician instructing a mother to discontinue bottle feedings. If bottle feeding her infant were more reinforcing to the mother than requiring her child to drink from a cup (perhaps due to the ease of bottle feeding), the mother may postpone compliance in order to avoid the aversive consequences of messy and time-consuming feeding. However, discussion of specific procedures for making drinking from a cup less aversive (e.g., allowing bottles at times when it is inconvenient for the parent to supervise drinking) may be much more likely to produce compliance. Being able to adequately assess the contingencies maintaining target responses requires many skills. In addition to a thorough understanding of behavioral principles and procedures, health care personnel must exhibit interviewing skills that encourage parents to provide accurate answers to questions.

Adolescent health education. Compared to efforts to educate parents during well child visits, only minimal discussion and research has been devoted to the education of adolescents by health care personnel. However, the health care needs of adolescents are great given the rapid rise in eating disorders, suicide attempts, and actual suicides, drug and alcohol abuse, and teenage pregnancies (e.g., Cohen, 1984; Eisenberg, 1984). Although the potential role of health care personnel in preventing adolescent health problems has received greater emphasis in recent years, the importance of this role has not yet been fully appreciated. In part, this probably is due to the fact that adolescent medicine is a relatively new emphasis within pediatrics. The following sections discuss three important educational topics for adolescents. The three topics—sex, drugs, and developmental education—are intended to illustrate the role of health care personnel as educators rather than provide an exhaustive account of adolescent health care needs.

Adolescent sex education. Approximately 25 percent of all reported cases of gonorrhea occurred in adolescents aged 15–19 (Cohen, 1984). Cohen estimated that approximately 5,000 girls are absent from school daily due to gonorrhea. Given the preponderance of venereal disease as well as the high and escalating rates of pregnancy and abortions in adolescents (Fielding & Williams, 1991), the importance of sex education is apparent. Additionally, adolescents are at risk for exposure to the AIDS virus (Olson, Huszti, Mason, & Seibert, 1989). However, the actual process can be difficult for both the adolescent and health care provider. For example, adolescents may be very reluctant to discuss their sexual behavior for fear that the content of their disclosures will be revealed to their parents (Resnick, Blum, & Hedin, 1980). The process can be made easier if pediatricians and other health care providers assure confidentiality. Of course, the legal limits of confidentiality must be outlined prior to the discussion (Felice & Friedman, 1982).

Educational efforts should be geared toward assuring that the adolescent accurately understands how pregnancy occurs and is prevented. For example, many sexually active teenagers lack knowledge about reproduction and contraceptives (Fielding & Williams, 1991). Health care personnel should reinforce adolescents' expressed beliefs about self-imposed limitations (Neinstein, 1984; & Shen, 1980). However, discussion of the fact that their beliefs may change and that the health care provided would be available for further discussion in the future may prevent an unwanted pregnancy. For example, in our experience numerous adolescent females have suggested that they believed it was not appropriate to be sexually active at their age. Although we reinforced this view, we emphasized that should they begin to feel differently, we were available.

Drug education. The importance of educating adolescents about the dangers of drug abuse has received increasing emphasis in the pediatric literature (Coupey & Schonberg, 1982; MacDonald, 1986). However, it is not clear whether physicians routinely provide this education to adolescent during office visits. As with sex education, physicians and health care providers are in a unique position to answer questions about drug use and to assist adolescents in generating methods of avoiding drug and alcohol use (MacDonald, 1986; Neinstein, 1984).

Adolescent development. Adolescents are very frequently concerned and distressed about the many changes that take place during puberty. Rapid changes in physical development often are accompanied by increased emphasis on peer evaluation and acceptance as well as a tendency toward self-deprecation. Consequently, many adolescents report being unhappy with aspects of their appearance. This problem is sometimes amplified in late or early maturing teenagers. In fact, poor body image has been shown to be highly correlated with both male and female adolescents' scores on the Beck Depression Inventory (Teri, 1982).

Given the emphasis on appearance evidenced by many adolescents, the potential role of health care personnel in allaying adolescents' fears about the maturational process as well as educating them about their bodies and normal development appears great. For example, a physician may be in a unique position to educate adolescents about skin care and other aspects of body care.

Educational strategies for adolescents. Effectively educating adolescents is likely to be much more difficult than that with parents of young children. In addition, very little research has been conducted on the effectiveness of educational programs as a part of well adolescent care. Several authors have emphasized the importance of scheduling lengthier visits than that typically provided to young children (Felice & Friedman, 1982). Lengthy visits allow for an opportunity to build rapport and to answer adolescents' questions in a less hurried fashion. In addition, it is recommended that adolescents be seen without their parents present so that confidentiality can be assured. Finally, dealing with adolescents' tendency to be noncommunicative should not be dealt with in an impatient manner. Rather, as Felice and Friedman (1982) recommend, healthcare providers are more likely to obtain cooperation from adolescents if they communicate in an empathetic, and supportive manner.

Many questions remain regarding the impact of educational efforts by health care providers on adolescents' behavior. As with parents, it is likely that the physicians' oral representation of information will be inadequate; thus the use of brochures may allow adolescents the opportunity to review the information presented by the pediatrician. For example, pediatricians could routinely provide handouts that discuss methods of refusing alcohol. Older, sexually active adolescents might be given material on the prevention of venereal disease and AIDS. Likewise, brochures that discuss normal development during adolescence may help allay teenagers' fears and concerns about their bodies. It may be that presentation of material to groups of adolescents could facilitate open discussion among peers.

The need for additional research aimed at the development and evaluation of educational interventions for adolescents is evident. Future efforts should be directed toward delineating the health needs of adolescents and developing and evaluating the effects of various educational strategies. For example, additional research is needed on the effects of education about normal development during well care visits on adolescents' satisfaction with their bodies.

Early Detection of Behavior Problems

As discussed earlier in this chapter, parents have many concerns about their children's behavior and routinely seek advice from pediatricians on how to deal with behavior problems. However, many parental concerns about behavior go undetected (Starfield & Barkowf, 1969, as discussed in Christophersen, 1983a). Although responsiveness to parental concerns may have improved since 1969, our experience suggests otherwise. For example, one of the authors recently began asking parents attending well child care visits at a charity hospital to complete a questionnaire that screened for the presence of behavior problems important to them. Approximately 40 percent of the mothers indicated the presence of one or more significant behavior problems. In talking with these mothers, very few of them had brought the problem to the attention of their pediatrician, or, if they had, did not feel that the problem had been satisfactorily addressed. Although not conclusive, these data suggest that the detection of behavior problems by pediatric residents was inadequate despite the frequent and unanimous support of supervising pediatric faculty. Additional support for improving detection of behavior problems by pediatricians comes from the fact that parents are unlikely to bring minor problems to mental health personnel and that it would be impractical if not impossible for qualified professionals to treat the number of individuals in need of such services (Christophersen, 1982).

Prevalence of behavior problems in children. Several studies have been conducted on the types and prevalence of problems parents report experiencing with their young children. For example, Richman, Stevenson, and Graham (1975) reported that 15 percent of a randomly selected population of 3-year-old children exhibited mild and 6 percent exhibited moderate-to-severe behavior problems. In another study more than 20 percent of 2-, 3-, and 4-year-old males and 2-year-old females exhibited high levels of oppositional behavior. Over 20 percent of all 2- and 3-year-old males were viewed as excessively inattentive and demanding of adults (Crowther, Bond, & Rolf, 1981). Although oppositional behavior tends to decrease substantially by the time children are 4 or 5 years old, approximately 33 percent of these children do not show acceptable levels of improved behavior with time (Crowther et al., 1981). This figure is higher for children from lower socioeconomic families. However, which children will and will not improve is difficult to determine and, thus, recognition and treatment of behavior problems in young children may serve to educate parents about effective parenting procedures as well as prevent future problems.

With regard to the types of behavior problems, parents reported that 3-year-old children frequently exhibited night and day wetting, sleeping and eating problems, oppositional behavior, and were excessively active and difficult to manage (Richman et al., 1975). In another study, Kanoy and Shroeder (1985) surveyed parents who had received short-term counseling by psychologists who were a part of a large pediatric private pratice. As a part of this study, the topics of discussion (n = 2008) were rank-ordered. In order, the most common concerns of parents about their children were negative behavior, toileting, personality or emotional problems, school difficulties, sleeping disturbances, developmental delays, sibling/peer problems, divorce/separation, family concerns, and infant management. Differences in parental concerns obtained in Kanoy and Shroeder's (1985) study and Richman et al. (1975) study are likely to be due to sample characteristics in that the former surveyed parents of children from a broader age range than did the latter.

Methods of detecting behavior problems in children. Perhaps the most common method of detecting behavior problems in children is through interviewing their parents. In order for health care personnel to conduct adequate interviews it appears that they must be familiar with problems that are typically encountered by parents and normal child development. For example, approximately 45 percent of all preschool children exhibit some mealtime behavior problems (Bentovin, 1970). They may misbehave during meals, dawdle, or refuse to eat many foods. In order to effectively recognize mealtime problems, pediatricians should be aware of the prevalence of the problem and schedule discussion about the mealtime routine into the well child visit. To aid the interview process, Christophersen (1982) suggests that pediatricians not simply ask parents whether they are having difficulty with their children's behavior, but instead he suggests asking a series of specific questions about commonly occurring problem areas such as bedtime problems, mealtime disturbances, and temper tantrums. For example, Christophersen (1982) recommends that parents be asked questions about bedtime such as: When does the child begin getting ready for and actually go to bed? How often does the child wake up? Where does the child fall asleep and wake up? Similar methods of structuring interviews with parents so that specific information is gathered have been presented elsewhere. Barkley (1990) also recommends a parent interview format that asks specific questions about behavior in 14 settings and methods used to correct problem behavior. The structured interview formats suggested by Christophersen and Barkley are intended to help pinpoint and operationalize specific problem behaviors. In addition, Barkley's format can be used to assist the interviewer in functionally analyzing the contingencies maintaining problem behavior.

Although physicians are likely to detect specific behavior problems through structuring their interview questions along the lines suggested by Christophersen and Barkley, we are not confident that a thorough understanding of the variables maintaining problem behavior is likely to consistently occur if health care personnel are not trained in applied behavior analysis. For example, a situation recently occurred in which a pediatric resident adequately obtained information about the contingencies maintaining overeating in a 20-month-old child. It appeared that, in part, the parent was giving in to the child's tantruming, hitting, biting, and demands for more food and other things. The resident's response was to provide nutritional information and to suggest that the mother hit or bite the child to teach him how it hurts. Although this is a simplistic account of the situation, it does highlight the fact that this resident failed to fully appreciate the contingencies maintaining both the mother's and the child's behavior even when adequate information to do so had been obtained. Furthermore, the resident's response also illustrates the "seat of the pants" approach to addressing parental concerns that is often used by physicians who feel pressured to provide answers.

Another method of detecting behavior problems during well child care is to ask parents to complete a questionnaire (Christophersen, 1982). Two such questionnaires, the Achenbach Child Behavior Checklist (Achenbach & Edelbrock, 1981) and the Eyberg Child Behavior Inventory (Eyberg & Ross, 1978) contain items that emphasize overt behavior and are developmentally normal. The Achenbach Child Behavior Checklist is a 118-item instrument that includes both internalizing and externalizing behavior problems and is intended for use with children age 4–16. The Eyberg Child Behavior Therapy is a 36-item instrument which emphasizes externalizing behavior disturbances. The Eyberg is intended for use with children aged 2–16. Although both instruments are well normed, the language may be too difficult for poorly educated parents.

Although questionnaires can be used to aid in the efficient detection of behavior problems, it is important that health care personnel be trained to understand the psychometric characteristics of the instruments and adhere to the ethical guidelines for test administration. Physicians and other health care personnel tend to be very test-oriented and to view test results as definitive, diagnostic indicators of pathology. Training in the importance of reliability and validity is necessary to pediatricians properly weighing information gained through the use of tests.

Prevalence of behavior problems in adolescents. To many adults, the term adolescence is often synonymous with behavior problems. In contrast to this commonly held belief, behavior problems generally decrease as the child gets older, including through the teenage years (Achenbach & Edelbrock, 1981). Not surprisingly, two problems that show a substantial increase during adolescence are truancy and drug and alcohol abuse (Achenbach & Edelbrock, 1981). In addition, several other problems are quite prevalent during adolescence including anorexia and bulimia, depression, suicidal behavior and actual suicides, and parent-adolescent conflict (Neinstein, 1984). For example, bulimia often begins with the occurrence of weight gain during or following puberty (DuPont, 1984). Estimates of the prevalence of the disorder in high school females have averaged 8 percent with a much lower prevalence rate in males (Johnson, Lewis, Love, Stuckey, & Lewis, 1983). With regard to depression, approximately 10 percent of all adolescents report experiencing significant levels of dysphoria and depressive symtomatology. Suicide represents the third leading cause of death in adolescents; suicide attempts are 10 times more common than actual suicides (Eisenberg, 1984). Thus, although behavior problems generally may occur less frequently as children get older, adolescents often experience very significant problems. Given that many adolescent problems are associated with physical symptomatology (e.g., depression and anorexia) pediatricians may very well be one of the first professionals seen by some disturbed adolescents.

Methods of detecting behavior problems in adolescents. The interview is likely to be the most useful method of obtaining accurate information from adolescents during well care visits. As stated earlier, adequate time for establishing rapport with the client must be provided and confidentiality should be assured. As many adolescents are reticent about disclosing personal information, health care providers must be well trained in interviewing skills. Although it is important to obtain specific information about problem behavior and the contingencies maintaining the behavior, health care providers must also be aware of the physical and behavioral symptoms of specific problems as the adolescent may be secretive and evasive (DuPont, 1984). For example, many bulimic individuals do not readily disclose their problem. However, the physical symptoms include sore throat, swollen glands, and fluctuating weight. Behavioral symptoms of an eating disorder include an intense fear of weight gain, distorted body image, and uncontrolled eating binges coupled with restricted eating at other times (Williamson, Kelley, Cavell, & Prather, 1987). Health care personnel could easily ask questions regarding diet and satisfaction with weight. Adolescents' answers to such questions could provide important clues to the presence of problem eating and facilitate the adolescent answering more direct questions about their eating behavior.

Given the high incidence of suicide attempts and depression in adolescents, the presence of these disorders should always be assessed. Again, indirect strategies such as asking questions about the presence of specific depressive syptomatology may encourage the adolescent to respond accurately.

Physicians should be aware of behavior associated with adolescent drug abuse (e.g., disinterest in school, decline in school grades) and question the adolescent directly about drug use, particularly if associated problems are present (MacDonald, 1986). Physicians are in a unique position to conduct drug screens and to detect drug use in their adolescent patients.

Although the interview is likely to be the primary method used by health care personnel to screen for behavior problems, objective assessment techniques also can be useful. Although few questionnaires are available for adolescents, there is a self-report form of the Achenbach Behavior Checklist for adolescents aged 12–16. Use of the Achenbach Youth Report (Achenbach & Edelbrock, 1983) may be most helpful in detecting minor problems that would be disclosed more readily by adolescents. Another advantage of the Achenbach is the availability of the parent form which would allow for comparison of adolescent and parent responses.

The role of health care providers in detecting behavioral disturbances in adolescents is only beginning to be fully recognized. Likewise, the contributions of psychologists to improving health care providers' ability to detect behavior problems in this population is very small in comparison to those made in well child care. Although the psychological literature has much to offer well adolescent care, the transfer of this information to pediatric settings has not taken place to any large degree. In part this is due to the relatively new emphasis on adolescent health care in pediatrics (Neinstein, 1984).

With the increasing emphasis on the health needs of adolescents, many research and clinical opportunities appear to exist for psychologists and other professionals operating in the field of behavioral pediatrics. For example, very little is known about the effectiveness of health care personnel in detecting behavior problems in adolescents or the best strategies for gathering information during well adolescent visits. What seems very apparent, however, is that the field of behavioral pediatrics potentially has much to offer the adolescent patient.

Treatment of minor behavior problems in children. Many of the problems seen during well child care visits are considered to be within the domain and expertise of pediatricians. For example, many of the common behavior problems exhibited by children that were mentioned earlier (e.g., enuresis and other toileting problems, oppositional behavior in toddlers) are typically addressed by pediatricians during well child care visits (Christophersen, 1982). Pediatricians' familiarity with behavioral procedures for treating common problems may greatly facilitate the early treatment of these problems and thereby prevent future, difficult-to-treat disturbances of behavior. For example, parents of two-year-old children spend much of their time trying to stop misbehavior and to shape new, more appropriate behavior. As anyone who has ever been in a grocery store can attest, parents often do so in an unsystematic and ineffective manner. Pediatricians are in a unique position to routinely provide instruction in timeout, giving appropriate instructions, and shaping appropriate behavior during well child visits.

If pediatricians are to recommend use of behavioral interventions to parents, they must be able to do so in a time-efficient manner. Accordingly, Christophersen (1982) and his colleagues have developed treatment protocols for managing specific, common problems. Although a number of the protocols, such as the one for handling bedtime crying, have been evaluated experimentally, a number of them have not. The following sections discuss two problem areas commonly addressed by pediatricians. The two areas, mealtime problems and oppositional behavior, were chosen to illustrate the procedures recommended by Christophersen and others. A more detailed presentation of the treatment of minor behavior problems by health care providers is presented in Christophersen (1982).

Mealtime problems. Eating and mealtime behavior problems are quite prevalent in young children and are a frequent concern of many parents (Christophersen & Hall, 1978; Hertzler, 1983). Common problems exhibited by children include dawdling, playing with food, food refusal, tantruming, and oppositional behavior (Williamson, Prather, Heffer, & Kelley, 1987). In response to parents' difficulty in managing mealtime behavior, Christophersen and Hall (1978), Christophersen (1982), and Finney (1986) developed several treatment protocols for use by health care professionals during well child care visits. Specific protocols for managing oppositional, unmannerly mealtime behavior, and food refusal were developed for pediatricians as hand outs for parents. For example, Christophersen and Hall (1978) discussed the importance of introducing new food textures (e.g., textured foods) at the appropriate time and to avoid backtracking when a new food is introduced. Christophersen's treatment protocols are based on behavioral principles and reflect common practices in the management of mealtime problems. The recommendations are clear and appear easy to follow. Although many mealtime problems may be easily corrected through the use of treatment protocols, Christophersen emphasizes the need to conduct follow-up consultation to ensure treatment adherence and success. In addition, he suggests that health care personnel assess for the presence of significant family or child problems as use of these protocols in more disturbed families is inappropriate.

In spite of the face validity of the recommendations, the procedures have not been evaluated adequately. Thus, it is not known whether the recommendations are effective or whether alternative procedures would be more effective.

Oppositional behavior. Very frequently, pediatricians are asked by parents to recommend procedures for disciplining children. Likewise parents' most common complaints to mental health care personnel are concerned with their children's oppositional behavior (Atkeson & Forehand, 1981). Fortunately, very effective, thoroughly researched strategies for dealing with noncompliance are available (Forehand & McMahon, 1981). We recommend that pediatricians routinely provide parents with information on these effective child management strategies. For example, Drabman and Jarvie (1977) provided pediatricians with detailed instruction in the use of time out. Likewise, Christophersen (1982) presented a parent handout on time-out procedures for use by pediatricians during well child care visits.

The use of handouts and verbal descriptions of child management procedures by pediatricians is likely to result in improved child behavior. However, many questions regarding the efficacy of health care providers as teachers remain unanswered. For example, few if any studies have evaluated the effects of parent training by health care personnel on children's behavior. In addition, very little has been written on the efficacy of various training strategies. For instance, little is known on whether physician's use of roleplay of the recommended techniques would substantially impact treatment effectiveness.

Problems also exist with using techniques with young, average children that have been evaluated primarily with clinical samples. For example, it typically is recommended that parents avoid providing children with a rationale for compliance when giving instructions (e.g., It is time to get out of the car. It is time to take your bath. You need to finish your dinner now.) It is hypothesized that by lengthening instructions, compliance may be reduced. However, short instructions may not be necessary for normal families. It may even be that eliminating rationales may actually reduce compliance in normal children. In addition, very little is known about the use of time-out with very young children (18 months–two years). However, it is during this time that parents begin to complain about their children's behavior. Perhaps modifications of the typical time out or very short periods of time-out procedures, such as a playpen time out, would be more appropriate for young children. It also may be that alternatives to time out, such as distracting the child from engaging in forbidden activities, would be an effective strategy for parents to use with young children. Thus, many research questions are unanswered regarding the effectiveness and appropriateness of currently recommended child management procedures with young children.

Educational strategies. As emphasized throughout this chapter, pediatricians' ability to functionally analyze the contingencies maintaining problem behavior appears integral to their potential effectiveness as instructors in child management procedures. Although Christophersen (1983) and others (Schmitt, 1985) recommend the use of handouts for dealing with common childhood problems and outline what should be contained in each protocol, pediatricians must be able to determine whether such handouts are appropriate and likely to produce behavior change. To be a good problem solver requires a very thorough understanding of the principles of behavior. Without such an understanding, pediatricians may be unlikely or unable to appropriately modify treatment protocols to fit the specific circumstances of the problem behavior. For example, reward procedures are often effective in decreasing nighttime wetting. Aware that psychologists' initial treatment efforts commonly begin with the use of a star chart and overcorrection procedures, a pediatric resident followed suit and recommended use of the procedures to one of his patients. The procedure failed to work and thus the resident referred the case to the first author's psychology consultative service. Although the resident had concluded that an alternative technique was necessary, in actuality he had failed to use the procedures appropriately. Specifically, he had failed to establish rewards that were available to the child only when he did not wet the bed. With simple modifications, the reward and overcorrection procedure was effective. Thus, in this instance, the resident assumed the procedure was inappropriate when it was not the procedure, but his inability to functionally analyze the situation that produced the failure.

Treatment of behavior problems in adolescents. Very little has been written about the management of adolescents' behavioral disturbances during well care visits. The emphasis in the literature appears to have been on education, particularly in the areas of sex education and contraception. However, there appear to be several areas in which pediatricians and other health care professionals might provide useful information to the management of minor problems exhibited by adolescents. For example, pediatricians could routinely provide adolescents and their parents with information on effective strategies for resolving minor parent-adolescent conflicts. Relatively minor eating problems such as poor nutrition or inappropriate eating habits could be addressed as a part of well adolescent care.

It is recommended that the intervention strategies employed with adolescents require the teenager to manage his or her own behavior, rather than relying primarily on parents as change agents. However, for health care providers to effectively design and monitor self-management interventions for adolescents requires more than a cursory familiarity with the technology—a familiarity often lacking in most training programs.

As with the prevention and detection of behavior problems in adolescents, the treatment of teenagers as a part of their well care has not been fully realized. Future research is needed that addresses the feasibility and effectiveness of behavioral interventions for adolescents as a component of the pediatric care.

REFERRAL AND COLLABORATION

The determination of what type of patients are best referred to psychologists or other mental health professionals has not been adequately addressed. It is unlikely that psychologists could possibly treat all the potential referrals of minor behavior problems (Christophersen, 1982). However, minor problems commonly treated by pediatricians should be referred if significant adult psychopathology exists in either parent, or when several children in the family exhibit behavior problems (Christophersen, 1982). Additionally, cases in which the occurrence of problem behaviors either are frequent, occur across many situations, are enduring, or significantly interfere with the child's functioning probably are best referred to psychologists or other mental health personnel (Phillips, Sarles, & Friedman, 1980). However, given the lack of familiarity many pediatricians have with behavioral assessment and treatment, there may be behavior problems that are not treated as effectively as possible. In addition, it is unclear to what degree pediatricians and other health care providers are able to accurately distinguish mild from more severe problems.

The problem of determining who is best treated by professionals outside of a pediatrician's office appears even less clear for adolescents. Although it is true that adolescents may outgrow many of their problems of moodiness, secrecy, and argumentativeness, these behavior problems may reflect other significant problems such as depression, drug abuse, or intense parent-adolescent conflict. Much more research is needed on the extent to which pediatricians are able to detect significant disturbances of behavior in adolescents and how such recognition might be improved.

Another issue that is perhaps more relevant to the field of behavioral pediatrics is that of pediatricians' collaboration with psychologists and other professionals in the treatment of children and adolescents. For example, there has been an increase in the number of children with Attention Deficit Hyperactivity Disorder (ADHD) referred to psychologists by pediatricians. These cases offer an opportunity to engage in collaborative treatment efforts. Such collaboration can only work, however, if psychologists are aware of the impact of medical, as well as behavioral, treatments for children with ADHD and are willing to empirically evaluate the effects of various treatment modalities on the behavior of the individual child. This requires the increased use of single-case methodology in evaluating treatment outcome and the carefully orchestrated collaboration between professionals. Although many examples of such collegial collaboration exist in the literature, the degree to which psychologists and pediatricians routinely accomplish this task is difficult to determine. Future research is needed that examines the separate and additive impact of psychological and medical treatments on children's functioning.

MODELS OF WELL CHILD CARE SERVICE DELIVERY

The aforementioned discussion advocated incorporating relevant psychological knowledge (e.g., treatment techniques) into day-to-day pediatric practice. The pediatric literature reflects a growing emphasis on the prevention, detection, and management of behavior and developmental problems by pediatricians and auxiliary staff. There are at least three ways in which pediatricians might effectively incorporate psychological procedures into their delivery of well child services. First, as was emphasized in this chapter, pediatricians, along with other health care professionals, could provide these services themselves. To do so would require increased training in the application of behavior analysis and psychological techniques by knowledgeable professionals. Behavioral psychologists appear well suited to provide this training to pediatric residents. A second model for addressing the psychological needs of pediatric patients and their families would be for psychologists to alter their clinical practices to address the types of behavior and developmental problems encountered in primary pediatric care. For example, psychologists, perhaps along with ancillary health care personnel such as nurses, could conduct classes for parents of young children as a part of well child care. Such classes could include discussion of common behavior problems and techniques for preventing or managing these problems. Alternately, psychologists could establish screening procedures within pediatric practices and routinely schedule sessions with parents experiencing problems in managing their children. A third model for addressing the psychological needs of children and adolescents within the context of primary pediatric care is one in which psychologists are housed within pediatricians' offices and are a part of pediatric practices. Examples of this type of collaboration exist, and preliminary evaluations support the efficacy of the approach (Kanoy & Schroeder, 1985; Schroeder, 1979). This service was developed because the pediatricians with whom Schroeder worked believed that time constraints limited their ability to effectively address the psychological needs of patients. Thus, in spite of the growing emphasis in pediatrics on the importance of addressing patients' behavioral and developmental problems, it may simply be that the realities of pediatric practice deem this task inappropriate, unreasonable, or inefficient.

The ways in which psychologists participate in primary pediatric care are diverse and range from indirect consultation through teaching to more interdependent, cooperative service delivery. Irrespective of the manner in which psychological and medical personnel collaborate, it seems apparent that for psychologists to become an integral part of primary pediatric care many changes within the field of psychology must occur (Drotar, 1982). For example, psychologists must become familiar with very short-term delivery of services and the management of minor behavior problems in young children.

SUMMARY

The field of pediatrics has rapidly changed in the last several decades from a field that primarily focused on the treatment of acute illness to one which emphasizes a physician's role in promoting optimal cognitive, social, and physical development (Richmond, 1985). Quite predictably, this change in focus has been accompanied by the development and growth of behavioral pediatrics. This chapter has emphasized the application of behavioral principles to well child and adolescent care. Although many accomplishments have been made, a host of clinical, research, and training issues have not been addressed adequately.

Changes in the training of psychologists and pediatricians appear necessary to improve well child care. Clearly, there is a need to ensure that pediatricians as well as other health care providers are trained in the principles of and technology associated with behavioral psychology. It is our contention that training in behavioral principles, behavior therapy, and the techniques of applied behavior analysis may be one of the greatest and most important ways psychologists can affect large numbers of children. In turn, psychologists must familiarize themselves with the logistics and goals of pediatric practice and adapt their procedures to achieving these goals (Drotar, 1982).

The need for psychologists and pediatricians alike to receive additional training in normal child development and the treatment of minor behavior problems is evident. For example, in our experience students in clinical psychology are not typically taught to assess and treat minor behavior problems such as bedtime problems, finicky eating, or methods of improving relatively normal parent–toddler interactions. Rather, training emphasis is on the assessment and treatment of significant behavior disturbances in children and adolescents—the types of problems typically encountered in clinical settings. The psychology students that we encounter tend to be unfamiliar with practical aspects of child development, such as the age at which children should be toilet trained or expected to identify colors and shapes. Thus, for psychologists to contribute to the training of physicians and collaborate in the treatment of minor behavior problems, they themselves must become more knowledgeable of the answers to problems encountered in well child and adolescent care (Drabman, 1985).

Many research possibilities exist within the domain of primary pediatric care. The development and evaluation of treatment regimens offered to parents, children, and adolescents during well care visits is clearly needed. For example, little has been done to develop and evaluate educational interventions for improving parent–adolescent communication in relatively normal families. Very little research has been conducted on the efficacy of health care providers as instructors in behavior management techniques. Studies examining the physicians'[1] effectiveness in detecting behavior problems are also needed. In general, the prevention, assessment, and treatment of behavioral disturbances in adolescents has only recently been an area of focus in behavioral pediatrics. Many questions regarding adolescent care remain unanswered. Numerous other areas for future research were suggested throughout this chapter.

---

[1] Throughout this chapter the term *pediatricians* is used interchangeably with pediatric personnel or pediatric care unit. We fully appreciate the fact that many aspects of behavioral counseling are performed by nurses and pediatric care unit members other than pediatricians. For the sake of brevity, however, the term pediatricians often is used to connote all members of the pediatric care unit.

In part, the intent of this chapter was to stimulate interest in the potential role of behavioral psychologist in well child and adolescent care. The impact of behavioral psychology on well child care potentially is a very significant avenue for improving family relationships and optimal child development in many families. To do so, however, requires changes in the curriculum in which pediatrics and psychologists are trained and greater emphasis on the empirical validation of assessment and treatment procedures adapted to well child care.

REFERENCES

Achenbach, T. M., & Edelbrock, C. S. (1981). Behavioral problems and competencies reported by parents of normal and disturbed children aged four through sixteen. *Monographs of the Society for Research in Child Development, 46*, 1–181.

Achenbach, T. M., & Edelbrock, C. (1983). *Manual for the Child Behavior Checklist and Revised Child Behavior Profile.* Queen City Printers.

American Academy of Pediatrics. (1978). Pediatric practice patterns. *Pediatrics, 62*, 625–680.

Atkeson, B. M., & Forehand, R. (1981). Conduct disorders. In E. J. Mash & L. G. Terdol (Eds.), *Behavioral assessment of childhood disorders* (pp. 185–219). New York: Guilford Press.

Barkley, R. A. (1990). *Attention Deficit Hyperactivity Disorder: A handbook for diagnosis and treatment* (pp. 246–247). New York: Guilford Press.

Bentovin, A. (1970). The clinical approach to feeding disorders of childhood. *Journal of Psychosomatic Research, 14*, 267–276.

Bergman, A. B. (1982). Use of education in preventing injuries. *The pediatric clinics of North America, 29*, 331–338.

Bijou, S. W., & Baer, D. M. (1978). *Behavior analysis in child development.* Englewood Cliffs, NJ: Prentice-Hall.

Casey, P. H., Bradley, R. H., Caldwell, B. M., & Edwards, D. R. (1986). Developmental intervention: A pediatric clinical review. *The Pediatric Clinics of North America, 33*, 889–923.

Christopherson, E. R. (1982). Incorporating behavioral pediatrics into primary care. *The pediatric clinics of North America, 29*, 261–296.

Christopherson, E. R. (1983a). Behavioral pediatrics: An overview. In D. J. McGrath & P. Firestone (Eds.), *Pediatric & adolescent behavioral medicine* (pp. 1–12). New York: Springer.

Christophersen, E. R. (1983b). Behavioral analysis of well baby and well child care. *Advances in Developmental and Behavioral Pediatrics, 4*, 109–123.

Christopherson, E. R. (1986). Anticipatory guidance and discipline. *The Pediatric Clinics in North America, 33*, 789–798.

Christophersen, E. R., Barrish, H. H., Barrish, I. J., & Christophersen, M. R. (1984). Continuing education of parents of infants and toddlers. In R. F. Dangel & R. A. Polster (Eds.), *Parent training: Foundations of research and practice* (pp. 127–143). New York: Guilford.

Christopherson, E. R., & Gyulay, J. (1981). Parental compliance with car seat usage: A positive approach with long term follow-up. *Journal of Pediatric Psychology, 6*, 301–312.

Christopherson, E. R., & Hall, C. L. (1978). Eating patterns and associated problems encountered in normal children. *Issues in Comprehensive Pediatric Nursing, 3*, 1–16.

Christophersen, E. R., & Rapoff, M. A. (1979). Behavioral pediatrics. In O. Pomerlau & J. Brady (Eds), *Behavioral medicine: Theory & practice* (pp. 99–123). Baltimore: Williams & Wilkins.

Christopherson, E. R., & Rapoff, M. A. (1980). Biosocial pediatrics. In J. M. Ferguson & C. B. Taylor (Eds.), *The comprehensive handbook of behavioral medicine* (pp. 3–21). Jamaica, NY: Spectrum.

Cohen, M. I. (1984). The society for behavioral pediatrics: A new portal in a rapidly moving boundary. *Pediatrics, 73*, 791–798.

Coupey, S. M., & Schonberg, S. K. (1982). Evaluation and management of drug problems in adolescents. *Pediatric Annals, 11*, 653–658.

Crowther, J. H., Bond, L. A., & Rolf, J. E. (1981). The Incidence, prevalence, and severity of behavior disorders among preschool-aged children in day care. *Journal of Abnormal Child Psychology, 9*, 23–42.

Drabman, R. S. (1985). Graduate training of scientist-practitioner-oriented clinical psychologist: Where we can improve. *Professional Psychology: Research & Practice, 16*, 623–633.

Drabman, R. S., & Jarvie, G. (1977). Counseling parents of behavior problem children: Use of timeout and extinction procedures. *Pediatrics, 59*, 78–85.

Drotar, D. (1982). The child psychologist in the medical system. In P. Karoly, J. J. Sleffen, & D. J. O'Grady (Eds.), *Child health psychology: Concepts and issues* (pp. 1–28). New York: Pergamon Press.

Drotar, D. (1985). Responses to Dr. Friedman: Discussants' remarks and group discussion summaries. *Developmental and Behavioral Pediatrics, 6*, 207–208.

DuPont, R. L. (1984). Bulimia: A modern epidemic among adolescents. *Pediatric Annals, 13*, 908–914.

Eisenberg, L. (1984). The epidemiology of suicide in adolescents. *Pediatric Annals, 13*, 47–53.

Eyberg, S., & Ross, A. W. (1978). Assessment of child behavior problems: The validation of a new inventory. *Journal of Clinical Child Psychology, 7*, 113–116.

Felice, M. E., & Friedman, S. B. (1982). Behavioral considerations in the health care of adolescents. *The Pediatric Clinics of North America, 33*, 399–413.

Fielding, J. E., & Williams, C. A. (1991). Adolescent pregnancy in the United States: A review and recommendations for clinicians and research needs. *American Journal of Preventive Medicine, 7*, 47–52.

Finney, J. W. (1986). Preventing common feeding problems in infants and young children. *The Pediatric Clinics of North America, 33*, 775–788.

Finney, J. W., & Christophersen, E. R. (1984). Behavioral pediatrics: Health education in pediatric primary care. In M. Hersen, R. M. Eisler, & P. M. Miller (Eds.), *Progress in behavior modification: Volume 16* (pp. 185–229). Orlando FL: Academic Press.

Forehand, R. L., & McMahon, R. J. (1981). *Helping the noncompliant child: A clinician's guide to parent training*. New York: Guilford Press.

Friedman, S. B. (1985). Behavioral pediatrics: Interaction with other disciplines. *Developmental and Behavioral Pediatrics, 6*, 202–207.

Glenn, N. D., & Weaver, C. N. (1978). A multivariate, multisurvey study of marital happiness. *Journal of Marriage and Family, 40*, 269–282.

Green, M. (1985). The role of the pediatrician in the delivery of behavioral services. *Developmental & Behavioral Pediatrics, 6*, 190–201.

Hertzler, A. A. (1983). Children's food patterns. A review (I): Food preferences and feeding problems. *Journal of the American Dietetic Association, 83*, 555–560.

Hobbs, S. A., Beck, S. J., & Wansley, R. A. (1984). Pediatric behavioral medicine: Directions in treatment and prevention. In M. Hersen, R. M. Eisler, & P. M. Miller (Eds.), *Progress in behavior modification: Volume 16* (pp. 1–29). Orlando, FL: Academic Press.

Homer, C., & Ludwig, S. (1981). Categorization of etiology of failure to thrive. *American Journal of Disease of Children, 135*, 848–851.

Johnson, C. L., Lewis, C., Love, S., Stuckey, M., & Lewis, S. (1983). A descriptive survey of dieting and bulimic behavior in a female high school population. In *Understanding anorexia and bulimia* (Report on the Fourth Ross Conference on Medical Research). Columbus, OH: Ross Laboratories.

Jones, R. T., Kazdin, A. E., & Haney, J. I. (1981). Social validation and training of emergency fire safety skills for potential injury prevention and life saving. *Journal of Applied Behavior Analysis, 14*, 249–260.

Kanoy, K. W., & Schroeder, C. S. (1985). Suggestions to parents about common behavior problems in a pediatric primary case office. Five years of follow-up. *Journal of Pediatric Psychology, 10*, 15–30.

LaGreca, A., & Stone, W. L. (1985). Behavioral pediatrics. In N. Schneiderman & J. T. Tapp (Eds.), *Behavioral medicine: The biosocial approach* (pp. 225–290). Hillsdale, NJ: Erlbaum.

MacDonald, D. A. (1986). *Prevention of Adolescent Smoking and Drug Use, 33*, 995–1003.

MacPhee, D. (1984). The pediatrician as a source of information about child development. *Journal of Pediatric Psychology, 9*, 87–100.

Mastria, M. A., & Drabman, R. S. (1979). The development of behavioral competence in medical settings. In J. R. McNamara (Ed.), *Behavioral approaches to medicine: Application and analysis* (pp. 33–63). New York: Plenum.

Mesibov, G. B. (1983). Evolution of pediatric psychology: Historical roots to future trends. *Journal of Pediatric Psychology, 9*, 3–11.

Namerow, P. B., & Philliber, S. G. (1982). The effectiveness of contraceptive programs for teenagers. *Journal of Adolescent Health Care, 2*, 190–198.

Neinstein, L. S. (1984). *Adolescent health care: A practical guide*. Baltimore: Urban & Schwarzenberg.

Olson, R. A., Huszti, H. C., Mason, P. J., Seibert, J. M. (1989). Pediatric AIDS/HIV Infection: An emerging challenge to pediatric psychology. *Journal of Pediatric Psychology, 14*, 1–21.

Phillips, S., Sarles, R. M., & Friedman, S. B. (1980). Consultation and referral: When, why, and how. *Pediatric Annals, 9*, 36–45.

Redd, W. H., & Rusch, F. R. (1985). Behavioral analysis in behavioral medicine. *Behavior Modification, 9*, 131–154.

Reisinger, K. S., & Bires, J. A. (1980). Anticipatory guidance in pediatric practice. *Pediatrics, 66*, 889–892.

Resnick, M., Blum, R. W., & Hedin, D. (1980). The appropriateness of health services for adolescents. *Journal of Adolescent Health Care, 1*, 137–141.

Richman, N., Stevenson, J. E., & Graham, P. J. (1975). Prevelance of behavior problems in 3-year old children: An epidemiological study in a London borough. *Journal of Child Psychology & Psychiatry, 16*, 277–287.

Richmond, J. B. (1967). Child development: A basic science for pediatrics. *Pediatrics, 31*, 649–658.

Richmond, J. B. (1985). Coming of age: Developmental pediatrics in the late twentieth century. *Developmental and Behavioral Pediatrics, 6*, 181–187.

Roberts, M. D., & Maddux, J. E. (1982). A psychosocial conceptualization of nonorganic failure to thrive. *Journal of Clinical Child Psychology, 11*, 216–226.

Rosenbaum, M., Creeden, D., & Drabman, R. S. (1981). Training preschool children to identify emergency situations and make emergency phone calls. *Behavior Therapy, 12*, 425–435.

Russo, D. C., & Varni, J. W. (1982). Behavioral pediatrics. In D. C. Russo & J. W. Varni (Eds.), *Behavioral pediatrics: Research & practice* (pp. 3–24). New York: Plenum Press.

Schmitt, B. D. (1985, May). When baby just won't sleep. *Contemporary Pediatrics*, pp. 38–52.

Schroeder, C. S. (1979). Psychologists in a private pediatric practice. *Journal of Pediatric Psychology, 4*, 5–18.

Schwartz, D. M., Tapp, J. T., Brucker, B. (1985). Behavioral assessment in medical settings. In N. Schneiderman & J. Tapp (Eds.), *Behavioral medicine: The biophysical approach* (pp. 159–191). Hillsdale, NJ: Erlbaum.

Shen, J. T. Y. (1980). *The clinical practice of adolescent medicine.* New York: Appleton-Century-Crofts.

Starfield, B., & Barkowf, S. (1969). Physicians' recognition of complaints made by parents about their children's health. *Pediatrics, 43*, 168–172.

Teri, L. (1982). Depression in adolescent: Its relationship to assertion and various aspects of self-image. *Journal of Clinical Child Psychology, 11*, 101–106.

Varni, J. W. (1983). Behavioral pediatrics: Historical perspective and current definition. *Clinical behavioral pediatrics: An interdisciplinary biobehavioral approach* (pp. 3–15). New York: Pergamon Press.

Varni, J. W., & Dietrich, S. L. (1981). Behavioral pediatrics. Toward a reconceptualization. *Behavioral Medicine Update, 3*, 5–7.

Williams, Foreyt, & Goodrick. (1981). Introduction. *Pediatric behavioral medicine* (pp. 1–19). New York: Praeger.

Williamson, D. A., Kelley, M. L., Cavell, T. A., & Prather, R. C. (1987). Eating and eliminating disorders. In C. L. Frame & J. L. Matson (Eds.), *Handbook of assessment in child psychopathology: Applied issues in differen-*

tial diagnosis and treatment evaluation (pp. 461–507). New York: Plenum Press.

Witt, J., & Cavell, T. A. (1986). Psychological assessment. In D. L. Wodrich & J. E. Joy (Eds.), *Multidisciplinary assessment of children with learning disabilities and mental retardation* (pp. 31–75). Baltimore: Paul H. Brooks Publishing Co.

Wright, L. (1967). The pediatric psychologist: A role model. *American Psychologist, 22*, 323–325.

9

Psychological and Behavioral Sequelae in Children with Chronic Disease: An Interactional Model

Amy J. Ginsberg and Elizabeth A. Klonoff

Case Western Reserve University School of Medicine and University Hospitals of Cleveland

Dennis C. Russo

Children's Hospital and Harvard Medical School

In reviewing the psychological literature on chronic childhood illness, two distinct and dichotomous approaches appear. Historically, the literature focused on the identification of personality traits and psychiatric characteristics of a child and his or her family that presumably predisposed that child to illness. This psychopathology model evolved directly from traditional, dynamic approaches to mental illness. In contrast, more recent studies have utilized an interactional or biopsychosocial model to explain the impact of chronic illness on children and families. Rather than focusing on identifying a psychiatric abnormality, this model assumes that the child with chronic illness has the potential to develop normally. Failure to do so is the result of specific, learned, maladaptive behaviors, as opposed to personality traits, that impact subsequent developmental tasks.

The current chapter is an attempt to delineate in more detail the potential impact of this interactional model. First, a brief review of the traditional pediatric psychology literature is provided. This review attempts to address some of the weaknesses in the traditional "psychosomatic model." Following this, we address the empirical support for an interactional or biopsychosical model of chronic disease in children. we use a few specific chronic disease conditions as examples, but we argue that the constructs presented are generalizable across a wide variety of illnesses. In addition, we review data to support our contentions that, beyond limitations imposed directly by the disease itself, there exists no a priori basis on which to rule out developmental normalcy in children with chronic disease. Finally, we address the implications for treatment and research that derive from this interactional model.

TRADITIONAL APPROACHES IN PEDIATRIC PSYCHOLOGY

Traditional psychological research in childhood illness has tended to fall into one of two major categories. One approach has emphasized the particular psychiatric substrates that predispose a child and his or her family to specific illnesses, especially those illnesses that have been hypothesized to have a significant psychological component. An alternative approach has emphasized the reactions to, or changes commensurate with, the acquisition of a chronic illness. Both approaches have focused on disease-specific psychopathology and have emphasized the delineation of specific psychological traits or attributes (e.g., intrapsychic conflicts, low self-esteem) that correlate with a chronic disease.

Psychosomatic Approach

The literature on psychopathological variables predisposing an individual to a chronic physical illness is problematic as diagnostic labels are often confusing and/or overlapping. Although recent attempts to revise diagnostic criteria have focused on more accurately discriminating among psychiatric illnesses involving a physical component (Hyler

& Spitzer, 1978), major difficulties still exist with respect to the use of the term *psychosomatic illness*. The exact meaning of this term remains unclear as it has been applied to a range of presentations including hysteria, hypochondriasis, and conversion disorders. Traditionally, an illness has been labeled *psychosomatic* if: (a) no clear etiology or pathogen is identified, (b) specific treatments typically utilized for similar symptoms are ineffective, (c) the illness occurs temporally contiguous to some major life event, or (d) the illness appears in an individual with obvious psychopathology. For many years, the field was guided either by Alexander's concept that psychophysiological disorders were each a product of a different unconscious emotional state (Alexander, 1950) or by the specific attitude theory that held that specific patterns of attitudes, rather than chronic emotional states, were associated with specific illnesses (Grace & Graham, 1952).

The literature to date has not consistently supported either of these psychosomatic theories. With respect to Alexander's theory, one major criticism is that supportive evidence has always been retrospective, typically stemming from extensive psychoanalytic work with an individual who has already been diagnosed with a "psychosomatic" illness. This research seems to ignore other data that suggest a more physiological basis to the problem. For example, Rees (1964) found that psychological factors were a dominant cause of asthma, long believed to be a "psychosomatic" illness, in only 37% of his sample, with infection generally being the most common etiological factor. Psychosomatic theories are also weak in empirical validation as much of the supportive literature has been correlational in nature. Thus, whereas certain personality traits may have been shown to be related to certain physical illnesses, it is impossible to know the direction of this relationship, that is, whether these personality traits prompt the illness in question, are the result of the illness, or are an artifact of the assessment procedure itself. In sum, the search for intrapsychic or intrafamilial processes leading to the development of specific disorders has not yielded significant results. Rather, these processes have been inferred, rather than demonstrated, from retrospective, uncontrolled case analyses.

Disease-Specific Coping Approach

The second major focus of traditional pediatric psychology has been in the area broadly conceptualized as the impact of chronic illness. Research on the impact of chronic illness has typically taken one of two directions: Either an attempt has been made to identify disease-specific psychopathology, or emphasis has been placed on describing the process of coping with a chronic illness.

Research in the first area—focusing on the identification of changes in psychological traits accompanying chronic disease—has been overwhelming. The methodology employed usually involves measurement of one or more trait variables hypothesized to covary with the illness in question. The relative presence or absence of these traits in ill subjects is then compared with its presence in either healthy controls or individuals with a different illness. For example, compared to normal peers, certain specific traits such as body image, self-concept, and independence (Bakwin & Bakwin, 1972) are thought to be at very high risk for disruption in chronically ill children. In terms of specific illnesses, diabetes has been found to be correlated highly with personality problems including aggressiveness, low self-concept, and peer isolation (e.g., Swift, Sidman, & Stein, 1967). Similarly, asthma has been found to correlate with increased psychopathology, maternal emotional disturbance, and abnormal parenting (Werry, 1972). In predicting psychopathology, the traditional chronic illness literature has focused on identifying variables specific to each illness as a unique entity. For example, whereas family functioning variables and maternal emotional disturbance, independent of illness severity, were determined to be the best predictors of psychopathology in asthmatic children, the severity of the disease itself was identified as the most important predictor of psychopathology in children with cystic fibrosis (Steinhausen, Schindler, & Stephan, 1983). Unfortunately, most of these data are correlational, making it impossible to ascertain if the emotional psychopathological response actually produces the illness or is in itself a product of the illness.

The second disease-specific research approach has focused on the description of coping mechanisms used to handle the stress associated with a chronic illness. Again, this approach has emphasized stresses unique to each disease. For example, whereas fears of suffocating were commonly reported in children with asthma, children with cystic fibrosis were most preoccupied with concerns regarding flatulence and stool odor (Mattsson, 1972). *Coping*, according to this model, has generally been conceptualized in terms of global personality variables and psychological defenses utilized to master distressing emotions. For example, in one study, coping styles characterized by anger, rather than by depression and anxiety, were identified as the most maladaptive, often leading to a need for psychosocial care (Shady, 1978). Drotar (1981) noted that this traditional view of *coping* is troublesome in that it seems to imply that adjustment to a chronic illness is synonymous with the absence of severe psychopathology. Conversely, failure to adequately cope or adjust appears synonymous with deviant personality functioning. These conclusions may be invalid, however, as the norms for adaptive behavior in healthy children are not necessarily applicable to chronically ill children (Drotar, 1981). Thus, behavior that is labeled as psychopathological in the absence of a chronic illness may constitute normal or predictable adjustment to a chronic illness.

Research has suggested that chronically ill children in general are no more at risk for psychopathology or maladjustment than their healthy peers (Tavormina, Kastner, Slater, & Watt, 1976). Although chronic illness may at times correlate with maladaptive behaviors, several studies have documented that children with chronic illness demonstrate relatively more strengths overall than weaknesses (Drotar, 1981; Tavormina et al., 1976). Controlled studies of children with juvenile-onset diabetes mellitus revealed that no personality traits, in and of themselves, were correlated with the illness, and that emotional disturbances in diabetic children were no more or less prevalent than emotional disturbances in the general population (Dunn & Turtle, 1981; Johnson, 1980). With respect to children with other chronic diseases, studies have failed to reveal either evidence for psychopathology or significant differences between healthy and ill adolescents on measures of depression, trait anxiety, and self-esteem (Kellerman, Zeltzer, Ellenberg, Dash, & Rigler, 1980; Sullivan, 1978).

Conclusions

Overall, traditional models of pediatric psychology, derived from psychodynamic theory, appear to be too simplistic from a number of perspectives when applied to children with chronic illness. First, an empirically validated mechanism for the etiology of psychosomatic or psychophysiological disorders has not been identified. Second, consistent factors that reliably discriminate either among various illness groups or between an illness group an a healthy control group have not been identified. Both of these endeavors may have been hampered by the inability to adequately demonstrate enduring psychological traits across time and across illnesses. Third, no clearly identifiable, empirically based intervention has developed from this approach for either the direct amelioration of psychosomatic symptoms or improved coping methods for children with psychophysiological illnesses. Finally, this approach has not proven overwhelmingly helpful either in the prevention of illness in children considered to be at risk or in decreasing the direct effects of the illness itself.

AN INTERACTIONAL MODEL OF DISEASE

Several researchers have suggested that, rather than focusing on the specific symptoms of each distinct chronic illness, a noncategorical approach across diseases should be utilized (Pless & Pinkerton, 1975; Starfield & Pless, 1980; Stein & Jessup, 1982). Such a model assumes psychological normalcy in chronically ill children (Kellerman et al., 1980; Russo, 1986) and focuses on the commonalities among diseases. Diseases are viewed as sharing features or burdens in, for example, disrupting family life, requiring increased time for health care, or impacting school attendance and social interactions. According to this conceptualization, a disease-specific diagnostic label (e.g., *diabetic*, *asthmatic*, *cystic fibrotic*) is inappropriate and irrelevant in that it provides no information about the stress or burden that the illness imposes on a given child and his or her family. Diagnostic labels communicate disease-specific differences only with respect to biomedical aspects of the disease (Stein & Jessup, 1984).

Children with chronic illness can be described noncategorically along a variety of discrete dimensions, including age at onset of illness, prognosis, course of disease, and visibility of disease (Pless & Pinkerton, 1975). These dimensions may be relevant in an analysis of the impact of disease on development. For example, the age at onset of a chronic illness may be related to specific developmental disruptions; that is, a congenital anomaly may affect early attachment behavior (Drotar, Baskiewicz, Irvin et al., 1975), whereas a chronic illness that develops during adolescence may affect adolescent tasks such as the development of autonomy and independence (Pless & Pinkerton, 1975). These developmental disruptions are directly linked to the stress imposed by an illness rather than to an inherent psychopathology that is somehow related to the specific disease itself.

The noncategorical approach represents a move away from the measurement of psychological traits variables toward a multivariate model of specific and measurable biological and environmental events. Such a biopsychosocial multifactorial model of illness (Engle, 1977; Varni, 1983) considers the "whole child" as a system, including internal and external stimuli. In order to better illustrate this, we identified at least four factors that may interact to increase the probability that normal behavior or development will be impeded in children with chronic illness. These factors include: (a) specific characteristics of the disease itself, (b) possible iatrogenic effects resulting from the medical procedures used to treat the disease, (c) changes in reinforcement patterns for the child when compared to preillness reinforcer patterns;

and (d) other life stressors. We discuss the impact of each of these factors separately.

Characteristics of the Disease

Specific aspects of the disease itself may have direct negative effects on the child who would otherwise develop normally. These effects range from significantly decreased life expectancy to decreased energy that may be a function of the illness itself or of its treatment. A variety of tasks of normal development may be affected *directly* by the symptoms of a chronic disease or *indirectly* as a consequence of learning or secondary to treatment intervention. For example, cerebral palsy may directly impede the development of some self-help skills such as feeding and dressing. In contrast, even when the disease itself is not inherently responsible for inhibiting normal development, specific learning mechanisms may interact with a chronic disease to produce iatrogenic developmental interference. For example, children who survive cancer may suffer neuropsychological deficits or conditioned food aversions as a function of chemotherapy and radiation treatments, and these "side effects" of treatment may lead to additional difficulties.

The nature of the developmental task that is negatively influenced by learning may sometimes be related to the type of disease but, at other times, may be related to the age of the child at the onset of the disease. That is, oftentimes the chronically ill child is most at risk for delayed development in upcoming developmental tasks and/or tasks that have not already been mastered. For example, whereas some gastrointestinal disorders, such as ulcerative colitis, may result in increased risk for feeding difficulties, any child with a chronic disease at a very early age may be at risk for delays in the areas of feeding and self-help skills, particularly if these skills have not already been acquired prior to the development of the disease. When a chronic disease develops in a school-age child who likely has already mastered self-help skills, other age-appropriate developmental tasks such as school attendance, school achievement, and the development of peer relations may be negatively impacted (Weitzman, 1984). Certain illnesses, such as asthma, have been associated with high rates of school absenteeism (Bharani & Hyde, 1976). Failure to attend school may lead to delayed acquisition of social skills that subsequently may further impact one's ability to cope with stress and thereby exacerbate symptoms of chronic illness.

The adolescent who develops a chronic disease may be at increased risk for developmental delay in areas relating to independence and separation from family, areas generally viewed as tasks of adolescence. Delays in some minor areas, such as obtaining a driver's license, may lead to other difficulties such as problems in balancing the demand for adolescent conformity with the need for skill development in resisting peer pressure. However, regardless of the child's age at the time of diagnosis, the chronic disease in and of itself does not necessarily directly result in delayed development. Rather a chronic disease may put a child at risk in that it sets the occasion for learning maladaptive responses with respect to developmental tasks.

An acute illness in a child with a chronic disease may also set the occasion for maladaptive behaviors. For example, children with organically based feeding difficulties, who successfully learn to accept a variety of tastes and textures, may temporarily "relapse" during an acute illness (Ginsberg, in press; Ginsberg & Klonoff, 1985). Ginsberg and Klonoff (1985) described their treatment of a 4-year-old girl with organic feeding difficulties secondary to the treatment of pulmonary disease. Although the child successfully learned to accept oral feeds, she would reliably take several steps back following an acute illness such as the flu or pneumonia. At these times, it was necessary to reimplement earlier stages of the feeding program to reshape appropriate behaviors, although the duration of each stage became shorter each time. Acute illnesses may also serve as discriminative stimuli for the development of maladaptive responses in children without previous chronic disease (Klonoff, Knell, & Janata, 1984).

Disease-Associated Iatrogenic Effects

The medical procedures typically administered in the course of treatment for a chronic illness may have inherently negative side effects associated with them. Oftentimes these secondary negative effects become symptoms in their own right, requiring treatment concurrent with, or even long after, treatment of the primary disorder. These secondary problems are essentially iatrogenically induced as they result indirectly from the therapeutic effort itself.

Conditioned nausea and vomiting in children undergoing chemotherapy is one well-documented example of an iatrogenically induced problem caused by the treatment of cancer (Morrow & Morrell, 1982; Redd & Andrykowski, 1982; Zeltzer, LeBaron, & Zeltzer, 1984). Emetic-inducing drugs may become either inadvertently paired—temporally or spatially—or cognitively associated with other environmental stimuli that subsequently serve as conditioned stimuli to elicit nausea and vomiting. Particular smells, sights, and sounds present at the time of the chemotherapy administration often become classically conditioned in this fashion, thus eliciting nausea and vomiting in the absence of medication.

Feeding delays in children with chronic disease may similarly be iatrogenically induced. Although gastrointestinal disease may directly result in eating difficulties, feeding delays may be associated with any chronic illness. Regardless of the patient's age, the treatment of certain illnesses, such as chemotherapy for cancer, may result in iatrogenic feeding difficulties. A young child who has not yet mastered feeding skills may be particularly vulnerable. Consider the child who is born prematurely and with chronic lung disease and respiratory distress syndrome (RDS). This child may be at particular risk for later feeding difficulties not directly due to the illness itself, but rather due to learning associated with the medical procedures and interventions (Ginsberg & Klonoff, 1987). The child with RDS often requires mechanical respiratory or ventilatory assistance and will likely not have the strength to eat. This may necessitate the use of parenteral feeds such as nasogastric tube feedings, gastrostomy tube feedings, or the use of arterial hyperalimentation. As a result, this child will have decreased experiences with food and thus fewer opportunities to acquire food-related skills at an early age. This, in and of itself, may place the child at risk for significant long-term delays in feeding as it has been suggested that there is a "critical" period in which to develop appropriate feeding skills (Illingsworth & Lister, 1964).

In addition to lack of experience and lack of physical strength, which contribute to feeding delays, the chronically ill infant may develop an iatrogenic conditioned aversion to food. At least four mechanisms can be identified for the development of food aversions in infants with RDS and other chronic diseases. First, the treatment of RDS, particularly the use of respirators, may result in additional (iatrogenic) difficulties such as bronchopulmonary dysplasia, ulcers, and oral malformations (Peabody & Lewis, 1985). These conditions may impede appropriate eating and lead to conditioned aversion to food as the ingestion of food may be associated with physical discomfort. A second mechanism involved in the development of a conditioned food aversion relates to the incompatibility of oral feeding and swallowing with mechanical breathing. That is, a respirator or ventilator may "force" a breath at the exact point in time at which the child has prepared for a swallow. As swallowing at this time may result in great discomfort, food-related anxiety and avoidance responses may be learned. Third, sustaining sucking may be especially difficult for the infant with RDS as sucking may impede air flow, particularly if the child breathes orally rather than nasally, causing the child to gasp.

Sucking and attempting to take food orally may thus be punishing for the child. Finally, environmental stimuli may play a role in the negative conditioning process. The child who experiences many aversive and intrusive medical procedures by the nursing staff may later reject food offered by the same staff. That is, the staff themselves may become negatively conditioned stimuli that signal to the child that an aversive task is forthcoming. Visual, auditory, and tactile stimuli associated with discomfort may similarly serve as negative conditioned stimuli that strengthen the food aversion, resulting in avoidance of food in their presence. For example, if a child received all of his or her medical care in the confines of the infant's crib, it is possible that he or she will later refuse feedings that are also offered in this crib. A separate feeding room might be necessary to avoid contact with conditioned stimuli that elicit food avoidance and to decrease the probability of response generalization (Ginsberg & Klonoff, 1987).

In sum, iatrogenic aspects of the treatment of many diseases may interact with the disease itself to produce another set of symptoms or behaviors. As is the case with iatrogenically induced food refusal, these behaviors may prove as serious or even life-threatening as the original disease, and behavioral intervention may be effective in ameliorating or even preventing their occurrence.

Changes in Reinforcement Patterns

The occurrence of a major illness may produce many significant changes in the life of a child. Parents may treat him or her differently, being more attentive to the child's needs and desires. Certain life responsibilities, such as school attendance and household chores, may be curtailed because of the child's condition. For some children these changes may be experienced as desirable, resulting in inadvertent positive reinforcement for illness-related behaviors. There is strong evidence that operant processes, including positive and negative reinforcement, can affect the probability and/or perception of a physical symptom. For example, Klonoff and Biglan (1987) demonstrated that hypoglycemic-like symptoms were susceptible to reinforcement and increased in probability when the subject consumed food contingent on symptom occurrence.

Several studies with asthmatic children have lent support for the role of social reinforcement and avoidance of aversive tasks in maintaining asthmatic symptoms. For example, Shepard and Hockstadt (1978) identified a subset of asthmatic patients believed to be "overusers" of hospitalization. Based on these patients' behavior, including their tendency to have exacerbations of asthma symptoms contingent on being told that discharge was imminent, it was hypothesized that being in the hospital was experienced as more "reinforcing" than being out of the hospital. This hypothesis was supported by the effective use of a time-out procedure that both reduced the time spent in the hospital and increased the time between hospitalizations. Similarly, Creer (1970; Creer, Weinberg, & Molk, 1974) demonstrated that removing positive reinforcers, such as staff attention and television, was effective in decreasing the frequency and duration of hospitalizations of asthmatic children.

Chronic pain behavior is another potential example of reinforced symptoms. Children with a potentially life-threatening condition, such as cancer, often receive increased social attention concurrent with the diagnosis. Increases in pain behavior associated with medical treatment are further accompanied by increases in social attention. As a result, pain behaviors inadvertently may be reinforced such that, when the disease is in remission and/or pain has stabilized, the child continues to emit pain-related behavior that is no longer appropriate or adaptive (Fordyce, Shelton, & Dundore, 1982; Masek, Russo, & Varni, 1984). That is, consistent with a process of response generalization, the child may continue to emit verbal complaints of pain, to decrease activity levels, and to be overly whiny or dependent in the absence of identifiable pain. Parents or caretakers, lacking the ability to empirically measure pain, may accidentally provide positive reinforcement for these pain responses, thereby maintaining the maladaptive behaviors. Other iatrogenic effects of treatment may similarly maintain in the absence of pain due to learning mechanisms other than positive reinforcement from parents. For example, the child with chronic pain may also experience depression, and both the pain and pain-related depression may lead to temporary withdrawal from social activities. Social withdrawal from peers may further increase depression and increased dependence on parents, both of which may further contribute to social avoidance. Consequently, a negative cycle may be created such that when the pain has subsided, social withdrawal maintains due to depression and learned avoidance.

In addition, frequent or prolonged hospitalizations, which may be a common experience for the chronically ill child, may contribute to social skill delays as a consequence of decreased contact with age-appropriate peers. This may lead to increased anxiety for the child when he or she returns to school and contacts increased pressures (Weitzman, 1984) and, this anxiety, which may be related to fear of failure, fear of rejection, and social-skill deficits, may further contribute to learned school or task avoidance. A negative reinforcement cycle or trap thus ensues in which the anxiety and skills deficits are strengthened over time as a function of avoidance. Although negative reinforcement principles may be initially operative in the development of school avoidance, this behavior may subsequently come under the control of various sources of positive reinforcement, including access to television and toys while at home.

Modeling and social learning may also function as learning mechanisms that interact with a chronic disease to maintain illness-related behaviors. Exposure to parents' modeling of avoidant or maladaptive behaviors may result in an increased probability of the chronically ill child emitting similar behaviors. For example, Turkat (1982) demonstrated that diabetic children of mothers who modeled eating sugar-based snacks had higher glucohemoglobin levels than diabetic peers not exposed to modeling effects.

As described earlier, positive reinforcement, negative reinforcement resulting in escape and/or avoidance behaviors, and modeling may be significant factors in facilitating maladaptive behavior in children with chronic illness. An example may help to clarify the interactional impact of positive and negative reinforcement.

Case illustration. Jerome was a 12-year-old boy who had undergone surgery, radiation treatment, and chemotherapy for a brain tumor (medulobalstoma) diagnosed 6 months earlier. In response to chemotherapy and radiation treatments, Jerome developed nausea and vomiting that eventually became anticipatory in nature such that, on days on that Jerome was scheduled for treatment, he began to feel nauseous upon awakening, and he began to vomit upon entering the hospital. This led to conditioned anorexia, which was thought to be related to drug and treatment effects rather than to the location of the tumor itself (i.e., the tumor was not thought to have affected the hypothalamic center that regulates appetite).

When cancer treatment was successfully terminated, Jerome continued to avoid eating and 6 weeks after the termination of radiation therapy was hospitalized due to significant weight loss. Jerome reported that he could not eat because all food smelled aversive to him and reminded him of the smell of the hospital basement in which the radiation treatment room was located. Thus, he had developed a conditioned aversion to certain smells that he associated with the aversiveness of radiation. Over time, this aversion generalized such that Jerome reported nausea in the presence of a variety of odors, dissimilar to the odors experienced in the radiation room, including gasoline and pizza. As Jerome considered himself to be overweight prior to his craniotomy, his pleasure in his weight loss, as well as praise from peers, further reinforced his food avoidance. Finally, Jerome's refusal to finish all of his meals was very upsetting to his mother, and food refusal, one of the few ways in which Jerome could exert control, may have further served as an "acting out" behavior maintained by his mother's reaction.

In sum, the treatment of Jerome's illness led to iatrogenic effects in the form of food refusal, a learned maladaptive behavior that was maintained by classical and operant conditioning processes. Treatment was successfully derived from an understanding of these mechanisms and thus included systematic desensitization to olfactory stimuli, behavioral contracting for weight gain, and parental contingency management.

Other Life Stresses

Experimental investigations have been directed increasingly toward the identification and assessment of variables that might increase the likelihood that an individual will acquire a chronic illness. One area that continues to receive significant attention is the impact of stress on the emergence of physical illness. Stress may serve as a predisposing factor in the development of a disease by increasing one's susceptibility to illness (Shapiro, 1983). Just as the disease process occasions learning (Russo, 1986), learning mechanisms associated with stress may also impact the disease process. For example, experimental studies have revealed that animals may develop changes in immune functions via learning (e.g., Adler, 1971; Anderson & Brady, 1979; Russo, 1986). It has repeatedly been demonstrated that stress may modify somatic functioning (Locke, 1982; Russo, Tarbell, & Follansbee, in press), and responses to environmental stress, including one's beliefs, may directly impact physiology (Levine, Gordon, & Fields, 1978; Russo, 1986). In one study, stress and environmental influences were shown to be directly related to an increase in the frequency of acute symptoms associated with a chronic illness (Bedell, Giordani, Amour, Tavormina, & Boli, 1977). However, this study failed to identify the mechanisms by which environmental stimuli and illness behaviors interact, and increased specificity of environmental variables perceived as stressful would be necessary to allow for experimental comparisons of "stress" levels across studies.

A variety of life stressors that impact illness behaviors have been identified in the literature. Although the age of the child at the time of diagnosis does not appear to be a risk factor per se, some researchers have suggested that children undergoing developmental transition periods, such as entering school and adolescence, may be at highest risk for the maintenance of illness behaviors (Klonoff, Knell, & Janata, 1984). Life stresses may make these children more vulnerable to the effects of adventitious reinforcement for disease symptoms. Thus, developmental transitions, psychosocial stressors, and reinforcement may be interactive in the etiology and/or maintenance of illness behavior. Some researchers have suggested that ordinary life events may interact with a chronic disease in such a way a to have a greater impact on the ill child, who may be more vulnerable to stress, than the healthy child (Stein & Jessop, 1984). For example, common environmental changes such as changing schools, moving to a new home, and the birth of a sibling may further impede the acquisition of developmental tasks in the chronically ill child and increase the probability that maladaptive behaviors will be learned. In general, it has been documented that stress and other social environmental factors that interact with a disease are the most important variables in predicting the impact of a chronic illness (Bedell et al., 1977; Orr, Weller, Satterwhite, & Pless, 1984).

The age of the child may be relevant in the identification of those developmental tasks for which the child will be particularly vulnerable if maladaptive learning occurs. As noted earlier, the young child may be at risk for delays in self-help skills, whereas the adolescent may be at risk for delays in exhibiting social skills. In addition, if the child is exposed to a significant other who has modeled maladaptive behaviors in the past, the risk of the child imitating these maladaptive responses increases (Turkat, 1982). Also, if a child exhibits certain skill deficits, such as inadequate social skills, prior to the development of a chronic disease, he or she may be particularly susceptible to negative reinforcement in the face of a chronic illness. This child may be at greater risk for the development of maladaptive behaviors, such as social avoidance, following diagnosis and for the maintenance of these maladaptive behaviors once the original disease symptoms have subsided.

Family stress may also increase the risk that the chronically ill child will develop maladaptive coping responses. In families in which marital conflict exists (unrelated to the child's illness), the necessity of cohesiveness when making treatment decisions may serve as positive reinforcement for the chronically ill child such that he or she continues to maintain illness responses in the absence of demonstrable illness (presumably in an effort to facilitate the reconciliation of his or her parents). For example, maintenance of abdominal pain behaviors in a young adolescent, in the absence of identifiable organic disease, was attributed to the decreased parental fighting that coincided with increased reports of pain (Klonoff, Ginsberg, & Janata, 1985). It is also likely that a family experiencing other sources of stress will predispose an ill child to increased risk of maladaptive behavior (Bedell et al., 1977; Orr et al., 1984). Families with high levels of stress may be inconsistent in applying behavioral contingencies to the chronically ill child, and lack of discipline may lead to the child learning a new array of developmentally unhealthy behaviors.

Research with children who suffer from insulin-dependent-diabetes mellitus (IDDM) has explored the impact and the interaction of stressors on the course of the disease. A variety of factors have been determined to interact to influence diabetic compliance, including the complexity of the treatment, the degree of behavior change demanded by the medical regimen, and the child's cognitive level (Johnson, 1986; Surwit, Scovern, & Feinglos, 1982). Some researchers have documented that stress, behavior, and physiology interact in IDDM to create a vicious interactive cycle in which stress leads to poor compliance, which leads to subsequent deterioration in vision, which correlates with an increased refusal of dialysis, which subsequently leads to greater physiological deterioration, and so on (Fisher, Delameter, Bertelson, & Kirklay, 1982). A case presentation will illustrate the impact of stress in a case of juvenile-onset diabetes.

Case illustration. Sandi was a 16-year-old adolescent referred for treatment of diabetic noncompliance complicated by an eating disorder. Her history contained several major stressful life events, including the precipitous death of her biological father, cataract surgery, and multiple hospitalizations. Several other significant events including missing a great deal of school, being given major responsibility for her own diabetic are at too early an age, and gaining weight in response to her initial insulin regimen, interacted to produce later maladaptive behaviors. Sandi developed social anxiety, presumably as a result of frequent school absences, as well as social skills deficits with respect to dealing with normal adolescent pressures. These social difficulties led to peer rejection, contributing even further to Sandi's perception to herself as different from her peers and setting the stage for Sandi's noncompliance in an attempt to "ignore" her disease and increase her sense of similarity to her peers. In addition, Sandi's insulin-induced weight gain resulted in an iatrogenically induced eating disorder in the form of anorexia nervosa with bulimic symptoms. As has been documented elsewhere (e.g., Ginsberg & Janata, 1986, 1987), insulin manipulation in weight-conscious diabetic patients may serve as a bulimic or purging function as underinjection of insulin may result in glucose and, indirectly, calories being "spilled" in the urine.

Sandi's maladaptive behaviors were thus maintained by a number of interactive environmental variables. The effects of diabetes set the stage for an iatrogenic eating disorder that resulted in insulin manipulation and poor diabetic control. Resulting hospitalizations exacerbated Sandi's social deficits, thereby increasing her social anxiety and school avoidance, which contributed to further diabetic noncompliance. Treatment required a functional analysis of all of these maintaining variables and was directed at the synergistic cycle of these interactive factors rather than at the individual factors themselves (Ginsberg & Janata, 1987).

Conclusions

In sum, if certain learning mechanisms are operative, the four factors outlined earlier, specifically, characteristics of the disease, iatrogenic aspects of treatment, changes in parental and social reinforcement patterns, and life stresses, may increase the probability that maladaptive illness behaviors will be maintained in children with chronic disease. A variety of learning mechanisms, as described in this chapter, may be involved in this process including: (a) decreased opportunity for appropriate skill acquisition and experiences; (b) positive reinforcement for maladaptive behaviors in the form of increased social attention; (c) vicarious or imitational learning as a result of exposure to modeling of inappropriate behaviors; (d) negative reinforcement via anxiety reduction associated with decreased family conflict and school or task avoidance; (e) classical conditioning of physiological and/or overt behavioral responses in the form of conditioned aversions and anxiety; (f) known iatrogenic effects of treatments and procedures utilized for chronic disease; and (g) operant control of pain-related responses. Although some experimental investigations have focused on an analysis of some of these individual factors, the interaction of these variables is difficult to demonstrate empirically and is most often hypothesized retrospectively. That is, once maladaptive behaviors are exhibited, identification of the controlling variables occurs similar to a post-hoc analysis. The interactive model presented here synthesizes this process and can be applied prospectively rather than retrospectively.

IMPLICATIONS OR TREATMENT AND RESEARCH: FUTURE DIRECTIONS

It was our intention in this chapter to critically review the literature in the area of pediatric behavioral medicine, and then propose an interactional model that could account for the various problems clinicians encounter. This proved to be an extremely difficult task. Although research and clinical practice have identified certain variables that interact to increase the probability of maladaptive illness behaviors, the specific nature of these interactions are, as yet, not well understood. The field of pediatric health psychology must move away from the mere documentation of such interactions toward a model that will assist us in predicting children at high risk for the development or maintenance of illness behaviors so that intervention may be facilitative in reducing both morbidity and psychosocial dysfunction. Continued emphasis on the interaction of variables ultimately may necessitate the utilization and development of more complex research and intervention designs. Increased reliance on mathematical or statistical model building might prove to be fruitful.

Despite the current conceptual limitations of the interactional model, various treatments derived from these models have been documented to be effective in decreasing illness behaviors. In this last section, treatments that have been used in the context of interactional models of chronic illness are briefly described. Then, directions for future research are discussed.

Treatment Directions

An interactional analysis of the maintaining variables of maladaptive behaviors is critical to the development of the most effective treatment program. Hovanitz, Gerwell, and Russo (in press) proposed a model for determining the maintaining variables of illness behaviors and for developing subsequent treatment suggestions. For example, if the observed symptom is a direct physiological outcome of a chronic disease and the behavior worsens under stress, the maintaining variables may be hypothesized to be physiological in nature. Cognitive and physiological regulatory techniques are likely to be most effective for the treatment of these conditioned physiological responses, particularly if the child can adequately self-monitor. Biofeedback has also been documented to be effective for patients with somatic complaints who are reluctant to accept psychological interventions (Klonoff & Moore, 1986; Klonoff, Youngner, Moore, & Hershey, 1983). If the behavior becomes more frequent when contingent attention is provided, or if the behavior results in decreased contact with aversive stimuli (such as cessation of parental conflict or avoidance of aversive activities such as school), then positive and negative reinforcement, respectively, may be maintaining the illness behaviors. In these cases, operant and social learning techniques may be the recommended treatment approach.

Klonoff, Ginsberg, and Janata (1985) proposed an age-dependent model for the treatment of pain-related behaviors. Relaxation and self-control strategies were found to be most effective for children over the age of 10 years, whereas parental contingency management training, focusing on shifting reinforcement toward nonillness behaviors, was generally most effective for younger children. Parental modeling of adaptive responses can also be employed to facilitate the child's acquisition of these responses; at other times, videotaped modeling may be effective in teaching appropriate coping responses (e.g., Melamed & Siegel, 1975).

For the child who develops school avoidance secondary to the treatment of a chronic disease, an educational evaluation may be helpful to rule out a learning disability. Social skills training may also be employed to remediate social anxiety and social delays such that the child can successfully accomplish the developmental task of acquiring an age-appropriate peer group. When skill deficits are compounded by conditioned aversions, as in the case of organic or iatrogenically induced feeding difficulties, a complex shaping program augmented by desensitization and contingency management procedures has proven effective (Ginsberg & Klonoff, 1985, 1987; Handen, Mandel, & Russo, 1986).

In sum, a variety of behavioral treatment approaches for illness-maintained maladaptive behaviors have been utilized successfully including contingency management, extinction procedures, skills training, modeling, systematic-desensitization, and cognitive and physiological regulatory techniques. The development of an appropriate treatment plan is facilitated by an experimental analysis of the interaction of controlling variables in maintaining illness behaviors. Under such a strategem, each case must be considered an independent analysis with disease factors, child development considerations, and family variables all contributing to the assessment and design of treatment.

Research Directions

Although the child with chronic disease may be at two to three times greater risk for the development of mental health problems in comparison to their physically healthy peers (Pless & Pinkerton, 1975), the presence of a chronic disease alone is insufficient to explain the development of maladaptive responses. Although we have introduced four factors that may be related to the emergence or maintenance of problem behaviors (characteristics of the illness itself, iatrogenic aspects of treatment, changes in reinforcement patterns, and life stresses), continued study is necessary to determine the relative contribution of each. In this section, suggestions for future research specific to each of these four factors are considered.

Characteristics of the disease. As commented on previously, a disease-specific approach has not consistently yielded helpful information. An interactional model emphasizes the need for research to be more functional in orientation. Thus, for example, investigators may choose to look at the emergence of maladaptive behavior in children who miss a certain amount of school, or who are diagnosed coincidental with certain developmental milestones. This functional approach places emphasis on understanding the increased probability of maladaptive behaviors, irrespective of the specific disease entity.

In addition, future research might focus on the measurement and assessment of physiological responses that covary with various disease states as these may be relevant to an analysis of the presenting problem. This may be a particularly fruitful area of investigation when dealing with children with organic feeding difficulties as their physiological distress is not clearly understood. Physiological and biochemical measures, such as glycosylated hemoglobin in diabetic children, can also be especially useful indicators of compliance, another topic with clear interactional components.

Iatrogenic effects. Another area requiring continued investigation in children with chronic illness is the role of iatrogenic effects of treatment in the development of maladaptive responses. A functional analysis should focus on the identification of the learning mechanisms responsible for the development of these responses once they are overtly exhibited. In addition, much work is needed to identify those children with chronic disease who are at relatively greater risk for iatrogenic effects that impact developmental tasks. It is generally assumed that chronic illness may predispose a child to negative learning effects by increasing his or her vulnerability to the potentially negative impact of stressful life events. The environmental variables that interact to "trigger" maladaptive responses in the predisposed child require further evaluation in an effort to identify high-risk children and promote the development of prevention and early intervention strategies. For example, it is not clear whether all children who receive prolonged parenteral feeds are at equal risk for the development of alter feeding delays if they encounter additional psychosocial or physiological stress. The mechanisms that control successful adaptation of learning also warrant elucidation. That is, it is unclear why, for some children with chronic disease, normal developmental tasks are not impeded.

Changes in reinforcement patterns. Here again, broad-scale psychological research is needed. More information is needed to identify and predict which parents change their behavior toward their child when their child becomes ill, how that behavior change is manifested, and what the long-term implications of changes in parental reinforcement patterns might be. In order to better understand this process, large-scale studies investigating parental responses to acute versus chronic childhood illness are needed.

In addition, the intensive study of children with chronic illnesses who do not present any additional maladaptive behaviors may be an important area of investigation. A thorough analysis of parental and child responses might yield useful information that could enable health professionals to better predict who might be susceptible to adventitious reinforcement of maladaptive responses. Again, an interactional approach argues for a prospective methodology, that is, one that begins no later than the point in time at which the illness is diagnosed.

Life stresses. Much research is currently being conducted on the effects of life stresses on illness. Large-scale prospective studies are needed to determine who will develop what illness under what set of stressful circumstances. These studies should begin with the occurrence of the stress, and then follow the child and his or her family across time.

Finally, future research in the field of pediatric behavioral medicine should consider a developmental perspective in education, prevention, and health promotion (Roberts, Maddux, & Wright, 1984). Typically, research on behavioral correlates of health has been concerned with adults (Matarazzo, 1982), and childhood behavior is studied in terms of its ramifications for later adult health (Roberts et al., 1984). Research that focuses on child health behaviors for the sake of the child is generally lacking, and future research should take into account children's concepts of illness in terms of their developmental level (Bibace & Walsh, 1978).

CONCLUSION

In this chapter, we outlined recently emerging data that suggest that an interactive analysis of childhood chronic illness may serve as the most fruitful model to increase our abilities to predict, identify, and treat the child which chronic disease. Inherent in such a model are two major assumptions: that problems are best addressed by first assuming psychological normalcy, as opposed to deviancy, of the child/family system; and that solutions are often best produced by a thorough understanding of the process of learning and the process of change induced by the interaction of a chronic illness with the environment.

In its search for metavariables, such as personality traits, psychology has for many years failed to appreciate the potency and richness of the ubiquitous and ongoing effects of learning. This chapter underscores our contention that an understanding of learning principles is absolutely critical to the study of chronic illness in children and provides a scientifically and clinically rewarding basis for experimental investigations.

REFERENCES

Adler, R. (1971). Experimentally induced gastric lesions. *Advances in Psychosomatic Medicine*, *6*, 1–39.

Alexander, F. (1950). *Psychosomatic medicine*. New York: Norton.

Anderson, D. E., & Brady, J. V. (1979). Experimental analysis of psychosomatic interactions: Behavioral affluences upon physiological regulations. In R. S. Davidson (Ed.), *Modification of pathological behavior* (pp. 198–231). New York: Gardner Press.

Bakwin, H., & Bakwin, R. M. (1972). *Behavior disorders in children*. Philadelphia: W.B. Saunders.

Bedell, J. R., Giordan, F. B., Amour, J. L., Tavormina, J., & Boll, T. (1977). Life stress and the psychological and medical adjustments of chronically ill children. *Journal of Psychosomatic Research*, *21*, 237–242.

Bharani, S. N., & Hyde, J. S. (1976). Chronic asthma and the school. *Journal of School Health*, *46*, 24–30.

Bibace, R. H., & Walsh, M. E. (1978). Developmental conceptions in children's conceptions of illness. In G. Stone, F. Cohen, & N. Adler (Eds.), *Health psychology: A handbook*. San Francisco: Jossey-Bass.

Creer, T. L. (1970). The use of a time-out from positive reinforcement procedure with asthmatic children. *Journal of Psychosomatic Research*, *14*, 117–120.

Creer, T. L., Weinberg, E., & Molk, L. (1974). Managing a problem hospital behavior: Malingering. *Journal of Behavior Therapy and Experimental Psychiatry*, *5*, 259–262.

Drotar, D. (1981). Psychological perspectives in chronic childhood illness. *Journal of Pediatric Psychology*, *6*, 211–228.

Drotar, D., Baskiewicz, A., Irvin, N., et al. (1975). The adaptation of parents to the birth of an infant with congenital malformation: A hypothetical model. *Pediatrics*, *56*, 710–717.

Dunn, S. M., & Turtle, J. R. (1981). The myth of the diabetic personality. *Diabetes Care*, *4*, 640–646.

Engle, G. L. (1977). The need for a new medical model: A challenge for biomedicine. *Science, 196*, 129–136.

Fisher, E. B., Jr., Delamater, A. M., Bertelson, A. D., & Kirkley, B. G. (1982). Psychological factors in diabetes and its treatment. *Journal of Consulting and Clinical Psychology, 50*, 993–1003.

Fordyce, W. E., Shelton, J. L., & Dundore, D. E. (1982). The modification of avoidance pain behaviors. *Journal of Behavioral Medicine, 5*, 405–414.

Ginsberg, A. J. (in press). Feeding disorders in developmentally disabled populations. *Analysis and Intervention in Developmental Disabilities.*

Ginsberg, A. J., & Janata, J. W. (1986, November). *Insulin mismanagement as a purging technique for diabetics with eating disorders.* Paper presented at the Annual Meeting of the Association for Advancement of Behavior Therapy, Chicago, IL.

Ginsberg, A. J., & Janata, J. W. (1987). *A treatment model for the synergistic coexistence of insulin-dependent-diabetes-mellitus and eating disorders.* Manuscript submitted for publication.

Ginsberg, A. J., & Klonoff, E. A. (1987). *Early intervention in organic feeding disorders: A behavioral conceptualization.* Manuscript submitted for publication.

Ginsberg, A. J., & Klonoff, E. A. (1985, November). Treatment of oral feeding difficulties associated with gastrointestinal, respiratory, and cardiac disorders. In E. A. Klonoff (Chair), *Behavioral treatment of organic and non-organic feeding difficulties in children.* Symposium presented at the Annual Meeting of the Association for Advancement of Behavior Therapy, Houston, TX.

Grace, W. J., & Graham, D. T. (1952). Relationship of specific attitudes and emotions to certain bodily diseases. *Psychosomatic Medicine, 14*, 243–251.

Green, M. (1965). The management of long-term nonlife-threatening illnesses. In M. Green & R. S. Haggerty (Eds.), *Ambulatory pediatrics.* Philadelphia: W. B. Saunders.

Handen, B. L., Mandel, F., & Russo, D. C. (1986). Feeding induction in children who refuse to eat. *American Journal of Diseases in Children, 140*, 52–52.

Hovanitz, C., Gerwell, E., & Russo, D. C. (in press). Behavioral methods in chronic illness.

Hyler, S. E., & Spitzer, R. L. (1978). Hysteria split asunder. *American Journal of Psychiatry, 135*(12), 1500–1504.

Illingsworth, R. S., & Lister, J. (1964). The critical or sensitive period with special reference to certain feeding problems in infants and children. *Journal of Pediatrics, 65*, 839–848.

Johnson, S. B. (1986). Knowledge, attitudes and behavior: Correlates of health in childhood diabetes. *Clinical Psychology Review.*

Johnson, S. B. (1980). Psychosocial factors in juvenile diabetes: A review. *Journal of Behavioral Medicine, 5*, 95–116.

Kellerman, J., Zeitzer, L., Ellenberg, L., Dash, J., & Rigler, D. (1980). Psychological effects of illness in adolescence: Anxiety, self-esteem, and perception on control. *Journal of Pediatrics, 97*, 126–131.

Klonoff, E. A., & Moore, D. J. (1986). Conversion reactions in adolescents: A biofeedback-based operant approach. *Journal of Behavior Therapy and Experimental Psychiatry, 17*(3), 179–184.

Klonoff, E. A., Ginsberg, A. J., & Janata, J. W. (1985, August). Out-patient treatment of pediatric pain. In D. C. Russo (Chair), *Outpatient management of pediatric pain and neurological dysfunction*. Symposium presented at the Annual Meeting of the American Psychological Association, Los Angeles, CA.

Klonoff, E. A., Knell, S. M., & Janata, J. W. (1984). Fear of nausea and vomiting: The interaction among psychosocial stressors, developmental transitions, and adventitious reinforcement. *Journal of Clinical Child Psychology, 13*, 263–267.

Klonoff, E. A., Youngner, S. J., Moore, D. J., & Hershey, L. A. (1983). Chronic factitious illness: A behavioral approach. *International Journal of Psychiatry in Medicine, 13*, 173–183.

Levine, J. D., Gordon, N. C., & Fields, H. L. (1978). The mechanisms of placebo analgesia. *Lancet, 8091*(2), 654–657.

Locke, S. (1982). Stress, adaptation and immunity: Studies in humans. *General Hospital Psychiatry, 4*, 49–58.

Masek, B. J., Russo, D. C., & Varni, J. W. (1984). Behavioral approaches to the management of chronic pain in children. *Pediatric Clinics of North America, 31*, 1113–1131.

Matarazzo, J. D. (1982). Behavioral health's challenge to academic, scientific, and professional psychology. *American Psychologist, 37*, 1–14.

Mattsson, A. (1972). Long-term physical illness in childhood: A challenge to psychosocial adaptation. *Pediatrics, 50*, 801–811.

Melamed, B. G., & Siegel, L. J. (1975). Reduction of anxiety in children facing hospitalization and surgery by use of filmed modeling. *Journal of Consulting and Clinical Psychology, 43*, 511–521

Morrow, G. R., & Morrell, C. (1982). Behavioral treatment for the anticipatory nausea and vomiting induced by cancer chemotherapy. *The New England Journal of Medicine, 307*, 1476–1478.

Orr, D. P., Weller, S. C., Satterwhite, B., & Pless, I. B. (1984). Psychosocial implications of chronic illness in adolescence. *Journal of Pediatrics, 104*, 152–157.

Peabody, J. L., & Lewis, K. (1985). Consequences of newborn intensive care. In A. W. Gottfried & J. L. Gaiter (Eds.), *Infant stress under intensive care: Environmental neonatology*. Baltimore: University Park Press.

Pless, I. B., & Pinkerton, P. (1975). *Chronic childhood disorder: Promoting patterns of adjustment*. Chicago: Yearbook Medical Publishers.

Redd, W. H., & Andrykowski, M. A. (1982). Behavioral intervention in cancer treatment: Controlling aversion reactions to chemotherapy. *Journal of Consulting and Clinical Psychology, 50*, 1018–1029

Rees, L. (1964). The significance of parental attitudes in childhood asthma. *Journal of Psychosomatic Research, 7*, 253–262.

Roberts, M. C., Maddux, J. E., & Wright, L. (1984). Developmental perspectives in behavioral health. In J. D. Matarazzo, S. M. Weiss, J. A. Herd,

N. E. Miller, & S. M. Weiss (Eds.), *Behavioral health: A handbook of health enhancement and disease prevention*. New York: Wiley.

Russo, D. C. (1986). Chronicity and normalcy as the psychological basis for research and treatment in chronic disease in children. In N. Krasnegor, J. Arestch, & M. Cataldo (Eds.), *Child health behavior: A behavioral pediatrics perspective* (pp. 521–536). New York: Wiley.

Russo, D. C., Tarbell, S. E., & Follansbee, D. J. (in press). Learning and the modification of somatic function. In A. Brownstein & P. Harzem (Eds.), *Progress in behavioral studies*. Hillsdale, NJ: Erlbaum.

Shady, G. (1978). Coping styles of patients with life-threatening illness. A literature review. *Essence, 2*, 149–154.

Shapiro, J. (1983). Family reactions and coping strategies in response to the physically ill or handicapped child: A review. *Social Science Medicine, 17*, 913–931.

Starfield, B., & Pless, I. B. (1980). Physical health. In O. G. Brim & J. Kagan (Eds.), *Constancy and change in human development* (pp. 272–324). Cambridge, MA: Harvard University Press.

Stein, R. E. K., & Jessop, D. J. (1984). General issues in the care of children with chronic physical conditions. *Pediatric Clinics of North America, 31*, 189–198.

Stein, R. E. K., & Jessop, D. J. (1982). A noncategorical approach to chronic childhood illness. *Public Health Reports, 97*, 354–362.

Steinhausen, H. C., Schindler, H. P., & Stephen, H. (1983). Correlates of psychopathology in sick children: An empirical model. *Journal of the American Academy of Child Psychiatry, 22*(6), 559–564.

Sullivan, B. J. (1978). Self-esteem and depression in adolescent diabetic girls. *Diabetes Care, 1*, 18–22.

Surwit, R. S., Scovern, A. W., & Feinglos, M. N. (1982). The role of behavior in diabetes care. *Diabetes Care, 5*, 337–342.

Swift, C. R., Sidman, F., & Stein, H. (1967). Adjustment problems in juvenile diabetes. *Psychosomatic Medicine, 29*, 555–571.

Tavormina, J. B., Kastner, L. S., Slater, P. M., & Watt, S. L. (1976). Chronically ill children: A psychologically and emotionally deviant population? *Journal of Abnormal Child Psychology, 4*, 99–110.

Turkat, I. D. (1982). An investigation of parental modeling in the etiology of diabetic illness behavior. *Behavior Research and Therapy*.

Varni, J. W. (1983). *Clinical behavioral pediatrics: An interdisciplinary biobehavioral approach*. New York: Pergamon Press.

Weitzman, M. (1984). School and peer relations. *Pediatric Clinics of North America, 31*, 59–69.

Werry, J. S. (1972). Psychosomatic disorders. In H. C. Quay & J. S. Werry (Eds.), *Psychopathological disorders of childhood*. New York: Wiley.

Zeltzer, L. K., LeBaron, S., & Zeltzer, P. M. (1984). A prospective assessment of chemotherapy-related nausea and vomiting in children with cancer. *The American Journal of Pediatric Hematology/Oncology, 6*, 5–16.

10

Attention Deficit Disorder

William E. Pelham

Western Psychiatric Institute and Clinic
University of Pittsburgh, School of Medicine

Debra Murphy

Medical College of Wisconsin

Attention Deficit Disorder (ADD), also commonly referred to as hyperactivity, is a disorder of childhood believed to affect approximately 3–5 percent of the elementary-aged population of North America. Children with this disorder comprise the largest category of child referrals to mental health professionals (Ross & Ross, 1982). From an early age, ADD children exhibit symptoms of inattention, impulsivity, and overactivity that result in extreme disruption in daily living and severe deficits in such areas as academic performance, relationships with parents, teachers, peers, and siblings, and self-concept. The high referral rate, poor prognosis, and refractoriness of ADD make it a challenging treatment problem for professionals. It is one of the most relevant childhood disorders for clinicians and researchers interested in behavioral medicine because the disorder spans both medical and psychological disciplines. Efficacious treatment requires knowledge of both behavioral assessment and therapy, as well as pediatric psychopharmacology. The purpose of this chapter is to provide information regarding ADD that will be of use to clinicians and researchers from both medical and psychological disciplines. Given space limitations, the chapter focuses on recent issues and developments in four areas of primary interest for a behavioral medicine text: (a) diagnosis, (b) prognosis, (c) pharmacological treatment and its assessment, and (d) combined pharmacological and behavioral treatments.

DIAGNOSIS

Although the term "hyperactivity" has been widely used and commonly accepted as a synonym for ADD, the earliest descriptions of the disorder included symptoms of short attention span, poor concentration, unpredictable/explosive behavior, and impulsivity, in addition to excessive motor activity (Laufer, Denhoff, & Solomon, 1957). Similarly, following considerable research (see Douglas & Peters, 1979, for a review), the 1980 revision of the Diagnostic and Statistical Manual of Mental Disorders (DSM III; American Psychiatric Association, 1980) relabeled "hyperkinetic reaction of childhood" as "attention deficit disorder," and defined ADD in terms of developmentally inappropriate degrees of inattention, impulsivity, and hyperactivity, with the emphasis placed on the first two and with the presence of excessive motor activity not required for diagnosis.

Although there is general agreement regarding the core characteristics of inattention and impulsivity in ADD, there is considerable controversy regarding how they should be operationalized. In the DSM-III, behavioral descriptors were listed for each of the three core symptoms (attention, impulsivity, and hyperactivity), and a child had to exhibit a specified number of the items for a core symptom to be determined present. However, despite the attempt of operational criteria, many of the DSM III descriptors are subjective and ambiguous (Pelham, 1982), and they show poor discriminant validity. That is, factor analyses have not revealed separate factors reflecting three core symptoms and have not always shown that DSM III symptoms of ADD load with other ADD symptoms rather than symptoms of conduct disorder (e.g., Lahey et al., 1988a; Murphy, Pelham, Atkins, & Murphy, 1987).

Rather than separating the behavioral descriptors into the three core symptoms groups, the DSM-III-R (American Psychiatric Association, 1987) lists 14 symptoms of ADD, which it relabels as "attention deficit hyperactivity disorder (ADHD)," and requires that any 8 of the 14 be present for a child to be diagnosed. Nine of the 14 items were listed in DSM III. Even though they are not separated into symptom clusters, the descriptors continue to tap inattention, impulsivity, and overactivity. Compared to DSM III, some of the additional DSM III-R items are less subjective, more easily operationalized, and based on findings from controlled studies. For example, "has difficulty organizing work (not due to cognitive impairment)," was replaced with "often loses things necessary for tasks or activities at school or at home (e.g., toys, pencils, books, assignments)" (cf. Atkins, Pelham, & Licht, 1985). Whether the changes will improve diagnostic reliability and validity remains to be studied.

Although the DSM definitions of ADD are vast improvements over previous definitions, they are not without problems. In the DSMs the manner in which inattention, impulsivity, and hyperactivity have been operationalized is largely unempirical (Cantwell, 1987; Quay, 1986a). As a result there has been a great deal of debate (and too little research) regarding whether the changes made in DSM III-R are improvements. Further, because of the DSM procedure that lists diagnostic criteria and requires that an individual exhibit at least a minimum number from any of a longer list of symptoms, not all children diagnosed as ADD will exhibit the same type or degree of the core symptoms. The resulting diagnostic heterogeneity, as well as the lack of cross-situational consistency and the high behavioral variability that characterizes the disorder, have contributed to a relatively low reliability for the diagnosis (e.g., Kappas of only .5 to .6 were reported in the DSM III field trials) (APA, 1980). Although such findings have led some to question the validity of the diagnosis of ADD, it is important to emphasize that these difficulties are not unique to ADD, but are evident in most other areas of child psychopathology as well (Quay, 1986b). Excellent reviews of empirical and clinical factors involved in the assessment and diagnosis of ADD are available elsewhere (e.g., Barkley, 1982; Hinshaw, 1987a; Prinz, Moore, & Roberts, 1986; Sleator, 1986), and an extensive discussion is beyond our purpose. Instead, we shall briefly mention several of the most common and promising of the approaches that have been taken to operationalize the definition of ADD beyond a simple symptom list as provided in the DSMs.

Operationalizing the Definition of ADD

The most common procedures for operationalizing the definition of ADD in both clinical and research settings have been standardized parent and teacher rating scales, of which a number that assess multiple dimensions of psychopathology have been developed. Rating scales on which item clusters labeled "hyperactivity" or "inattention" have been identified in factor analyses (see Achenbach & Edelbrock, 1978, Hinshaw, 1987b, and Quay, 1986a, for reviews) included the Conners Teacher and Parent Rating Scales (Edelbrock & Achenbach, 1984; Goyette, Conners, & Ulrich, 1978), the Child Behavior Checklists (Achenbach, 1978; Edelbrock & Achenbach, 1984), and the revised Behavior Problems Checklist (Quay & Peterson, 1983).

In contrast to rating scales that tap a range of psychopathology, several rating scales have been developed exclusively to measure ADD. A parent-teacher rating scale on which a cutoff score of 15 has been the standard for diagnosing ADD for many years is the Abbreviated Conners Rating Scale or Hyperkinesis Index (ACRS) (Goyette et al., 1978). However, several problems have led to its fall from grace as a diagnostic tool (Prinz et al., 1986; Ullman, Sleator, & Sprague, 1985a). For example, the inclusion of items such as "temper outbursts, explosive and unpredictable behavior" led to misidentification of conduct-disordered children as ADD, and age interacts with ACRS score, with the result that a cutoff score of 15 identifies different levels of severity at different ages.

Other scales designed to measure ADD include two empirically derived scales—the ADD-H Comprehensive Teacher's Rating Scale (ACTeRS) (Ullman, Sleator, & Sprague, 1985b) and the IOWA Conners Rating Scale (Loney & Milich, 1982; Pelham, Milich, Murphy & Murphy, 1989); and two scales that are based on the DSM criteria for ADD—the Swanson, Nolan, and Pelham (SNAP) Rating Scale (Atkins, Pelham, & Licht, 1985) and the Disruptive Behavior Disorder (DBD) Rating Scale (Pelham, Gnagy, Greenslade, & Milich, in press). With the exception of the DBD, which is based on DSM III-R and therefore has not yet been widely studied, all of these rating scales have similar and adequate levels of reliability.

Although they are most commonly used as diagnostic instruments, there are a number of limitations in the use of rating scales. First, rating scales reflect the adult's perception of the child's behavior rather than the behavior itself. In addition, ADD children's behavior is highly variable across situations and raters. As a result, interrater agreement between teachers and/or parents rating the same child is relatively low, with correlations rarely exceeding .5 or .6 (e.g., Achenbach, 1978; Goyette et al., 1978). Further, although validity studies reveal that rating scale factors are correlated with direct observations and other measures of the behaviors that they are intended to reflect, these correlations are not nearly as high as one would hope (e.g., Abikoff, Gittelman, & Klein, 1980; Atkins et al., 1985; Atkins, Pelham, & Licht, 1989). Finally, it should be noted that rating scale *factors* rather than *items* form the basis for diagnostic decisions. Because factor scores are typically computed by adding the scores for all items loading on that factor, children can receive the same score with different combinations of symptom presence and severity. Therefore rating scales do not necessarily reduce the group heterogeneity that results from the DSM type of diagnostic procedure.

Given these limitations, rating scales should obviously not be used as the sole or definitive criteria in the diagnosis of ADD. In most studies of ADD, extreme scores on appropriate instruments, particularly teacher rating scales, are viewed as necessary but not sufficient criteria for diagnosis. Clinical judgment must be used in interpreting ratings and resolving discrepancies between different raters of the same child and between ratings and other sources of information. For example, a mother who has only one child may not have a good reference set as to how a typical child behaves. She may rate her truly ADD child as nonproblematic on a rating scale when his teacher, who has seen many children for extended time periods, rates the child as a severe problem. Good judgment, as well as DSM III (p. 43), suggests that weight should be placed on the teacher rating in such a case. Discussions of the process of integrating rating scale with other data in diagnosis are available (Achenbach, 1985; Cantwell, 1987; Conners, 1987).

A great deal of research has focused on the nature of ADD children's behavior and performance on measures other than rating scales for diagnostic purposes, including laboratory measures of inattention, impulsivity, and neurobiological functioning, as well as direct observations in the natural environment. Comprehensive reviews of these studies are available elsewhere (Campbell & Werry, 1986; Douglas, 1983; Ferguson & Rapoport, 1983; Milich & Kramer, 1984; Zametkin & Rapoport, 1987). Despite the consensus that ADD children have deficits in attention and impulsivity, there is little agreement regarding how these deficits are best measured in the laboratory. ADD children routinely exhibit performance deficits on vigilance tasks and often on measures of attentional capacity or effort, but they perform no worse than controls on selective attention tasks that measure distractibility. Similarly, ADD deficits are found on some but not all laboratory measures of impulsivity. For example, one of the most widely used but one of the *least* reliable and *least* valid tasks is the Matching Familiar Figures Test (Milich & Kramer, 1984). Even when reliable differences are found on laboratory tasks of inattention and impulsivity, however, they are not sufficiently large to be useful in diagnosis (Milich, Pelham, & Hinshaw, 1986). The same situation exists when studies of observations of ADD children in school settings are examined. Although there are often large mean differences between ADD and comparison groups (e.g., in off-task and disruptive behavior), the differences are not large enough to have diagnostic importance (e.g., Abikoff et al., 1980; Atkins et al., 1985). Unfortunately, no solution is offered by moving into the realm of biological measures. Recent reviews have shown quite convincingly that measures such as neurotransmitter metabolite levels, evoked cortical potentials, indices of peripheral or central arousal, and various neuroanotomical measures have revealed no consistent pattern of findings that are useful in the diagnosis of ADD.

Subgrouping Issues in the Definition of ADD

The realization that the ADD population is not homogeneous with respect to etiology, symptomatology, or prognosis has led in the past few years to research into possible subgroups of the disorder that might be homogeneous with respect to these dimensions. One attempt to deal with this issue was the separation in DSM III of ADD children into those with (ADD/H) and those without (ADD/Not H) deviant levels of motor activity.This dichotomy was not empirically based when DSM III was developed, but it has been the attention of recent research (Carlson, 1986). Although some research has supported the validity of the category (e.g., Lahey et al., 1988a), ADD/Not H was dropped from DSM-III-R because a majority of the subcommittee working on the ADD category believed that there was insufficient empirical support for it. Other subtyping approaches that have been investigated include presence of concurrent aggression, various measures of organicity, concurrent learning disabilities, and drug responsiveness. As we noted above, no biological measure has proven useful in subgrouping the disorder (Zametkin & Rapoport, 1986), including response to medication, which has been widely advocated as a promising subgroup approach (e.g., Swanson & Kinsbourne, 1979; Swanson, Sandman, Deutsch, & Baren, 1983). Further, no correlates of the presence of a concurrent learning disability besides the defining one have been discovered.

In contrast to these disappointing results, one approach to subgrouping that has been validated and is now widely accepted is the presence of concurrent aggression (Milich & Loney, 1979). Opinion regarding the independence or amount of overlap between the externalizing symptomatology of ADD and aggression has undergone a metamorphosis in the last decade. Because aggression or Conduct Disorder (CD) and hyperactivity or ADD rating scale factors share a large common variance, the relationship between aggression as the primary symptom of CD, and ADD has been a much debated subject. Various studies have shown that 25–60 percent of ADD children are rated as aggressive by parents, teachers, and peers (Stewart, Pitts, Craig, & Dieruf, 1966; Prinz, Conner, & Wilson, 1981; Pelham & Bender, 1982). From earlier views that proposed that these two disorders were basically the same (e.g., Quay, 1979), the consensus now appears to be that not only are the disorders distinct, but that valuable information is obtained by assessing both dimensions concurrently (see Hinshaw, 1987b, for a comprehensive review). In addition, there is growing evidence that those children who exhibit both ADD and aggression may constitute a diagnostic entity separate both from ADD and from conduct problems. Failure to differentiate ADD children with concurrent aggression from those without it obscures important differences between the subgroups.

In the seminal study, Loney and her colleagues conducted a factor analysis on psychiatric chart ratings of a number of symptoms of ADD and CD for a sample of outpatient hyperactive boys (Loney, Langhorne, & Paternite, 1978). They identified one factor on which the symptoms of ADD loaded (which they labeled "H" for hyperactivity) and a second factor on which symptoms of conduct disorder loaded (which they labeled "A" for aggression). Although the two factors were correlated, they showed evidence of differential validity in this and subsequent studies. For example, differential patterns of correlations were found with a number of familiar measures, suggesting that high levels of aggression were associated with low SES, hostile fathers, and undercontrolling mothers—associations that were not found for the hyperactivity dimension (e.g., Milich, Loney, & Landau, 1982; Paternite & Loney, 1980). Similar findings have been reported in other studies (e.g., Werner, Bierman, & French, 1971).

Loney and Milich (1982) developed the IOWA Conners Teacher Rating Scale to operationally define their dimensions of hyperactivity and aggression. The I/O and A subscales were created by identifying those items from the CTRS that correlated most highly with either but not both of the Hyperactivity or Aggression chart rating factors, and children are given scores on both scales. In academic settings, the hyperactivity dimension has been found to be associated with such variables as observations of activity level, inattention, noncompliance, and daily academic productivity and accuracy (Loney & Milich, 1982); Milich & Fitzgerald, 1985; Roberts, 1987). The A scale has been found to be associated with verbal and physical aggression and verbal disruption in the classroom (Atkins et al., 1989; Milich & Pelham, 1985).

Subgroup differences have also been found in the critical area of peer relationships (see Campbell & Werry, 1986, Milich & Landau, 1990, Pelham & Milich, 1984, and Whalen, 1989, for reviews). Both ADD children and aggressive children are observed to engage in high rates of negative interaction with peers and receive high numbers of negative nominations from their peers on classroom sociometrics. However, subgroups differ in the style of their interactions, with HA boys generally showing more impulsive, aggressive, and bossy behavior than H or A boys (e.g., Pelham & Bender, 1982).

The differences that we have been discussing are found when formal diagnoses rather than ratings on H and A dimensions are considered. In one sample, 61 percent of hyperactive children were also given a concurrent diagnosis of aggressive CD, and within a CD group 67 percent were also given a diagnosis of hyperactivity (e.g., Stewart, Cummings, Singer, & deBlois, 1981). This high degree of co-occurrence necessitates studying the separate contributions of ADD and CD diagnoses in referred children (Milich & Loney, 1979). Recent studies that have done this have shown that measures of parental pathology are associated with a CD diagnosis rather than an ADD diagnosis, and that parents of children with both diagnoses exhibit the most severe pathology (Lahey et al., 1988b; Stewart, deBlois, & Cummings, 1980). This subgroup analysis thus clarified earlier studies that had associated parental pathology with a diagnosis of ADD (e.g., Cantwell, 1975).

Finally, it is worth noting that we have been discussing the utility of aggression/CD in subgrouping ADD as if aggression and CD are unitary constructs. As we discussed with ADD, CD can be diagnosed with a number of different patterns of symptoms, and these symptoms are not equivalent in their concurrent or prognostic correlates (Quay, 1986c). It appears likely that one clear area of future research will be the relative utilities of different types of aggression and conduct disorder in subgrouping ADD.

Summary

The problems of definition outlined in this section should alert the reader to the complexities involved in diagnosing ADD. Different patterns of symptoms can lead to the same diagnosis; rating scales are necessary but imperfect tools for operationalizing symptomatology; no useful neurobiological measure, laboratory task, or classroom observation has diagnostic utility, and, with the exception of aggression, subgrouping procedures are of limited utility. It is important to note, however, that most of these issues should be of primary concern for the researcher rather than the clinician. Diagnostic homogeneity and discriminant validity are quite important for researchers studying the nature, etiology, and prognosis of the disorder. However, the clinician's primary concern with an individual case should be an accurate and comprehensive clinical assessment rather than a diagnosis. Guidelines for such clinical assessments have been presented elsewhere (Sleator & Pelham, 1986).

It is important to note that, with few exceptions, knowing whether a child meets diagnostic criteria for ADD does not provide information relevant for that child's treatment—either pharmacological or psychosocial (Conners & Wells, 1986). Whether a child meets exact DSM criteria for ADD should therefore not be the critical variable in deciding whether that child should receive behavioral treatment or a trial of psychostimulant medication. Instead, the degree to which the child is experiencing dysfunction in daily living, the nature and frequency of the child's target symptoms, his educational placement, and the family situation—all information gathered during assessment—are more pertinent to the question of appropriate treatment than is whether the child meets diagnostic criteria for ADD.

As in most other areas of psychopathology, clinicians who need to make a diagnosis for administrative or clinical reasons should follow the procedures and recommendations made in the DSMs. In order to provide a comprehensive basis for diagnosis, information should be gathered from both parents and teachers, with weight given to teacher information, and using both interviews and standardized rating scales. As DSM III-R notes, the diagnosis must be based on the child's behavior in the natural environment and can neither be ruled in nor ruled out based on behavior in the clinician's office (Sleator, 1986).

PROGNOSIS

Although the follow-up studies have shown for at least five years that ADD children continue to have problems into adolescence and adulthood, it is still commonly believed outside of academic settings that ADD children outgrow their disorder when they reach puberty. In reality, at least two-thirds to three-quarters of children diagnosed as ADD exhibit a variety of serious problems when they reach adolescence and adulthood (Murphy & Pelham, 1988).

A major reason for the misbelief that the children outgrew their disorder is that the core symptoms of ADD all improve in absolute levels with age. Attentional abilities, impulsive control, and unrestrained activity each improve developmentally in all children—

normal as well as ADD. Thus 12-year-old ADD boys in fact have much longer attention spans than 7-year-old ADD boys. These improvements led parents and professionals to believe that the children were outgrowing their problems. However, when attention and impulsivity are measured in adolescence, it is clear that the differences between ADD and comparison children remain. For example, on laboratory measures of attention and impulse control, as well as upon parental and self-report, ADD adolescents exhibit deficits quite similar to those they showed in childhood (e.g., Gittelman & Mannuzza, 1985; Gittelman, Mannuzza, Shenker, & Bonagura, 1985; Hoy, Weiss, Minde, & Cohen, 1979; Klorman, 1986; Neuchterlein, 1983; Stewart, Mendelson, & Johnson, 1973).

Given that their core deficits remain and given that expectations and rules for appropriate behavior are more restrictive after than during childhood, it is not surprising that ADD children's difficulties continue. For adolescents and adults the range and number of areas of functioning that their ADD symptomatology affects broadens. For example, a young ADD child who impulsively pockets a candy bar in his mother's company at the local market is chastised by his mother or the clerk and punished at home. In contrast, when an adolescent ADD child impulsively pockets a cassette at a record store and is caught, he comes into contact with the legal authorities for shoplifting. Similarly, the consequences for misbehavior at school become more severe as a child moves from elementary to middle to high school. Thus, follow-up studies have reported that 67 percent of ADD adolescents are serious discipline problems in school, with high rates of school suspensions and expulsions found (Mendelson, Johnson, & Stewart, 1971; Weiss & Hechtman, 1986); and 50–70 percent of adolescent hyperactives have average failing grades in high school, and have failed at least one grade in school, and half of these have failed two grades (Dykman & Ackerman, 1980; Huessy & Cohen, 1976; Weiss, Hechtman, Perlman, Hopkins, & Wener, 1979; Weiss, Minde, Werry, Douglas, & Nemeth, 1971).

In addition to cognitive and academic deficits, follow-up studies have also focused on the rates of school dropout and criminal offenses, and rates of later referral for psychiatric care or institutionalization for delinquency or psychopathology. In the bleakest outcome yet reported for adolescent ADD children, Satterfield, Hoppe, and Schell (1982) followed 110 outpatient hyperactive boys and matched controls. At follow-up the mean age of the ADD adolescents was 17.3 (range 14–21). Arrests for serious crimes (robbery, burglary, grand theft, grand theft automobile, and assault with a deadly weapon) as obtained from court records was the measure of interest. Rates of both single and multiple arrests were significantly higher for the ADD group, as was institutionalization for delinquency. For lower, middle, and upper socioeconomic classes, the rates of at least one arrest were 58 percent, 36 percent, and 52 percent for the ADD children, respectively; and 11 percent, 9 percent, and 2 percent for the matched controls. Twenty-five percent of the ADD adolescents had been institutionalized compared to 1 percent of the controls.

In contrast to Satterfield et al.'s results, Weiss et al. (1979) reported a more benign outcome. At 10-year follow-up, their hyperactive subjects, aged 17 to 24 years, were interviewed and ratings were gathered from employers. They were found to have less education, a history of more motor vehicle accidents, a higher frequency of characterological and personality trait disorder diagnoses, and more geographical moves than matched controls. However, only a small percentage of the hyperactive group were still exhibiting antisocial behavior or severe psychopathology. Similar findings were reported by Borland and Heckman (1976), who examined adult adjustment of 20 men who had been seen at a child guidance clinic 25 years earlier and who were retrospectively diagnosed as hyperactive. Comparisons were made between the probands and their brothers. Percentages of probands and brothers, respectively, who reported the following psychological problems were: nervousness, 60 percent and 20 percent; restlessness 60 percent and 0 percent; difficulty with temper, 60 percent and 15 percent; impulsiveness, 40 percent and 10 percent; and lack of friends, 40 percent and 10 percent. Twenty percent of the targets were diagnosed as sociopathic, and 25 percent reported that they had sought professional help in the past. None of their brothers were given a diagnosis or reported ever having sought professional help. These investigators also reported that their subjects changed jobs more often than their brothers and achieved lower levels of vocational functioning than predicted based on their fathers' occupations. Other studies have also reported that hyperactive adults have more difficulties in carrying out assigned tasks at work and are laid off and quit jobs more frequently than controls (Weiss & Hechtman, 1986).

Finally, it should be noted that these studies have followed ADD individuals only to young adulthood, and they therefore underestimate the probability of adult problems in the ADD groups. When the likelihood of mental health difficulties across the entire life span is projected, there is evidence that children with ADD symptoms are at risk for, among other problems, alcohol abuse, and schizophrenia (Robins, 1966; Rieder & Nichols, 1979).

Although their average prognosis is poor, not all ADD children continue to have later difficulties. Not surprisingly, childhood aggressiveness has been implicated as a good predictor of later outcome among ADD children. Milich and Loney (1979) were the first to argue that the presence of concurrent aggression appeared to place ADD children at great risk for continued problems, and their conclusions have since been validated. Several prospective studies have shown that the level of aggression in ADD children predicts whether they will later show continued aggression, delinquency, and adult criminal behavior (August, Stewart, & Holmes, 1983; Farrington, Loeber, & van Kammen, 1987; Johnston & Pelham, 1986; Loney, Kramer & Milich, 1981). The implication of these studies is that Satterfield et al.'s group of ADD children must have been predominately aggressive ADD children and Weiss et al.'s must have been predominately nonaggressive. This is consistent with an earlier multivariate study (Loney, Kramer, & Milich, 1981), in which the single significant predictor of aggressive interpersonal behavior at adolescence was child aggression at referral; predictors of hyperactive symptoms at follow-up included hyperactivity, lower socioeconomic status, child aggression, and perinatal complications. However, one epidemiological study presents a slightly different picture (Farrington, Loeber, & van Kammen, 1987). In this study, both the hyperactive and the conduct problem groups were more likely than controls to be convicted of a juvenile crime, with children having both disorders having the highest conviction rate (i.e., the effects of H and A were additive). Only the conduct problem group had elevated rates of adult offending; but among offenders, hyperactivity predicted early conviction and *both* dimensions independently predicted chronic offending.

Particularly interesting is that the aggressive ADD subgroup appears to overlap considerably with extremely disturbed subgroups in other areas of child psychopathology in which prediction of adult outcome is being studied. Included are the prediction of criminal behavior (Loeber & Schmaling, 1985a) and of adult schizophrenia (Ledingham, 1981). It has long been known that a proportion of children with externalizing problems have highly probable psychopathological or criminal outcomes as adults (e.g., Robins, 1966), but it has not been known what beyond the early aggression that places them at risk insures that their adult outcome will be negative. There are striking similarities between aggressive ADD children and those children that Loeber and Ledingham have been studying. Research appears to be coalescing that shows that the children variously labeled as hyperactive/aggressive (as we have discussed), overt or versatile CD (Loeber & Schmaling, 1985a, 1985b), and aggressive/withdrawn (Ledingham,

1981; Milich & Landau, 1984) are the *same* children and form the core of that at-risk group.

Summary. It is apparent from the studies reviewed here that most ADD children do not outgrow their disorder. Their deficits as adolescents and adults include continued problems with the core symptoms of inattention, impulsivity, and restlessness; continued academic and later vocational adjustment difficulties; delinquency and later criminal behavior; and a variety of other mental health problems. There is a consensus that many children diagnosed as ADD will continue to have problems, with percentages ranging from 50–80 percent, although the severity of these problems vary across outcome studies. Those ADD children who are also aggressive appear to be at much greater risk for continuing to have serious problems than those who are not. There are numerous differences among the outcome studies—some are retrospective and sample inclusion criteria and informants differ—that limit drawing firm conclusions. A plausible summary of studies conducted thus far is that hyperactive children have a possibility for one of three adult outcomes, each of which are approximately equally probable: one-third of hyperactive children may be essentially normal as adults; one-third may exhibit a variety of mild to moderate adjustment difficulties that interfere with their interpersonal and vocational adjustment; and one-third are likely to be diagnosed as having serious psychopathology or to be in serious trouble with legal authorities.

PHARMACOLOGICAL INTERVENTION

Pharmacological intervention with one of the central nervous system (CNS) stimulant drugs has been the most common mode of treatment for ADD for the past 25 years. Although other classes of drugs have been evaluated for ADD, they have not been widely used, and they have not met with much success (Cantwell & Carlson, 1978; Gittelman & Kanner, 1986). In contrast, 80–90 percent of all ADD children have been treated with a CNS stimulant at some point in time (Bosco & Robin, 1980), and the drugs have been shown to be quite effective in the short-term management of the disorder. The purpose of this section is to describe the effects that stimulant drugs have on ADD children and their role in a comprehensive treatment for ADD. Because of the drugs' ubiquitous role in treatment of ADD, professionals interested in ADD from a behavioral medicine perspective need to be much more knowledgeable about stimulants than is typical and need to play a major role in both studying stimulant effects and collaborating with physicians in the drugs' use in treatment.

Basic Information

The three psychostimulants that are commonly employed with ADD children are methylphenidate (MPH; Ritalin), dextroamphetamine (Dexedrine), and pemoline (Cylert), with many more children receiving MPH than dextroamphetamine or pemoline. These drugs have relatively brief half lives; they take effect quickly and their effects wear off quickly. Behavioral effects are observed within 30 minutes (regular MPH and dextroamphetamine) to 90 minutes (pemoline) following ingestion (Swanson, Kinsbourne, Roberts, & Zucker, 1978; Stephens, Pelham, & Skinner, 1984). The behavioral effects of MPH and dextroamphetamine peak approximately 2 hours post ingestion and generally disappear 2 (MPH) to 4 (dextroamphetamine) hours later (e.g., Brown, Hunt, Ebert, Bunney, & Kopin, 1979; Solanto & Conners, 1982; Swanson et al., 1978). Pemoline has a later peak and its effects last for a total of 8 to 10 hours (Sallee, Stiller, Perel, & Bates, 1985), as do the effects of timed-release forms of dextroamphetamine and methyphenidate (Pelham et al, 1987, 1990). Both MPH and dextroamphetamine are typically given with both breakfast and lunch, while the timed-release preparations and pemoline are given only with breakfast. The maximum effects of MPH and dextroamphetamine are observed following the first dose, while pemoline requires two consecutive days of dosing before maximum effects are obtained (Stephens et al., 1984).

There is considerable controversy regarding what dose of stimulant is best for ADD children (see the following discussion). Generally, MPH is administered twice daily in doses that range from .25 to .75 mg/kg of body weight, with dextroamphetamine doses half this amount. Pemoline dosing levels are not as well determined as for the other stimulants, but it appears that doses 4 to 6 times those of a single dose of MPH are required to yield the same behavioral effect (Stephens et al., 1984; Pelham et al., 1990). The dose ranges for these drugs that are described in most standard pharmacology texts and ADD treatment articles are considerably higher than those typically used in actual practice (cf. Cantwell & Carlson, 1978; Dulcan, 1986). For example, doses on the lower end of the MPH range described above are much more common than doses in the higher end of that range.

The precise neural mechanisms of the stimulants' effects in humans are as yet unknown (Solanto, 1984). The drugs are presumed to enhance broadly the effects of CNS neurotransmitters (the catecholamines, dopamine and norepinephrine) by increasing their availability at the synapse. This action appears to be nonspecific to types of stimulant and catecholamine (Zametkin & Rapoport, 1986). Although at one time, stimulant effects on ADD children were thought to be different from those that would be obtained with normal children (thus the old notion of the paradoxical effect), it is now clear that stimulants affect normal children and adults in the same manner that they affect ADD children (e.g., Peloquin & Klorman, 1986; Rapoport et al., 1980). Specifically, on a variety of measures the drugs increase activity or arousal in the CNS and improve performance on various laboratory tasks of cognitive functioning (Solanto, 1984). As at the neurochemical level, these changes appear to be nonspecific, occurring on numerous measures of CNS function. How these changes in CNS activity are related to changes in ADD children's behavior is not yet well understood (Zametkin & Rapoport, 1986).

Cognitive and Behavioral Effects of Stimulants

Whatever the underlying physiological action of the stimulants, a great deal is known about their effects on cognitive and behavioral measures. On laboratory measures of sustained attention and impulsivity stimulants have routinely been found to improve ADD children's performance. On a typical sustained attention or vigilance task, relative to a placebo condition, medicated children make fewer impulsive responses to nontarget stimuli, and they maintain attention and miss fewer targets (e.g., Sykes, Douglas, Weiss, & Minde, 1971). Similarly positive effects of stimulants have been reported on a wide variety of laboratory tasks of information processing and learning (for reviews see Cantwell & Carlson, 1978; Conners & Rothschild, 1968, Pelham, 1986a; Swanson & Kinsbourne, 1979). For example, beneficial stimulant effects (approximately 25 percent average improvement) have been consistently reported on paired-associate learning tasks, nonsense word spelling tasks, and other measures of learning (Douglas, Barr, O'Neill, & Britton, 1986; Pelham, Milich & Walker, 1986; Swanson et al., 1978; Stephens et al., 1984). These positive medication effects on cognitive tasks are observed on concurrent electrophysiological measures of brain activity (e.g., Klorman, Salzman, & Borgstedt, 1988; Swanson et al., 1983).

Given the results from laboratory cognitive tasks—stimulant-induced reductions in impulsivity and increases in attention—it should not be surprising that beneficial stimulant effects have been observed in ADD children's classroom behavior and performance. These are observed most clearly as reductions in classroom disruptiveness and increases in on-task behavior. Relative to unmedicated ADD children, those receiving stimulants decrease the extent to which they (a) talk

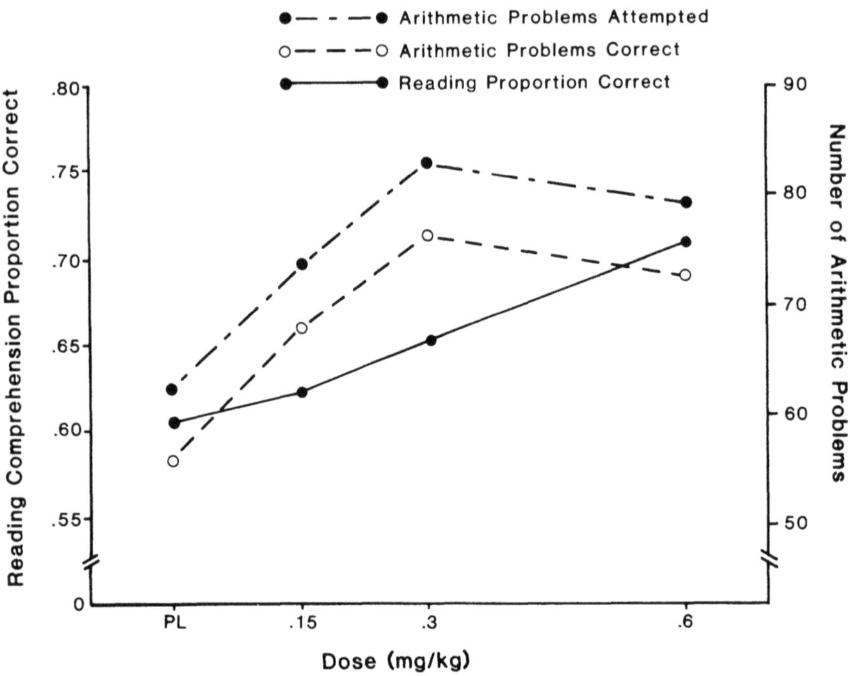

FIGURE 10.1 (Left panel:) Average number of arithmetic problems attempted and completed correctly during 15-minute period as a function of drug dosage. Proportion of reading problems completed correctly during 15-minute period as function of drug dosage. PL indicates placebo. (Right panel:) Frequency of negative behaviors during 30-minute classroom period as function of drug dosage. Proportion on task during 15-minute classroom observation as function of drug dosage. PL indicates placebo.

out inappropriately in class, (b) bother peers who are working, violate classroom rules or engage in other behaviors (e.g., noncompliance) that require teacher attention, and (d) interact aggressively and otherwise inappropriately with peers (e.g., Gittelman et al., 1980; Pelham & Bender, 1982; Pelham, Bender, Caddell, Booth, & Moorer, 1985; Whalen, Henker, Collins, Fink, & Dotemoto, 1979a). These effects, which have been reported in a very large number of studies and are among the most well documented treatment effects in child psychopathology, are clearly evident whether children are observed directly or rated by their teachers. Instead of engaging in inappropriate behaviors, ADD children medicated with stimulants spend more time on task and complete more of their assigned academic work, often with increased accuracy (e.g., Pelham et al., 1985, 1987, 1990; Rapport, Stoner, DuPaul, Birmingham, & Tucker, 1985). Medication effects on typical measures of behavior and academic performance in a recent study are shown in Figure 10.1.

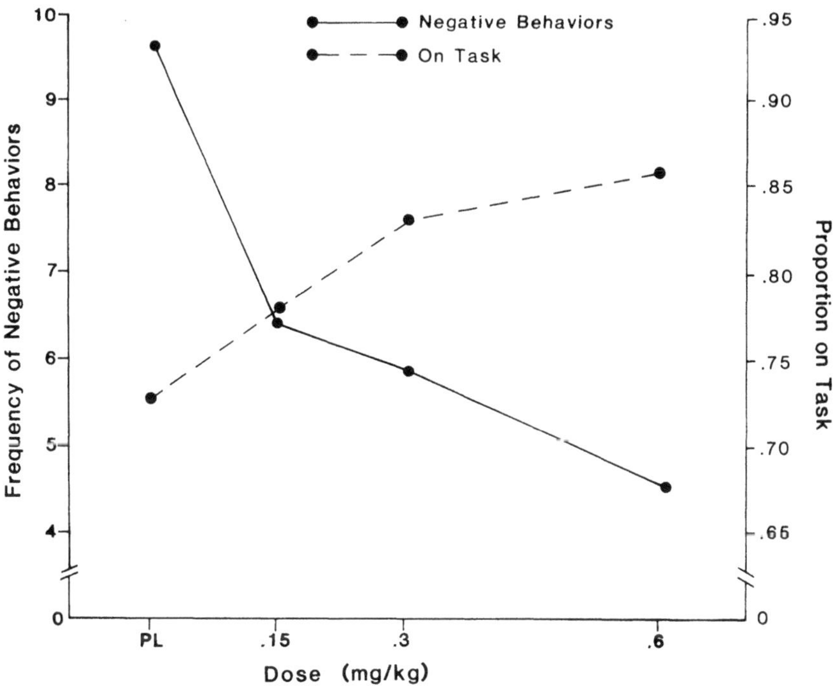

FIGURE 10.1. Cont.

It is quite important to note that drug-facilitated improvement in academic tasks or social behavior such as shown in Figure 10.1 will only be evident if children perform the academic tasks or engage in social interactions during the time when their medication is active. For example, for a child who takes his MPH at 7:00 a.m. and at noon, MPH will exert a clear effect on the child's behavior and academic performance between 8:00 a.m. and 10:00 a.m. (peak at 9:00 a.m.) and between 1:00 p.m. and 3:00 p.m. (peak at 2:00 p.m.). This medication schedule would not be expected to provide benefit on academic tasks or social behavior (e.g., during recess) that occurs between 10:00 and 1:00. The data reported in Figure 10.1 were gathered on average two hours after medication administration, during which time medication effects should have been at their peak.

There has been considerable debate regarding whether these salutary stimulant effects on classroom behavior and performance would be translated into long-term gains in academic achievement, an area in which most ADD children suffer (Gadow, 1986). To date, studies that have given stimulants to ADD children for as long as 18 weeks have failed to find significant drug effects on achievement (e.g., Gittelman, Klein, & Feingold, 1983). On the basis of negative results in early studies of 4 to 12 week drug trials, influential reviews concluded that stimulants did not affect academic achievement but affected only attention in the classroom (Barkley & Cunningham, 1978). However, those early studies have been severely criticized on methodological grounds, and an alternative interpretation of their failure to yield positive medication effects is that it results from flaws in the studies rather than a failure of medication (Pelham, 1983, 1986a). Because daily productivity and accuracy on academic assignments are among the best predictors of long-term achievement, it can be reasonably argued that ADD children who show stimulant-facilitated improvement in daily academic performance will have long-term gains in achievement (see Pelham, 1986a, for further discussion of this point). Because the relevant, controlled, outcome study has not yet been conducted, however, this hypothesis is at present unsupported by data. Further, because the nature of school settings and school work change in middle and junior high schools, it is not clear whether medication will result in long-term achievement changes for medicated children in those placements (Clampit & Pirkle, 1983; Murphy & Pelham, 1988; Pelham et al., 1991).

Studies in laboratory analogue settings have shown that stimulant drugs positively affect ADD children's behavior during structured parent-child interactions in the same way that the drugs affect the children's behavior at school. Medicated children are less disruptive and more compliant that nonmedicated children (e.g., Barkley, Karlsson, Strzelecki, & Murphy, 1984). Because medication is typically not given in the evenings, and the daytime doses have worn off by evening, however, these potentially beneficial effects on parent–child interactions are rarely realized in practice. Unless a third dose of medication is given in the late afternoon, parents usually will not see drug-related behavior changes and thus cannot be relied upon to detect them.

Although early studies suggested that medication did not have beneficial effects on ADD children's interaction with peers (see Pelham & Bender, 1982, for a review and examples), subsequent studies have contradicted those results. Acute dose studies have shown that for many ADD children moderate doses of methylphenidate both decrease aggression and increase prosocial interactions with peers in play settings (Hinshaw, Henker, & Whalen, 1984; Pelham & Hoza, 1987; Pelham et al., 1987; Whalen et al., 1987). Several qualifications of these effects need to be noted, however: (a) the beneficial effects of medication are much more evident when the medicated children are in groups of peers rather than in dyads (cf. Cunningham, Siegel, & Offord, 1985; Whalen, Henker, Collins, McAuliffe, & Vaux, 1979b); (b) reductions in aggression are clearest for those children who were most aggressive prior to medication (Murphy, Pelham, & Lang, in press; Pelham & Bender, 1982); and (c) these medication effects may depend on the presence of concurrent interventions, being most evident in settings in which concurrent behavioral interventions are in effect (e.g., Hinshaw et al., 1984; Pelham & Hoza, 1987; Whalen et al., 1987). Along with the drug effects noted above on parent–child interactions, these apparently beneficial stimulant effects on peer interactions have contributed to a recent trend to provide a third daily dose of medication and to medicate on weekends in order to affect children's behavior when they are with peers in both organized and sandlot activities. Although both clinical anecdotes (see Gadow, 1986, p. 56) and recent empirical evidence (Pelham, McBurnett, Harper, Murphy, Milich, Clinton, & Thiele, 1990) provide some support for the notion that stimulants improve ADD children's performance in sports activities, the incremental value of such a regimen beyond twice-daily dosing is to date uninvestigated. The increased risk of side effects generated by the increase in dose (see discussion below) may outweigh any added benefit of medication.

We have been discussing stimulant effects as if an average effect was characteristic of all ADD children. Unfortunately, not all ADD children show positive responses to stimulant drugs, and there are considerable individual differences in the size of the drug effect for those who do respond. Approximately 70 percent of ADD children respond positively to a stimulant regimen, but the remaining 30 percent show either an adverse response or none. Of those who do respond, only a minority show sufficient improvement for their behavior to fall entirely within the normal range; the rest are improved but their behavior is not normalized (e.g., Abikoff & Gittelman, 1985a; Sleator & von Neumann, 1974). For example, the average rating on the ACTRS for a group of unmedicated ADD children is often 20. In many drug studies, this mean rating decreases to 10, a 50 percent reduction. This compares with a score of only 2 or 3 that nondeviant children receive on this scale ($SD = 5$). Even for the majority of positive medication responders, then, ADD children are not "normalized" by medication even after it has been administered for up to 2 years (e.g., Riddle & Rapoport, 1976; Sleator & von Neumann, 1974). Interventions in addition to medication are required to maximize treatment efficacy for most medicated ADD children (Pelham & H. A. Murphy, 1986).

One variable on which the degree of a child's response to a stimulant drug depends is the administered dose. Generally, the larger the dose, the larger the drug effect, and the dose-response relationship is usually linear up to .6 mg/kg or slightly higher (Douglas et al., 1986; Rapport et al., 1985; Whalen et al., 1987). An example of this pattern can be seen in Figure 10.2 from Pelham et al. (1985); only the linear component of the dose effect was significant on all four dependent measures. Some authors have reported, however, dose-response curves that vary over tasks and are not linear. For example, in a widely cited study Sprague and Sleator (1977) presented data showing that maximal improvement on a cognitive, laboratory measure was obtained with .3 mg/kg of MPH, whereas maximal improvement in teacher ratings on the ACTRS was not apparent until the dose was 1.0 mg/kg, at which level children's performance on the cognitive task was impaired relative to placebo. However, Sprague and Sleator did not administer a dose between .3 and 1.0 mg/kg, and numerous studies including those cited above that have administered MPH doses up to .75 mg/kg have found improvement on cognitive tasks. Although most professionals agree with Sprague and Sleator's conclusion that classroom disruptiveness may require higher doses of stimulants to be corrected than cognitive deficits require, the precise point at which stimulants have adverse effects on cognition is not yet determined.

The fact that drug-related improvement is found on group data through .75 mg/kg, however, does not mean that this dose is appropriate for all children. There are large individual differences in the size and topography of the drug response among the 70 percent of ADD children who respond to stimulants. Although this fact has been known for some time (e.g., Conners, 1972), its profound implications for research and treatment have not been appreciated. Response to stimulants varies both across and within children and depends on dose, dependent measure, and the child's target symptoms (e.g., Conners & Wells, 1986; Pelham & Hoza, 1987). For example, in a partial replication and extension of the results presented in Figure 10.2, data were gathered and analyzed in such a way that single subjects' dose response functions could be plotted in addition to the group average. On many dependent measures, the group data did not accurately reflect dose effects for the individuals who made up the group (Pelham et al., 1992). Unfortunately, as noted above, no measures have been discovered that enable reliable prediction of drug response in individuals (e.g., Pelham & Milich, 1991). It is worth noting that this extends to commonly accepted diagnostic variables. Although some reviewers have argued that deficits on measures of attention predict drug response, and although a diagnosis of ADD is generally considered a prerequisite for a stimulant trial, neither of these common beliefs is supported by data (Conners & Wells, 1986).

In addition to the salutary main effects of stimulant drugs, other side effects or treatment emergent symptoms (TES) are sometimes associated with stimulant treatment (see Conners & Werry, 1979, and Gittelman & Kanner, 1986, for reviews). For example, long-term stimulant treatment (2 to 4 years) with average doses of 40 mg of MPH per day results in a reduction in the rate of weight gain and to a lesser extent height gain in treated children (Mattes & Gittelman, 1983). This effect is dependent on the total cumulative dose that the child takes, however, and can be avoided by keeping the dose low, medicating during school hours only, and by discontinuing medication on weekends and holidays (Gittelman-Klein & Mannuzza, 1988). Although not known for certain, this reduction in growth may result from the anorectic effect of stimulants. Medicated children usually have a reduced appetite and eat less at meals compared to placebo days. Stimulants can also cause socially withdrawn behavior in treated children (Pelham & Hoza, 1987), and as discussed above cognitive improvement occurs in some children at some doses (Sprague & Sleator, 1977; Swanson et al., 1978). Finally, stimulants have been reported to exacerbate motor tics when present in treated children, with some professionals even suggesting that stimulants can precipitate Tourette's syndrome. Although many of the most serious TES are rare, and although irreversible side effects are extremely rare, their potential impact means that medicated children should be very carefully monitored to insure that these adverse side effects are not caused or exacerbated by stimulant therapy. Several standard rating scales for evaluation of TES are available (Rapoport, Conners, & Reatig, 1985).

Clinical Assessment of Pharmacotherapy

The question facing every practitioner is how to decide whether a stimulant should be used with a child and what the correct dose should be. Our discussion of individual differences in response should alert the reader to the fact that a diagnosis of ADD does not convey automatic information about drug response. The "whether to medicate" decision is rarely made systematically in practice. Most often, parents contact their child's physician at the insistence of the school, and the physician prescribes medication (or does not) based on his or her knowledge and beliefs regarding the role of stimulants in the treatment of ADD. A starting dose is selected and increases are made based on parental reports until optimal drug response is presumably obtained and no adverse side effects are apparent. Neither drug response nor TES are measured systematically, and only rarely does the physician obtain information systematically about the child from the setting that initiated the referral—the school (Gadow, 1981, 1986). This procedure, which is fairly standardly recommended in pediatric psychopharmacology, has numerous shortcomings: it fails to gather systematically the information that should form the basis of a decision regarding whether to medicate (i.e., whether the medication has beneficial effects on the symptoms that prompted the referral and does not have adverse effects on other important domains of functioning); it confounds increasing medication dose with events that may be changing over time (e.g., improvement in the teacher's behavioral management of the child); and it results in children receiving the highest possible dose of stimulant (i.e., the dose is increased until side effects are observed).

Because of these shortcomings, alternative procedure for determining the utility of stimulant therapy for a child and for selecting the proper dose have been advocated in recent years (e.g., Barkley, Fischer, Newby, & Breen, 1988; Pelham & Hoza, 1987; Swanson et al., 1978). Because of their short half-lives and the fact that they do not require days of successive dosing to yield therapeutic effects, stimulants can be alternated frequently with placebo for brief periods of time (days or weeks) in a short-term, clinical trial designed to determine a child's response to medication. The assessment may take a total of 2 to 5 weeks, depending on the number of drugs or doses evaluated. All of the investigators currently conducting and writing about systematic medication assessments employ this alternating drug-condition protocol as well as placebo-controlled, double-blind procedures.Thus, what is essentially a single-subject study using an alternating treatments design is used to evaluate an individual child's response to medication. The information gathered in the assessment is used to make data-based recommendations concerning the utility of stimulant medication in a referred child's treatment. A variety of different types of medication assessments have been described, using different dependent measures and conducted in settings ranging from inpatient to outpatient. Most employ some type of laboratory- or office-based cognitive testing (e.g., a paired-associates learning task or a vigilance task), and teacher and parent ratings of main effects and TES. Those conducted in settings that lend themselves to gathering objective data often extend the dependent measures to behavioral observations. The general goal is to gather information on as many measures as possible, tapping all important domains of function. Because drug response in the natural environment cannot be reliably predicted from a single laboratory task (Pelham & Milich, 1991), the emphasis in an assessment of medication effects should be on measuring effects on the target symptoms on which change is desired in the settings in which the symptoms occur.

Because pediatricians and psychiatrists are usually not trained in the range of assessment procedures needed to conduct a comprehensive evaluation of this nature, psychologists and educational personnel need to work collaboratively with prescribing physicians to conduct these assessments. Some time may need to be invested initially convincing a child's physician that a comprehensive medication evaluation is necessary. A pediatrician who is used to writing a prescription for MPH without follow-up may find unnecessarily cumbersome the prospect of referring his patient for an assessment that may take five weeks and cost $300. However, given that the child may take medication for years and given the complex nature of response to stimulants, such an initial evaluation is well worth the cost. It is worthwhile to note that a straightforward psychoeducational evaluation, for which physicians routinely refer patients suspected of learning problems, costs $300 to $500.

Consider the following example of a medication evaluation conducted in our clinic. The assessment was conducted on a child participating in a summer day treatment program (STP) using a double-blind, placebo-controlled protocol in which active drug and placebo are alternated daily (Pelham & Hoza, 1987). As others', our purpose is to determine whether stimulants have a beneficial effect on a child and how they should be used in the child's long-term treatment.

The results of an assessment on one child, Matt, from our 1985 STP are presented in Table 10.1 (Pelham, 1986b). Matt was a severely hyperactive, 8-year-old child who also met diagnostic criteria for conduct disorder and learning disability. He had a long history of behavior and learning problems in school, had been retained once, and had been referred to the STP by his school psychologist. Table 10.1 shows the effects of .3 and .6 mg/kg MPH b.i.d. on Matt's behavior and performance in a wide variety of domains, and it illustrates many of the points we noted above regarding stimulant effects on ADD children.

On the daily frequency counts of how often Matt followed the rules as well as the measure of following rules in the classroom, MPH resulted in substantial improvement. Further, Matt was on task more in the classroom while medicated, and he completed more of his seatwork and performed more math and reading problems in timed tasks. When medicated, his accuracy on both the reading and math tasks improved, and he made fewer errors in a nonsense spelling learning task. As the table indicates, his teacher's and his counselors' ratings of his behavior improved dramatically on medication days. When medicated, Matt was also more compliant with adult requests, as indicated by the 50 percent decrease in recorded noncompliance.

Table 10.1.
Matt's Medication Assessment Results

Variable Measured	Placebo (7 days) M	Placebo (7 days) SD	.3 mg/kg MPH b.i.d. (6 days) M	.3 mg/kg MPH b.i.d. (6 days) SD	.3 mg/kg MPH b.i.d. (6 days) % Change from PL	.6 mg/kg MPH b.i.d. (6 days) M	.6 mg/kg MPH b.i.d. (6 days) SD	.6 mg/kg MPH b.i.d. (6 days) % Change from PL
Daily Frequencies:								
Following Rules	14.9	4.8	18.3	2.5	23	19.7	1.5	32
Noncompliance	12.7	9.4	7.3	6.8	−42	5.8	2.7	−54
Positive Peer Behaviors	37.3	10.3	65.5	23.2	76	87	31.3	133
Conduct Problems	.7	.8	.2	.4	−77	.2	.4	−77
Negative Verbalizations	8.3	4.8	5.8	3.7	−30	3.8	2.5	−54
Time Outs:								
Number per day	1.7	1.4	.2	.4	−91	.3	.5	−81
Minutes per day	38	45.3	1.7	4.1	−96	2.7	4.6	−93
Average minutes per Time Out	16.9	11.9	10	0	−41	8	4.2	−53
Classroom:								
% On Task	80	23	94	9.8	18	94	10	18
% Following Rules	57	20	71	37	24	96	5	69
Timed Math:								
Number Attempted	11.4	3.0	12.4	3.4	9	14.6	3.4	28
Percentage Correct	76	36.6	91.1	11.2	20	80	27.6	5
Timed Reading:								
Number Attempted	14	6.1	18.5	11.6	32	15.3	7.7	9
Percentage Correct	63.8	24.3	78.5	9.1	23	78	28.9	22
Seatwork:								
% Completion	56	41	81	35	45	88	16	57
% Correct	75	16	71	22	−5	83	15	11
Nonsense Spelling:								
Number of Errors	70	—	46	0	−34	—	—	—
Teacher Rating:								
(Conners Short Form)	16.5	.7	5	6.2	−70	4	0	−76
Counselor Rating	179	25	101	0	−43	99	15	−45
Pos. Daily Report Card								
(% of Days Received)	50	54	100	0	100	100	0	100
Observed Interactions:								
Positive Peer	94.4	5.0	98.8	1.6	5	97	3.5	3
Negative Peer	5.2	5.5	.4	.9	−92	2.3	2.9	−57
No Interactions	.4	.9	.8	1.3	100	.8	1.5	88

Stimulant-induced changes in Matt's antisocial behaviors are shown by the decreases in daily occurrences of conduct problems (stealing, lying, aggression, and destruction of property), negative verbalizations (e.g., cursing, name-calling, talking back), and observed negative peer interactions on the playground. It is interesting to note that these decreases were accompanied by increases in both daily frequency counts of positive peer behaviors (e.g., helping, sharing, saying something nice) and in observed positive peer interactions on the playground.

The data presented in Table 10.1 show that there were many intraindividual differences in the shapes of Matt's dose-response curves on different measures. Although his response to the two doses of MPH continued to improve in a linear manner as dose was increased on some measures (e.g., positive peer behaviors, classroom following rules), maximal response was reached on other variables at the low dose, .3 mg/kg. Sometimes when maximal response was reached at .3 mg/kg, the higher dose yielded only slight incremental improvement (e.g., noncompliance, teacher rating), whereas the higher dose appeared to worsen behavior on the other measures (e.g., percentage correct on timed math, observed negative peer interactions). Finally, on several measures Matt showed maximal improvement only with the high dose (e.g., negative verbalizations). These positive main effects of MPH were not accompanied by parent- and teacher-rated TES at the low dose, but on days when Matt received the higher dose, he exhibited pronounced irritability and anorexia.

It is noteworthy that the basic treatment in the STP was a highly structured behavior modification program that included a point system, response cost, time out, and a variety of other components. The medication assessments were conducted while the behavioral intervention was in effect. Matt's behavior on placebo days was quite deviant and thus reflected deficits that were not corrected with as intensive and comprehensive a behavioral intervention as we could design. Matt appeared to need both medication and a behavior modification program in order to show maximal improvement in his behavior.

Given the TES observed on the higher dose and the clearly beneficial effects of .3 mg/kg MPH on many of the symptoms for which Matt had been referred, we recommended that Matt receive that dose of MPH b.i.d. in conjunction with a behavioral intervention in his classroom setting. For the year following his assessment, he received that treatment regimen as well as resource room help for his learning disability, and his mother continued to receive parent training. Matt's behavior in school was much improved during that year, compared to the previous year when he was not medicated.

Long-Term Effects

Despite the often dramatic salutary short-term effects of stimulants, there is as yet no evidence that long-term stimulant therapy modifies the dismal adolescent and adult prognoses of ADD children (see Weiss

& Hechtman, 1986, for a review). At best, several studies have shown very weak residual beneficial effects on a few outcome measures when the young-adult outcome of ADD children medicated in childhood is examined. There has been considerable debate regarding why these short-term benefits fail to translate into long-term changes. Excessive doses, lack of compliance with prescribed regimens, absence of an effect on critical behavioral domains, lack of necessary concurrent interventions, and presence of a persistent, underlying biological deficit are all reasons that have been postulated to account for this discrepancy, but none have been systematically evaluated in outcome studies. Some researchers have argued that the discrepancy is only apparent, and that the long-term studies have failed to show long-term benefits because the studies are not well controlled and are insensitive to the effects they seek to measure. Finally, the problem may lie with professionals' expectations rather than with stimulant therapy. Why should it be expected that as little as 2 or 3 years of treatment during the elementary-school years would have residual effects 15 years later on children who have a chronic disorder?

No resolution of this paradox—that the acute studies of stimulant effects yield such positive results compared to the long-term outcome studies—is currently evident. The hope is that the effectiveness of long-term stimulant therapy will be increased if children undergo a systematic, clinical assessment as described above prior to beginning a stimulant regimen and if adequate monitoring procedures are used to follow a medicated child (for example, reassessing with a placebo probe at yearly intervals to insure that a medicated child continues to respond positively), and if other variables such as compliance and concurrent interventions are controlled. Finally, there is widespread agreement that stimulants should not be used in isolation in the treatment of ADD. A number of studies have demonstrated quite clearly that the combination of behavioral and stimulant interventions are more effective in the short-term than either treatment alone (Pelham & H. A. Murphy, 1986). As it was for Matt in our case example, the combination of these two modalities is becoming the treatment of choice for ADD. Further, there is good reason to believe that potentially beneficial medication effects may actually *depend* on the presence of appropriate, concurrent educational placement and instruction and behavioral interventions (see Pelham, 1986a, and Pelham & Hoza, 1987, for reviews).

As we discuss below, the importance of concurrent intervention cannot be overemphasized. All too often an ADD child's dramatic, short-term improvement with medication removes pressure from parents and teachers to invest the necessary effort in concurrent, comprehensive treatments, such as behavioral interventions. Parents then rely on the medication alone to solve the problem. Mental health professionals, educators, and physicians need to be especially alert to this possibility and to take action to prevent it from happening.

A final question that merits attention is how long a child should receive stimulant therapy. One approach has been to use stimulants for limited time periods (e.g., 3 to 6 months) to stabilize a problematic situation and to facilitate the initiation of other treatments. Although this approach has been frequently advocated, there are no guidelines suggesting how it is to be done (e.g., how medication is to be withdrawn), and no data that conclusively demonstrate its effectiveness. Maintenance stimulant regimens are more common. Several years ago, the *zeitgeist* was the stimulant therapy needed to be terminated when the target child reached puberty, as the medication would lose its effectiveness after that point. Recent studies have suggested, however, that stimulants have beneficial effects both on some ADD adolescents (Coons, Klorman, & Borgstedt, 1987; Pelham et al., 1991; Varley, 1983) and on some adults who have residual ADD (Wender, Reimherr, Wood, & Ward, 1985). At present, then, there are no data that provide a definitive answer to the question of how long a child should receive a stimulant drug. One answer that emphasizes the importance of the kind of assessment we have described is "as long as periodic, systematic evaluations reveal a therapeutic effect."

COMBINED PHARMACOLOGICAL AND BEHAVIORAL INTERVENTIONS: TREATMENT OF CHOICE

During the past few years, it has become clear that the most effective short-term treatment for the majority of ADD children is an intervention that combines pharmacological and behavioral treatment (see Pelham & H. A. Murphy, 1986, for a review), and this approach is rapidly becoming the treatment of choice for ADD (Donnelly & Rapoport, 1989). Behavioral interventions and stimulant therapy are the only validated treatments for ADD. Despite the evidence for their separate efficacies, however, both behavior therapy and psychostimulant medication have limitations that mean that neither alone constitutes a sufficient or maximally effective treatment for ADD. Further, each modality offers something that improves the other's effectiveness.

Insufficiencies of Psychostimulant Therapy

We have discussed above the limitations inherent in pharmacotherapy with the stimulants, and they can be briefly summarized. First, even with drug responders, stimulant therapy is rarely sufficient to bring children into a normal range of academic and social functioning, leaving room for improvement with additional interventions. Second, psychostimulant effects are limited to the time when the drugs are physiologically active. Stimulants typically do not provide adequate control of the child's behavior throughout the entire day, and because of potential side effects the medications are typically not administered in the late afternoons and evenings. Therefore interventions during the daytime when the medication is not active and in the evenings when the child is home are necessary. A final limitation of psychostimulant therapy is that without exception studies that have followed children treated with psychostimulant medication for periods up to 15 years have failed to provide any evidence that the drugs improve ADD children's long-term prognosis. Although their methodological inadequacies require that these studies be interpreted cautiously, they nonetheless argue clearly that stimulant medication as typically administered is an insufficient long-term treatment.

These limitations of pharmacotherapy are the most salient of those discussed earlier. They led in the 1970s to a number of studies designed to evaluate the efficacy of behavior modification/therapy with ADD children. These studies focused on teaching parents and teachers to implement contingency-management programs with their children, and results consistently demonstrated that behavioral interventions could be used as an alternative to medication in the treatment of ADD (e.g., O'Leary, Pelham, Rosenbaum, & Price, 1976; O'Leary & Pelham, 1978; Rapport, Murphy, & Bailey, 1982). At the same time, however, it has become clear that behavioral interventions with ADD children also have limitations that restrict their usefulness.

Insufficiencies of Behavioral Interventions

The shortcomings of behavioral interventions with ADD children are similar to those of psychostimulant medication. First, although a growing number of studies have shown that behavior therapy is effective in improving parent and teacher ratings on standardized rating scales of ADD, posttreatment ratings are usually one SD above normative means, and direct observations of classroom behavior and classmate sociometric ratings usually reveal that children often continue to function well outside the normal range even after treatment (Abikoff

& Gittelman, 1984; O'Leary & Pelham, 1978; O'Leary et al., 1976; Pelham, Schnedler, Bologna, & Contreras, 1980; Pelham et al., 1988). As with psychostimulant medication, the short-term effects of behavioral interventions are limited to the period when the programs are actually in effect.

Further, a substantial number of children in these studies (comparable to the proportion cited for stimulant medication) fail to show improvement. In many cases this is no doubt because parents and teachers fail to implement the behavioral programs as directed. As anyone who has conducted many behavioral interventions in the schools knows, a major problem for behaviorally oriented child clinicians is that a large number of teachers, who are not obligated to cooperate with outside consultants, will not implement a behavioral intervention (Witt, 1986). In addition, many parents—up to half of those beginning treatment—discontinue parent training against therapeutic advice (Firestone, Kelly, Goodman, & Davey, 1981; Fleischman, 1981). Even when parents and teacher apparently comply with treatment, therapist contact in standard, clinical behavior therapy is typically limited to once per week, and manipulation checks of whether parents and teachers actually follow through with treatment are almost never conducted. Parents and teachers of children who failed to show maximum improvement in intervention studies may not have implemented the treatment programs appropriately, if at all (Atkins, Pelham, & White, 1989; Bernal, Kinnert, & Schultz, 1980; Flanagan, Adams, & Forehand, 1979). For example, single mothers with relatively lower levels of education, income, and contact with other adults have great difficulty implementing and maintaining behavioral treatment, and it is thus not particularly effective with children of such parents (Firestone & Witt, 1982; Wahler, 1980).

As some of the limitations of medication can be removed by increasing the dosage, the effects of behavior therapy can be maximized by increasing the power and comprehensiveness of the intervention. The standard approach to clinical behavior therapy that has been employed in most therapy studies has the therapist making once weekly contact with parents and teachers and focuses on relatively straightforward interventions. More frequent contact and more complicated programs would be more effective than this standard approach, but as with psychostimulant medication, this tactic introduces problems. For example, a highly structured, closely monitored, contingency-management program (e.g., including response cost) in effect throughout the school day results in greater improvement than a simple daily report card (Atkins, Pelham, & White, 1989). Because it is very time-consuming and difficult to conduct such a system unassisted, however, regular classroom teachers are much less willing to implement the more powerful of the two programs (Witt, Martens, & Elliott, 1984). Similarly, classroom behavioral programs that include some form of prudent negative consequences (e.g., verbal reprimands, withdrawal of privileges, time out) are considerably more effective with ADD children than those that do not (e.g., Rosen, O'Leary, Joyce, Conway, & Pfiffner, 1984), but teachers rate such programs as unacceptable and do not want to use them (Witt & Robins, 1985). In summary, behavior therapy depends on the motivation and capabilities of the significant adults in the child's life. If these adults are unwilling or unable to implement the interventions, and if the objections or obstacles to intervention cannot be overcome, then behavior therapy will not be effective.

A final possible limitation of behavior therapy with ADD children is the lack of evidence for long-term effects, studies of which have not been conducted. A number of studies with behavior problem children (in all likelihood a mixture of ADD, CD, and oppositional disorder diagnostic categories) have shown that a substantial number of treated children fail to maintain treatment gains for periods of time as short as one year following intervention (Bernal et al., 1980; Kent & O'Leary, 1976; Wahler, 1980). Demonstration of generalization over time is one of the major concerns of those employing behavioral interventions with children (Alexander & Malouf, 1983; Ollendick, 1986). Unfortunately, at our current stage of knowledge the best guess regarding the long-term effects of behavior therapy with ADD and CD children is that short-term effects will often fail to maintain. If this were true, then, as with psychostimulant medication, the absence of long-term effects would be the major limitation of behavior therapy with ADD children.

Benefits of a Combined Intervention

Both behavioral and pharmacological interventions have clear limitations, but the limitations that we have discussed can often be reduced by combining the two modalities. Theoretically, the effects of a combined pharmacological and behavioral intervention can differ from the effects of the component treatments in several different ways (Uhlenhuth, Lipman, & Covi, 1969). The two treatments can interact to potentiate one another, yielding a combined effect greater than the total of the two component effects, or they can interact to inhibit one another, yielding an effect that is less than the effects of either component. Alternatively, the combined effect can simply be additive, equaling the total of the components. Reciprocation can occur in which the combined outcome is the same as one or the other component. Finally, the two interventions can have complementary effects; that is, each treatment can affect different symptoms such that the combined intervention affects a greater range of symptomatology than either treatment alone. The major potential benefit of a combined behavioral and pharmacological approach to treatment of ADD appears to be that additivity, complementary effects, and (in some studies) potentiation occur, thus minimizing the shortcomings of both treatments and yielding an intervention that may come closer to maximal effectiveness than either component alone.

A recent review of the available literature in which a combination of behavioral and stimulant treatments was used with ADD children revealed 19 studies and drew several conclusions (Pelham & H.A. Murphy, 1986). First, 13 of the 19 independent studies (68%) showed superiority for a combined treatment on at least one classroom-based task, motor, or social measure. For those studies in which a behavioral or pharmacological effect was found, only very rarely was either of these treatments alone superior to their combination. In fact, if order of condition means, rather than statistical significance, were used to interpret results, the combination treatment was superior to component treatments to which it was compared in virtually every study reviewed. For the average ADD child treated in these studies, a combined behavioral and pharmacological intervention resulted in greater improvement than either treatment alone.

Consider, for example, the study reported by Gittelman et al. (1980). In an 8-week study, they compared a (a) clinical behavioral intervention (mainly teacher rather than parent training), (b) a stimulant treated group, and (c) a group that received both treatments. On a variety of measures they found that the combined treatment group came closer to normalization of functioning than either treatment alone, with stimulant treatment alone next in efficacy and behavioral treatment a far third. In another treatment outcome study, Pelham et al. (1988) examined the incremental effects of adding .3 mg/kg MPH b.i.d. to a 20-week behavioral intervention conducted with ADD children in classroom and home settings. On one key measure, the ACTRS, the children who received methylphenidate in addition to the behavioral intervention were rated at midtreatment by teachers as considerably better ($M = 6.5$, $SD = 2.9$) than children who received behavior therapy plus placebo ($M = 12.7$, $SD = 6.8$), both reductions from mean ratings of 19 before treatment. Eighty percent of the combined intervention children were "normalized" on this measure, compared to 30 percent of the behavior therapy plus placebo group. Of note is that this positive level of functioning was reached with a dose of MPH that was half that used by Gittelman et al. Other treatment studies have also shown that treated children are more likely to reach a "normalization" of functioning with a combined intervention than with the separate modalities (Hinshaw et al., 1984; Pelham et al., 1980). However, it is important to note that in all of these studies, the incremental beneficial effects of the combined treatments did not last after either component was withdrawn, at which point effects reduced immediately to those produced by the remaining component. Whether a systematic withdrawal and maintenance program could maintain the obviously beneficial effects of the combined treatment has yet to be investigated. No controlled, long-term outcome studies of combined interventions have been conducted.

As we noted, many combined treatment effects are additive. A graphic example of the additive effects of MPH and reinforcement is illustrated in Figure 10.2 (Pelham et al., 1986). In this acute dose study, .3 mg/kg MPH and reward (points earned in a token economy) yielded a combined effect on a laboratory learning task that was the sum of the the separate treatment effects. This incremental effect did not depend on whether the reward was delivered on a continuous or partial schedule. In a few other studies, potentiation has been observed

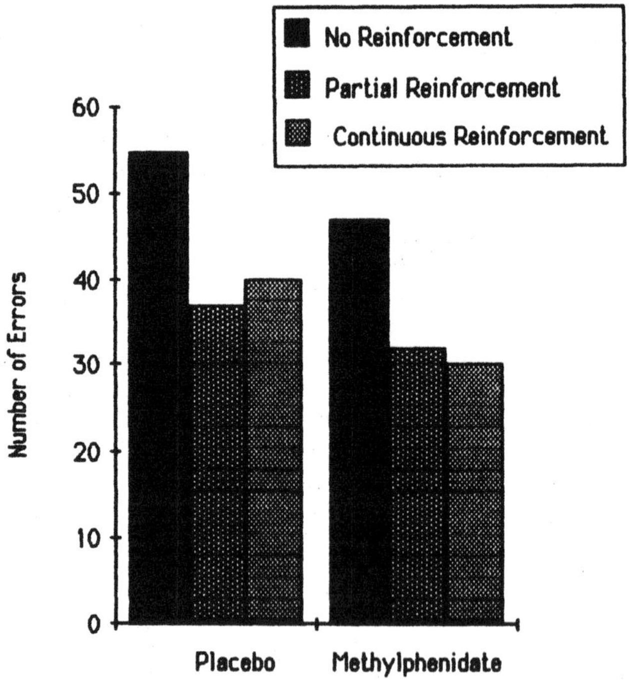

FIGURE 10.2. Mean number of errors on the nonsense-word spelling task by reinforcement and medication conditions.

on at least some measures such that a combined treatment was considerably more effective than the totaled effects of the behavioral and stimulant interventions (e.g., Pelham et al., 1980; Schell et al., 1986). In the Pelham et al. study, the interaction occurred with dose, such that the effects of a low dose of MPH were considerably enhanced by the behavioral intervention. Thus, an important result of combined treatments is that maximal improvement in behavior can be reached without resorting to high dosages of psychostimulant medication, which have adverse side effects discussed earlier. Atkins, Pelham, & White (1989) also demonstrated that a low dose of psychostimulant combined with a simple behavioral program was as effective as a response-cost behavioral intervention that worked well but that the target child's teacher refused to implement because of its time requirement. Because lower dosages and less restrictive behavioral interventions can be used, the risk/benefit ratio involved in combined treatments is decreased, and greater effects can be obtained with intervention levels—both pharmacological and behavioral—that carry fewer risks.

It is important to note, however, that there are large individual differences in response to medication, behavior therapy, and their combination. We have previously noted that if the children who respond to behavioral interventions and those who respond to medication are not the same children, then a combined treatment group study would yield evidence of combined treatment efficacy even though not a single individual had responded more positively to the combination than to the individual treatments (Pelham & H. A. Murphy, 1986). Although many ADD children respond best to a combined intervention, some children respond best to one or the other component treatment. Group studies that present only averaged data can be misleading, and the combined treatment must be examined in individuals, as well as in groups, in order to provide the most accurate analysis of its effects. As with medication, there is no way of predicting whether a child will have a positive response to a behavioral regimen. Other than by directly measuring the child's response in a short-term treatment trial, there is no way to predict which children will respond to a combined intervention. This highlights the importance of using comprehensive behavioral assessments in evaluating treatment effectiveness in combined behavioral and psychopharmacological interventions with ADD children.

One recent single-subject study illustrates how to evaluate the utility of a combined approach for one child (Schell et al., 1986). A multiply handicapped child (ADD, mentally retarded, dysphasic) was evaluated who had been referred by his pediatric neurologist for assessment of whether psychostimulant medication, behavior modification, or the combination of the two was most effective in improving his learning and behavior. Over a period of weeks the child learned lists of reading sight vocabulary words under different behavioral and drug conditions in an alternating treatments design (e.g., with and without reward, with placebo or 0.3 mg/kg MPH). The initial assessment revealed that the child improved both with medication and with a behavioral program, but the combined intervention was most effective. A combined treatment regimen was therefore recommended for the child, and he has been maintained on that treatment for the past six years as of this writing. Annual reassessments have demonstrated the continued incremental value of the combined pharmacological and behavioral treatment for him. It is interesting to note that this child showed additive, potentiated, and complementary effects of the combined treatment, depending on the dependent measure that was examined, a result that highlights the importance of multiple measures in evaluating combined treatment response, as we discussed earlier with regard to medication.

Because most studies of a combined approach to treating ADD have employed between-subject designs, beyond a few case studies there are few data available regarding what percentage of children actually respond best to a combined regimen. We presented data relevant to this question when we evaluated response to medication in the summer treatment programs attended by the child whose data were described in Figure 10.1 (Pelham & Hoza, 1987). Among that sample of ADD children, 44 percent were thought definitely to need medication beyond the highly structured behavioral day treatment program. An additional 25 percent showed an incremental response to medication beyond that shown to the behavioral treatment, but medication was recommended only if a behavioral intervention in the natural environment was insufficient.

One of the major advantages of a combined behavioral/pharmacological treatment for ADD is that the behavioral component of treatment can usually be reduced in scope and complexity if combined with low dosages of medication. Because less complex treatments are also less expensive, the cost-effectiveness of treatment is improved with a combined intervention. For example, a powerful, maximally effective, contingency management intervention in a referred child's classroom might require daily therapist trips to the school compared to the single weekly trip characteristic of clinical behavioral therapy. At $75 per visit, the more powerful behavioral intervention would cost an additional $300 per week. In contrast, the addition of a low dose of psychostimulant medication to a typical clinical behavioral intervention might also maximize improvement (cf. Atkins, Pelham, & White,

1989), but would cost less than $5 per week. Although such concerns are unimportant in research settings where costs are not born by a child's parents, in actual practice they are often one of the primary determinants of whether parents will seek out and follow through with treatment.

In addition to potential interactive or additive effects, behavioral therapy and psychostimulant medication each have areas of deficit and effectiveness that the other intervention can complement. For example, parent training is a standard component of a behavioral intervention for ADD, thus insuring that a treatment is available to the child and family's home programs that are typically not addressed by medication. Similarly, psychostimulant medication can reduce problematic behaviors that are very difficult to treat with practical behavioral programs, such as low-rate, peer-directed aggression that occurs in the absence of adult authority (e.g., on the school playground). An untested but intriguing possibility is that medication might facilitate behavioral treatment of other low-rate behaviors, such as stealing, that have been relatively unresponsive to behavioral interventions alone (Reid & Hendriks, 1973). As we noted earlier, medication effects on prosocial and antisocial behaviors appear to be facilitated when behavioral contingencies supporting social behavior are in effect. In several ways, then, a combined intervention is thus more comprehensive in coverage than either treatment alone.

Finally, there are several reasons to speculate that long-term maintenance of treatment effects might be improved with a combined intervention. First, it is clear that ADD children suffer from a lack of cognitive and behavioral skills that are necessary for academic and social adjustment (Douglas, 1983). To the extent that these skills must be acquired for successful long-term outcome, medication alone, which does not teach a child alternative behaviors for coping with problematic situations, would not be expected to be a sufficient treatment. The addition of a behavioral intervention that focused in part on teaching such skills might improve the long-term outcome that would be achieved with medication alone.

Similarly, one of the suggestions that has been made to facilitate maintenance of behavioral treatment effects is to make the intervention one that is likely to be continued by the child's parents or teachers for a long time and/or maintained by naturally occurring contingencies following therapy termination (Stokes & Baer, 1977). Because the addition of a low dose of psychostimulant medication enables relatively greater effects to be achieved with less restrictive and more natural behavioral programs, a combined intervention may be more likely to be maintained following termination of therapeutic contact than a behavioral intervention alone.

Summary and Future Directions

Although combined behavioral and stimulant interventions appear to be the emerging treatment of choice for ADD, that conclusion does have some limitations. One of them is that compared to the large numbers of subjects who have been studied over considerably longer time periods with separate behavioral and pharmacologic interventions, the combined intervention is relatively unstudied. Only 167 children were treated in the 19 studies that Pelham and H.A. Murphy reviewed, and the median duration of treatment was less than three weeks. Much more research needs to be conducted before we have adequate knowledge regarding the procedures and effects of combined behavioral and pharmacologic treatment for ADD. We have discussed in detail elsewhere the focus that future research needs to take (Pelham 1990; Pelham & H.A. Murphy, 1986), but a few final points are worth noting.

1. First, what is *not* worth investigating? Continued research into the efficacy of cognitive-behavioral interventions and their combination with medication does not appear warranted. Excellently conducted studies of combined treatments have failed to provide any evidence that cognitive interventions add to the effectiveness of medication (e.g., Abikoff & Gittelman, 1985b; Brown, Wynne, & Medenis, 1985). Presumably this is because the cognitive interventions are ineffective (Abikoff, 1985). Similarly, the studies showing that diet bears no relationship to ADD behavior (Milich, Woolraich, & Lindgren, 1986) argue that no effort should be invested in examining how dietary interventions might interact with other combined treatments. Similarly, the absence of any indication for (or evidence for the effectiveness of) individual, insight-oriented therapy with ADD children means that there is no point in adding such treatments to combined interventions.

2. On the positive side, additional research directed at the effects of combined treatments on peer relationships is sorely needed. This is a critical domain in which behavioral and social skills training interventions have had weak effects with ADD children (Krehbiel & Milich, 1986). The recent evidence that stimulants may result in improvement in this sphere highlight the need for additional research. It would be especially interesting to see such research conducted in settings as natural as possible and focusing as much on the development of sports skills as on the development of what are typically viewed as social skills.

3. There has been a great deal of discussion regarding the potential

negative attributions that ADD children make to their medication (e.g., Whalen, 1989). Although this discussion to date has been unsupported by hard evidence, if children did have attributions about medication that had untoward effects on the child's self-esteem, this would be a point of concern. It is quite reasonable to speculate that if medication is only administered in combination with a behavioral intervention, then unwanted attributions could be avoided. This area warrants additional research.

4. Given our discussion regarding the overlap between ADD and aggression, it should be clear that additional research is needed on the efficacy of combined intervention for the two subgroups of ADD children—those with and those without concurrent conduct problems. None of the studies conducted thus far have divided their subjects on the aggression dimension, and subgrouping analysis is needed.

5. A question of primary importance in school settings is whether an ADD child can be continued in a regular classroom placement (i.e., mainstreamed) or whether special class placement is necessary. The implication of our discussion is that a combined treatment may enable many children to be mainstreamed rather than placed in special classes. Since both legal guidelines and current educational philosophy strongly favor mainstreaming, this would appear to be an important advantage of a combined treatment approach. However, comparative outcome studies of special-class-placed versus combined-treatment-mainstreamed children have not yet been conducted and are necessary.

6. All of the combined treatment studies that have been conducted have involved ADD children of elementary school age. Studies of combined treatments for preschoolers are needed as a worthwhile focus on early intervention. In addition, studies with ADD adolescents who continue to exhibit both school- and home-based difficulties are needed.

7. Finally, research on the long-term effects of combined interventions needs to be conducted. ADD has been extremely refractory to treatment, and, as our discussion of prognosis made clear, it is a chronic disorder out of which most children do not grow. Professionals involved in treating ADD, as well as parents and school professionals, need to begin to think in terms of intervention strategies that will be conducted for years rather than weeks or months. For all of the reasons we have discussed, it is our firm belief that an intervention that combines behavioral and pharmacological modalities should be the strategy that is used, but research demonstrating its long-term effectiveness is required to validate that belief.

REFERENCES

Abikoff, H. (1985). Efficacy of cognitive training interventions in hyperactive children: A critical review. *Clinical Psychology Review, 5*, 479–512.

Abikoff, H., & Gittelman, R. (1984). Does behavior therapy normalize the classroom behavior of hyperactive children? *Archives of General Psychiatry, 41*, 449–454.

Abikoff, H., & Gittelman, R. (1985a). The normalizing effects of methylphenidate on the classroom behavior of ADDH children. *Journal of Abnormal Child Psychology, 13*, 33–44.

Abikoff, H., & Gittelman, R. (1985b). Hyperactive children treated with stimulants. *Archives of General Psychiatry, 42*, 953–961.

Abikoff, H., Gittelman, R., & Klein, D. F. (1980). Classroom observation code for hyperactive children: A replication of validity. *Journal of Clinical and Consulting Psychology, 48*, 555–565.

Achenbach, T. M. (1978). The child behavior profile: 1. Boys aged 6–11. *Journal of Consulting and Clinical Psychology, 46*, 478–488.

Achenbach, T. M. (1985). *Assessment of taxonomy of child and adolescent psychopathology*. Beverly Hills, CA: Sage.

Achenbach, T. M., & Edelbrock, C. S. (1978). The classification of child psychopathology: A review and analysis of empirical efforts. *Psychological Bulletin, 85*, 1275–1301.

Alexander, J. F., & Malouf, R. E. (1983). Intervention with children experiencing problems in personality and social development. In P. H. Mussen (Ed.), *Handbook of child psychology* (pp. 913–981). New York: John Wiley & Sons.

American Psychiatric Association. (1980). *Diagnostic and statistical manual of mental disorders* (3rd ed.). Washington, DC: Author.

American Psychiatric Association. (1987). *Diagnostic and statistical manual of mental disorders* (3rd ed. rev.). Washington, DC: Author.

Atkins, M. S., Pelham, W. E., & Licht, M. (1985). A comparison of objective classroom measures and teacher ratings of attention deficit disorder. *Journal of Abnormal Child Psychology, 13*, 155–167.

Atkins, M. S., Pelham, W. E., & Licht, M. (1989). The differential validity of teacher ratings of inattention/overactivity and aggression. *Journal of Abnormal Child Psychology, 17*, 423–435.

Atkins, M. S., Pelham, W. E., & White, K. J. (1989). Hyperactivity and attention deficit disorders. In M. Hersen & V. B. Van Hasselt (Eds.), *Psychological aspects of developmental and physical disabilities: A casebook* (pp. 136–156). Beverly Hills, CA: Sage.

August, G. J., Stewart, M. A., & Holmes, C. S. (1983). A four-year follow-up of hyperactive boys with and without conduct disorder. *British Journal of Psychiatry, 143*, 192–198.

Barkley, R. A. (1982). Guidelines for defining hyperactivity in children: Attention deficit disorders with hyperactivity. In B. B. Lahey & A. E. Kazdin

(Eds.), *Advances in clinical child psychology* (Vol. 5, pp. 4–175). New York: Plenum.
Barkley, R. A., & Cunningham, C. E. (1978). Do stimulant drugs improve the academic performance of hyperkinetic children? *Clinical Pediatrics, 17*, 85–92.
Barkley, R. A., Fischer, M., Newby, R. F., & Breen, M. J. (1988). Development of a multi-method clinical protocol for assessing stimulant drug response in ADD children. *Journal of Clinical Child Psychology, 17*, 14–24.
Barkley, R. A., Karlsson, J., Strzelecki, E., & Murphy, J. V. (1984). Effects of age and Ritalin dosage on the mother-child interactions of hyperactive children. *Journal of Consulting and Clinical Psychology, 52*, 739–749.
Bernal, M. E., Kinnert, M. D., & Schultz, L. A. (1980). Outcome evaluation of behavioral parent training and client-centered parent counseling for children with conduct problems. *Journal of Applied Behavior Analysis, 13*, 677–691.
Borland, B., & Heckman, K. (1976). Hyperactive boys and their brothers: A follow-up study. *Archives of General Psychiatry, 33*, 669–675.
Bosco, J., & Robin, S. (1980). Hyperkinesis: Prevalence and treatment. In C. Whalen & B. Henker (Eds.), *Hyperactive children: The social ecology of identification and treatment* (pp. 173–187). New York: Academic Press.
Brown, G. L., Hunt, R. D., Ebert, M. H., Bunney, W. E., & Kopin, I J. (1979). Plasma levels of d-amphetamine in hyperactive children: Serial behavior and motor responses. *Psychopharmacology, 62*, 133–140.
Brown, R. T., Wynne, M. E., & Medenis, R. (1985). Methylphenidate and cognitive therapy: A comparison of treatment approaches with hyperactive boys. *Journal of Abnormal Child Psychology, 13*, 69–88.
Campbell, S. B., & Werry, J. S. (1986). Attention deficit disorder (hyperactivity). In H. Quay & J. Werry (Eds.), *Psychopathological disorders of childhood* (3rd ed., pp. 111–155). New York: John Wiley & Sons.
Cantwell, D. P. (1975). Familial-genetic research with hyperactive children. In D. P. Cantwell (Ed.), *The hyperactive child: Diagnosis, management, current research* (pp. 93–105). Hollywood, NY: Spectrum.
Cantwell, D. P. (1987). How are DSM-III and DSM-III-R used to make the diagnosis of attention deficit disorder? In J. Loney (Ed.), *The young hyperactive child: Answers to questions about diagnosis, prognosis, and treatment* (pp. 5–18). New York: Haworth Press.
Cantwell, D. P., & Carlson, G. A. (1978). Stimulants. In J. S. Werry (Ed.), *Pediatric psychopharmacology: The use of behavior modifying drugs in children* (pp. 171–207). New York: Brunner/Mazel.
Carlson, C. L. (1986). Attention deficit disorder without hyperactivity: A review of preliminary experimental evidence. In B. B. Lahey & A. E. Kazdin (Eds.), *Advances in clinical child psychology* (Vol. 9, pp. 153–175). New York: Plenum.
Clampit, M. K., & Pirkle, J. B. (1983). Stimulant medication and the hyperactive adolescent: Myths and facts. *Adolescence, 28*, 811–822.

Conners, C. K. (1972). Psychological effects of stimulant drugs in children with minimal brain dysfunction. *Pediatrics, 49*, 702–708.

Conners, C. K. (1987). How is a teacher rating scale used in the diagnosis of attention deficit disorder? In J. Loney (Ed.), *The young hyperactive child: Answers to questions about diagnosis, prognosis, and treatment* (pp. 33–52). New York: Haworth Press.

Conners, C. K., & Rothschild, G. H. (1968). Drugs and learning in children. In J. Hellmuth (Ed.), *Learning disorders* (Vol. III, pp. 191–217). Seattle, WA: Special Child Publications.

Conners, C. K., & Wells, K. C. (1986). *Hyperkinetic children: A neuropsychosocial approach.* Beverly Hills, CA: Sage.

Conners, C. K., & Werry, J. (1979). Psychopharmacology. In H. Quay & J. Werry (Eds.), *Psychopathological disorders of childhood* (2nd ed., pp. 336–386). New York: John Wiley & Sons.

Coons, H. W., Klorman, R., & Borgstedt, A. D. (1987). Effects of methylphenidate on adolescents with a childhood history of attention deficit disorder: I. Clinical findings. *Journal of the American Academy of Child and Adolescent Psychiatry, 26*, 363–367.

Cunningham, C. E., Siegel, L. S., & Offord, D. R. (1985). A developmental dose-response analysis of the effects of methylphenidate on the peer interactions of attention deficit disordered boys. *Journal of Child Psychology and Psychiatry, 26*, 955–972.

Donnelly, M., & Rapoport, J. (1989). Treatment for disruptive behavior disorders. In B. Karasu (Ed.), *Treatment manual for psychiatric disorders.* Washington, DC: American Psychiatric Association.

Douglas, V. I. (1983). Attentional and cognitive problems. In M. Rutter (Ed.), *Developmental neuropsychiatry* (pp. 280–329). New York: The Guilford Press.

Douglas, V. I., Barr, R. G., O'Neill, M. E., & Britton, B. G. (1986). Short-term effects of methylphenidate on the cognitive learning and academic performance of children with attention deficit disorder in the laboratory and in the classroom. *Journal of Child Psychology and Psychiatry, 27*, 191–211.

Douglas, V. I., & Peters, K. (1979). Toward a clearer definition of the attentional deficits of hyperactive children. In G. Hale & M. Lewis (Eds.), *Attention and the development of cognitive skills* (pp. 173–246). New York: Plenum.

Dulcan, M. K. (1986). Comprehensive treatment of children and adolescents with attention deficit disorders. The state of the art. *Clinical Psychology Review, 6*, 539–569.

Dykman, R. A., & Ackerman, P. T., (1980). Long-term follow-up studies of hyperactive children. *Advances in Behavioral Pediatrics, 1*, 97–128.

Edelbrock, C., & Achenbach, T. M. (1984). The teacher version of the child behavior profile: I. Boys aged 6–11. *Journal of Consulting and Clinical Psychology, 52*, 207–217.

Farrington, D. P., Loeber, R., & van Kammen, W. B. (1987, October). *Long-term criminal outcomes of hyperactivity-impulsivity-attention deficit and conduct problems in childhood.* Paper prepared for the Society for Life History Research meeting on "Straight and Devious Pathways from Childhood to Adulthood." St. Louis, MO.

Ferguson, H. B., & Rapoport, J. L. (1983). Nosological issues and biological validation. In M. Rutter (Ed.), *Developmental neuropsychiatry* (pp. 369–384). New York: Guilford.

Firestone, P., & Witt, J. E. (1982). Characteristics of families completing and prematurely discontinuing a behavioral parent-training program. *Journal of Pediatric Psychology, 7*, 209–222.

Firestone, P., Kelly, M. J., Goodman, J. T., & Davey, J. (1981). Differential effects of parent training and stimulant medication with hyperactives. *Journal of the American Academy of Child Psychiatry, 20*, 135–147.

Flanagan, S., Adams, H. E., & Forehand, R. (1979). A comparison of four instructional techniques for teaching parents to use time-out. *Behavior Therapy, 10*, 94–102.

Fleischman, M. J. (1981). A replication of Patterson's "Intervention for boys with conduct problems." *Journal of Consulting and Clinical Psychology, 49*, 342–351.

Gadow, K. D. (1981). Drug therapy for hyperactivity: Treatment procedures in natural settings. In K. Gadow & J. Loney (Eds.), *Psychosocial aspects of drug treatment for hyperactivity* (pp. 325–380). Boulder, CO: Westview Press.

Gadow, K. D. (1986). *Children on medication: Hyperactivity, learning disabilities, and mental retardation* (Vol. 1). San Diego, CA: College Hill Press.

Gittelman, R., Abikoff, H., Pollack, E., Klein, D. F., Katz, S., & Mattes, J. (1980). A controlled trial of behavior modification and methylphenidate in hyperactive children. In C. K. Whalen & B. Henker (Eds.), *Hyperactive children: The social ecology of identification and treatment* (pp. 221–243). New York: Academic Press.

Gittelman, R., & Kanner, A. (1986). Psychopharmacotherapy. In H. Quay & J. Werry (Eds.), *Psychopathological disorders of childhood* (3rd ed., pp. 455–495). New York: John Wiley & Sons.

Gittelman, R., Klein, D. F., & Feingold, I. (1983). Children with reading disorders-II. Effects of methylphenidate in combination with reading remediation. *Journal of Child Psychology and Psychiatry, 24*(2), 193–212.

Gittelman, R., & Mannuzza, S. (1985). Diagnosing ADD-H in adolescents. *Psychopharmacology Bulletin, 21*, 237–242.

Gittelman, R., Mannuzza, S., Shenker, R., & Bonagura, N. (1985). Hyperactive boys almost grown up: I. Psychiatric status. *Archives of General Psychiatry, 42*, 937–947.

Gittelman-Klein, R., & Mannuzza, S. (1988). Hyperactive boys almost grown up III. Methylphenidate effects on ultimate height. *Archives of General Psychiatry, 45*, 1131–1134.

Goyette, C. H., Conners, C. K., & Ulrich, R. F. (1978). Normative data on revised Conners parent and teacher rating scales. *Journal of Abnormal Child Psychology, 6*, 221–236.

Hinshaw, S. P. (1987a). Hyperactivity, attention deficit disorders, and learning disabilities. In V. B. Van Hasselt & M. Hersen (Eds.), *Psychological evaluation of the developmentally and physically disabled* (pp. 213–260). New York: Plenum.

Hinshaw, S. P. (1987b). On the distinction between attentional deficits/hyperactivity and conduct problems/aggression in child psychopathology. *Psychological Bulletin, 101*, 443–463.

Hinshaw, S. P., Henker, B., & Whalen, C. K. (1984). Cognitive-behavioral and pharmacologic interventions for hyperactive boys: Comparative and combined effects. *Journal of Consulting and Clinical Psychology, 52*, 739–749.

Hoy, E., Weiss, G., Minde, K., & Cohen, N. (1979). The hyperactive child at adolescence: Emotional, social, and cognitive functioning. *Journal of Abnormal Child Psychology, 6*, 311–324.

Huessy, H., & Cohen, A. (1976). Hyperkinetic behaviors and learning disabilities followed over seven years. *Pediatrics, 54*, 4–10.

Johnston, C. J., & Pelham, W. E. (1986). Teacher ratings predict peer ratings of aggression at 3-year follow-up in boys with attention deficit disorder with hyperactivity. *Journal of Consulting and Clinical Psychology, 54*, 571–572.

Kent, R., & O'Leary, K. D. (1976). A controlled evaluation of behavior modification with conduct problem children. *Journal of Consulting and Clinical Psychology, 44*, 586–596.

Klorman, R. (1986). Attention deficit disorder in adolescence. *Advances in Adolescent Mental Health, 1*, 19–62.

Klorman, R., Salzman, L. F., & Borgstedt, A. D. (1988). Brain event-related potentials as a tool for evaluating cognitive deficits in attention deficit disorder and stimulant therapy. In L. Bloomingdale & R. Klorman (Eds.), *Attention deficit disorder* (Vol. 3). New York: Pergamon.

Krehbiel, G., & Milich, R. (1986). Issues in the assessment and treatment of socially rejected children. In R. Prinz (Ed.), *Advances in behavioral assessment of children and families* (Vol. 2, pp. 249–270). Greenwich, CT: JAI Press.

Lahey, B. B., Pelham, W. E., Schaughency, E., Atkins, M., Murphy, H., Hynd, G., Russo, M., Hartdagen, S., & Lorys-Vernon, A. (1988a). Dimensions and subtypes of attention deficit disorders. *Journal of the American Academy of Child and Adolescent Psychiatry, 27*, 330–335.

Lahey, B. B., Piacentini, J. C., McBurnett, K., Stone, P., Hartdagen, S., & Hynd, G. (1988b). Psychopathology in the parents of children with conduct disorder and hyperactivity. *Journal of the American Academy of Child and Adolescent Psychiatry, 27*, 163–170.

Laufer, M. W., Denhoff, E., & Solomons, G. (1957). Hyperkinetic impulse disorder in children's behavior problems. *Psychosomatic Medicine, 19*, 38–49.

Ledingham, J. E. (1981). Developmental patterns of aggressive and withdrawn behavior in childhood: A possible method for identifying preschizophrenics. *Journal of Abnormal Child Psychology, 9*, 1–22.

Loeber, R., & Schmaling, K. (1985a). The utility of differentiating between mixed and pure forms of antisocial child behavior. *Journal of Abnormal Child Psychology, 13*, 315–336.

Loeber, R., & Schmaling, K. (1985b). Empirical evidence for overt and covert patterns of antisocial conduct problems: A metaanalysis. *Journal of Abnormal Child Psychology, 13*, 337–352.

Loney, J., Kramer, J., & Milich, R. S. (1981). The hyperactive child grows up: Predictors of symptoms, delinquency and achievement at follow-up. In K. D. Gadow & J. Loney (Eds.), *Psychosocial aspects of drug treatment for hyperactivity* (pp. 381–415). Boulder, CO: Westview Press.

Loney, J., Langhorne, J., & Paternite, C. (1978). An empirical basis for subgrouping the hyperkinetic/MBD syndrome. *Journal of Abnormal Psychology, 87*, 431–439.

Loney, J., & Milich, R. (1982). Hyperactivity, inattention, and aggression in clinical practice. In M. Wolraich & D. K. Routh (Eds.), *Advances in behavioral pediatrics* (Vol. 2, pp. 113–147). Greenwich, CT: JAI Press.

Mattes, J. A., & Gittelman, R. (1983). Growth of hyperactive children on maintenance regimen of methylphenidate. *Archives of General Psychiatry, 40*(3), 317–321.

Mendelson, W., Johnson, N., & Stewart, M. A. (1971). Hyperactive children as teenagers: A follow-up study. *Journal of Nervous and Mental Disease, 6*, 483–492.

Milich, R., & Fitzgerald, G. (1985). A validation of inattention/overactivity and aggression ratings with classroom observations. *Journal of Consulting and Clinical Psychology, 53*, 139–140.

Milich, R., & Kramer, J. (1984). Reflections on impulsivity: An empirical investigation of impulsivity as a construct. *Advances in Learning and Behavioral Disabilities, 3*, 57–94.

Milich, R., & Landau, S. (1984). A comparison of the social status and social behavior of aggressive and aggressive/withdrawn boys. *Journal of Abnormal Child Psychology, 12*, 277–288.

Milich, R., & Landau, S. (1990). The social status and social behavior of hyperactive and aggressive children. In J. Swanson & L. Bloomingdale (Eds.), *Attention deficit disorders IV: Current concepts and emerging trends in the treatment of attention and behavior problems in children* (pp. 1–16). London: Pergamon.

Milich, R., & Loney, J. (1979). The role of hyperactive and aggressive symptomatology in predicting adolescent outcome among hyperactive children. *Journal of Pediatric Psychology, 4*, 93–112.

Milich, R., & Pelham, W. E. (1985, October). *Identifying the aggressiveness of hyperactive/aggressive boys.* Invited presentation to the sixth annual Bloomingdale conference on Attention Deficit Disorders, San Antonio, TX.

Milich, R., Loney, J., & Landau, S. (1982). Independent dimensions of hyperactivity and aggression: A validation with playroom observation data. *Journal of Abnormal Psychology, 91*, 183–198.

Milich, R., Pelham, W. E., & Hinshaw, S. (1986). Issues in the diagnosis of attention deficit disorder: A cautionary note on the Gordon Diagnostic System. *Psychopharmacology Bulletin, 22*, 1101–1104.

Milich, R., Wolraich, M., & Lindgren, S. (1986). Sugar and hyperactivity: Critical review of empirical findings. *Clinical Psychology Review, 6*, 473–513.

Murphy, D. A. & Pelham, W. E. (1988). Attention deficit disorder. In L. K. Hsu & M. Hersen (Eds.), *Recent developments in adolescent psychiatry* (pp. 234–267). New York: John Wiley & Sons.

Murphy, D. A., Pelham, W. E., Atkins, M. S., & Murphy, H. A. (1987, November). *Relationships between impulsivity and inattention, overactivity, and aggression on teacher and mother ratings.* Paper presented at the annual meeting of the Association for the Advancement of Behavior Therapy, Boston, MA.

Murphy, D. A., Pelham, W. E., & Lang, A. R. (in press). Aggression in boys with attention deficit hyperactivity disorder: Methylphenidate effects on naturalistically observed aggression, response to provocation, and social information processing. *Journal of Abnormal Child Psychology.*

Neuchterlein, K. H. (1983). Signal detection in vigilance tasks and behavioral attributes among offspring of schizophrenic mothers and among hyperactive children. *Journal of Abnormal Psychology, 92*, 4–28.

O'Leary, S. G., & Pelham, W. E. (1978). Behavior therapy and withdrawal of stimulant medication with hyperactive children. *Pediatrics, 61*, 211–217.

O'Leary, K. D., Pelham, W. E., Rosenbaum, A., & Price, G. H. (1976). Behavioral treatment of hyperkinetic children: An experimental evaluation of its usefulness. *Clinical Pediatrics, 15*, 510–515.

Ollendick, T. H. (1986). Behavior therapy with children and adolescents. In S. L. Garfield & A. E. Bergin (Eds.), *Handbook of psychotherapy and behavior change* (3rd ed., pp. 525–564). New York: John Wiley & Sons.

Paternite, C. E., & Loney, J. (1980). Childhood hyperkinesis: Relationships between symptomatology and home environment. In C. K. Whalen & B. Henker (Eds.), *Hyperactive children: The social ecology of identification and treatment* (pp. 105–141). New York: Academic Press.

Pelham, W. E. (1982). Childhood hyperactivity: Diagnosis, etiology, nature, and treatment. In R. Gatchel, A. Baum, & J. Singer (Eds.), *Behavioral medicine and clinical psychology: Overlapping disciplines* (pp. 261–327). (Volume 1 of A. Baum & J. Singer (Eds.), *Handbook of psychology and health.*) Hillsdale, NJ: Erlbaum.

Pelham, W. E. (1983). The effects of stimulant drugs on academic achievement in hyperactive and learning disabled children. *Thalamus, 3*, 1–47.

Pelham, W. E. (1986a). The effects of stimulant drugs on learning and achievement in hyperactive and learning-disabled children. In J. K. Torgesen & B. Wong (Eds.), *Psychological and educational perspectives on learning disabilities* (pp. 259–295). New York: Academic Press.

Pelham, W. E. (1986b). What we know about stimulant drug effects. *Journal of Children in Contemporary Society, 19*, 99–110.

Pelham, W. E. (1990). Behavior therapy, behavioral assessment, and psychostimulant medication in treatment of attention deficit disorders: An interactive approach. In J. Swanson & L. Bloomingdale (Eds.), *Attention deficit disorders, IV: Current concepts and emerging trends in the treat-*

ment of attention and behavior problems in children (pp. 169–195). London: Pergamon.

Pelham, W. E., & Bender, M. E. (1982). Peer relationships in hyperactive children: Description and treatment. In K. Gadow & I. Bialer (Eds.), *Advances in learning and behavioral disabilities* (Vol. 1, pp. 366–436). Greenwich, CT: JAI Press.

Pelham, W. E., Bender, M. E., Caddell, J., Booth, S., & Moorer, S. (1985). The dose-response effects of methylphenidate on classroom academic and social behavior in children with attention deficit disorder. *Archives of General Psychiatry, 42*, 948–952.

Pelham, W. E., Gnagy, E. M., Greenslade, K. E., & Milich, R. (in press). Teacher ratings of DSM-III-R symptoms for the disruptive behavior disorders. *Journal of the American Academy of Child and Adolescent Psychiatry.*

Pelham, W. E., Greenslade, K. E., Vodde-Hamilton, M. A., Murphy, D. A., Greenstein, J. J., Gnagy, E. M., & Dahl, R. E. (1990). Relative efficacy of long-acting CNS stimulants on ADHD children: A comparison of standard methylphenidate, Ritalin SR-20, Dexedrine Spansule, and pemoline. *Pediatrics*, 86, 226–237.

Pelham, W. E., & Hoza, J. (1987). Behavioral assessment of psychostimulant effects on ADD children in a summer day treatment program. In R. Prinz (Ed.), *Advances in behavioral assessment of children and families* (Vol. 3, pp. 3–33). Greenwich, CT: JAI Press.

Pelham, W. E., McBurnett, K., Harper, G. W., Murphy, D. A., Milich, R., Clinton, J., & Thiele, C. (1990). Methylphenidate and baseball playing in ADD children: Who's on first? *Journal of Consulting and Clinical Psychology, 58*, 130–133.

Pelham, W. E., & Milich, R. (1984). Peer relationships in hyperactive children. *Journal of Learning Disabilities, 17*, 560–567.

Pelham, W. E., & Milich, R. (1991). Individual differences in response to Ritalin in classwork and social behavior. In B. P. & L. Greenhill (Eds.), *Ritalin: Theory and patient management* (pp. 203–222). New York: Mary Ann Liebert.

Pelham, W. E., Milich, R., Murphy, D. A., & Murphy, H. A. (1989). Normative data on the IOWA Conners teacher rating scale. *Journal of Clinical Child Psychology, 18*, 259–262.

Pelham, W. E., Milich, R., & Walker, J. (1986). The effects of continuous and partial reinforcement and methylphenidate on learning in children with attention deficit disorder. *Journal of Abnormal Psychology, 95*, 319–325.

Pelham, W. E., & Murphy, H. A. (1986). Attention deficit and conduct disorders. In M. Hersen (Ed.), *Pharmacological and behavioral treatment: An integrative approach* (pp. 108–148). New York: John Wiley & Sons.

Pelham, W. E., Schnedler, R. W., Bender, M. E., Miller, J., Nilsson, D., Budrow, M., Ronnei, M., Paluchowski, C., & Marks, D. (1988). The combination of behavior therapy and methylphenidate in the treatment of hyperactivity: A therapy outcome study. In L. Bloomingdale & R. Klorman (Eds.), *Attention deficit disorders* (Vol. III, pp. 29–48). London: Pergamon.

Pelham, W. E., Schnedler, R. W., Bologna, N., & Contreras, A. (1980). Behavioral and stimulant treatment of hyperactive children: A therapy study with methylphenidate probes in a within-subject design. *Journal of Applied Behavior Analysis, 13*, 221–236.

Pelham, W. E., Sturges, J., Hoza, J., Schmidt, C., Bijlsma, J., & Moorer, S. (1987). Sustained release and standard methylphenidate effects on cognitive and social behavior in children with attention deficit disorder. *Pediatrics, 80*, 491–501.

Pelham, W. E., Vodde-Hamilton, M., Hoza, J., Milich, R., Greenslade, K. E., Gnagy, E. M., Greiner, A. R., Sturges, J., & Murphy, D. A. (1992). Individual differences in dose response effects of methylphenidate in ADHD boys. Manuscript under review.

Pelham, W. E., Vodde-Hamilton, M., Murphy, D. A., Greenstein, J., & Vallano, G. (1991). The effects of methylphenidate on ADHD adolescents in recreational, peer group, and classroom settings. *Journal of Clinical Child Psychology, 20*, 293–300.

Peloquin, L. J., & Klorman, R. (1986). Effects of methylphenidate on normal children's mood, event-related potentials, and performance in memory scanning and vigilance. *Journal of Abnormal Psychology, 95*, 88–99.

Prinz, R., Conner, P., & Wilson, C. (1981). The intertwined dimensions of aggression and hyperactivity in childhood. *Journal of Abnormal Child Psychology, 9*, 191–202.

Prinz, R. J., Moore, P. A., & Roberts, W. A. (1986). Measurement of childhood hyperactivity. In R. Prinz (Ed.), *Advances in behavioral assessment of children and families* (Vol. 2, 99–119). New York: JAI Press.

Quay, H. C. (1979). Classification. In H. C. Quay & J. S. Werry (Eds.), *Psychopathological disorders of childhood* (2nd ed., pp. 1–42). New York: John Wiley & Sons.

Quay, H. C. (1986a). Classification. In H. C. Quay & J. S. Werry (Eds.), *Psychopathological disorders of childhood* (3rd ed., pp. 1–34). New York: John Wiley & Sons.

Quay, H. C. (1986b). A critical analysis of DSM-III as a taxonomy of psychopathology in childhood and adolescence. In T. Millon & G. Klerman (Eds.), *Contemporary directions in psychopathology: Toward the DSM-IV* (pp. 151–166). New York: Guilford Press.

Quay, H. C. (1986c). Conduct Disorders. In H. C. Quay & J. S. Werry (Eds.), *Psychopathological disorders of childhood* (3rd ed., pp. 35–72). New York: John Wiley & Sons.

Quay, H. C., & Peterson, D. R. (1983). Interim manual for the *Revised Behavior Problem Checklist.* Box 248074, University of Miami, Coral Gables, FL 33124.

Rapoport, J. L., Buchsbaum, M. S., Weingartner, H., Zahn, P., Ludlow, C., & Mikkelsen, E. J. (1980). Dextroamphetamine: Cognitive and behavioral effects in normal and hyperactive boys and normal men. *Archives of General Psychiatry, 37*, 933–943.

Rapoport, J. L., Conners, C. K., & Reatig, N. (Eds.). (1985). Rating scales and assessment instruments for use in pediatric psychopharmacology research. *Psychopharmacology Bulletin, 21*, 713–1125.

Rapport, M. D., Murphy, H. A., & Bailey, J. S. (1982). Ritalin vs. response cost in the control of hyperactive children: A within-subject comparison. *Journal of Applied Behavior Analysis, 15*, 205–216.

Rapport, M. D., Stoner, G., DuPaul, G. J., Birmingham, B. K., & Tucker, S. (1985). Methylphenidate in hyperactive children: Differential effects of dose on academic, learning, and social behavior. *Journal of Abnormal Child Psychology, 13*, 227–244.

Reid, J. B., & Hendriks, A. F. (1973). Preliminary analysis of the effectiveness of direct home intervention for the treatment of delinquent boys who steal. In L. A. Hamerlyunck, L. C. Handy, & E. J. Mash (Eds.), *Behavior change: Methodology, concepts and practice.* Champaign, IL: Research Press.

Riddle, D., & Rapoport, J. (1976). A 2-year follow-up of 72 hyperactive boys. *Journal of Nervous and Mental Disease, 162*, 126–134.

Rieder, R., & Nichols, P. (1979). Offspring of schizophrenics III. *Archives of General Psychiatry, 36*, 665–674.

Roberts, M. A. (1987). How is playroom behavior observation used in the diagnosis of attention deficit disorder? In J. Loney (Ed.), *The young hyperactive child: Answers to questions about diagnosis, prognosis, and treatment* (pp. 65–74). New York: Haworth Press.

Robins, L. E. (1966). *Deviant children grown up.* Baltimore, MD: Williams & Wilkins.

Rosen, L. A., O'Leary, S. G., Joyce, S. A., Conway, G., & Pfiffner, L. J. (1984). The importance of prudent negative consequences for maintaining the appropriate behavior of hyperactive students. *Journal of Abnormal Child Psychology, 12*, 581–604.

Ross, D. M., & Ross, S. A. (1982). *Hyperactivity: Research theory, and action* (2nd ed.). New York: John Wiley & Sons.

Sallee, F. R., Stiller, R., Perel, J., & Bates, T. (1985). Oral pemoline kinetics in hyperactive children. *Clinical Pharmacological Therapy, 37*, 606–609.

Satterfield, J. H., Hoppe, C. M. & Schell, A. M. (1982). A prospective study of delinquency in 110 adolescent boys with attention deficit disorder and 88 normal adolescent boys. *American Journal of Psychiatry, 139*, 795–798.

Schell, R. M., Pelham, W. E., Bender, M. E., Andree, J., Law, T., & Robbins, F. (1986). The concurrent assessment of behavioral and psychostimulant interventions: A controlled case study. *Behavioral Assessment, 8*, 373–384.

Sleator, E. (1986). Diagnosis. In E. Sleator & W. Pelham (Eds.), *Dialogues in pediatric management: Vol. 1. Attention deficit disorder* (pp. 11–43). Norwalk, CT: Appleton-Century-Crofts.

Sleator, E., & Pelham, W. E. (Eds.). (1986). *Dialogues in pediatric management: Vol. 1. Attention deficit disorder.* Norwalk, CT: Appleton-Century-Crofts.

Sleator, E., & von Neumann, A. (1974). Methylphenidate in the treatment of hyperkinetic children. *Clinical Pediatrics, 13*, 19–24.

Solanto, M. V. (1984). Neuropharmacological basis of stimulant drug action in attention deficit with hyperactivity: A review and synthesis. *Psychological Bulletin, 95*, 387–409.

Solanto, M. V., & Conners, C. K. (1982). A dose-response and time-action analysis of autonomic and behavioral effects of methylphenidate in attention deficit disorder with hyperactivity. *Psychophysiology, 19*, 658–667.

Sprague, R. L., & Sleator, E. K. (1977). Methylphenidate in hyperkinetic children: Differences in dose effects on learning and social behavior. *Science, 198*, 1274–1276.

Stephens, R., Pelham, W. E., & Skinner, R. (1984). The state-dependent and main effects of pemoline and methylphenidate on paired-associates learning and spelling in hyperactive children. *Journal of Consulting and Clinical Psychology, 52*, 104–113.

Stewart, M. A., Cummings, C., Singer, S., & deBlois, C. S. (1981). The overlap between hyperactive and unsocialized aggressive children. *Journal of Child Psychology and Psychiatry, 22*, 35–45.

Stewart, M. A., deBlois, C. D., & Cummings, C. (1980). Psychiatric disorder in the parents of hyperactive boys and those with conduct disorder. *Journal of Child Psychology and Psychiatry, 21*, 283–292.

Stewart, M. A., Mendelson, W. B., & Johnson, N. E. (1973). Hyperactive children as adolescents: How they describe themselves. *Child Psychiatry and Human Development, 4*, 3–11.

Stewart, M. A., Pitts, F., Craig, A., & Dieruf, W. (1966). The hyperactive child syndrome. *American Journal of Orthopsychiatry, 36*, 861–867.

Stokes, T. F., & Baer, D. M. (1977). An implicit technology of generalization. *Journal of Applied Behavior Analysis, 10*, 349.

Swanson, J., & Kinsbourne, M. (1979). The cognitive effects of stimulant drugs on hyperactive (inattentive) children. In G. Hale & M. Lewis (Eds.), *Attention and the development of cognitive skills* (pp. 249–274). New York: Plenum.

Swanson, J., Kinsbourne, M., Roberts, W., & Zucker, K. (1978). Time-response analysis of the effect of stimulant medication on the learning ability of children referred for hyperactivity. *Pediatrics, 61*, 21–29.

Swanson, J. M., Sandman, E., Deutsch, C., & Baren, M. (1983). Methylphenidate (Ritalin) given with or before breakfast: Part I. Behavioral, cognitive & electrophysiological effects. *Pediatrics, 72*, 49–55.

Sykes, D. H., Douglas, V. I., Weiss, G., & Minde, K. K. (1971). Attention in hyperactive children and the effect of methylphenidate (Ritalin). *Journal of Child Psychology and Psychiatry, 2*, 129–139.

Uhlenhuth, E. H., Lipman, R. S., & Covi, L. (1969). Combined pharmacotherapy and psychotherapy: Controlled studies. *Journal of Nervous and Mental Disease, 148*, 52–64.

Ullmann, R. K., Sleator, E. K., & Sprague, R. L. (1985a). A change of mind: The Conners abbreviated rating scales reconsidered. *Journal of Abnormal Child Psychology, 13*, 553–566.

Ullmann, R. K., Sleator, E. K., & Sprague, R. L. (1985b) Introduction to the use of the ACTeRS. *Psychopharmacology Bulletin, 21*, 915–916.

Varley, C. K. (1983). Effects of methylphenidate in adolescents with attention deficit disorder. *Journal of the American Academy of Child Psychiatry, 22*, 351–354.

Wahler, R. G. (1980). The insular mother: Her problems in parent-child treatment. *Journal of Applied Behavior Analysis, 13*, 207–219.

Weiss, G., & Hechtman, L. (1986). *Hyperactive children grown up*. New York: Guilford Press.

Weiss, G., Hechtman, L., Perlman, T., Hopkins, J., & Wener, A. (1979). Hyperactives as young adults: A controlled prospective ten-year follow-up of 75 children. *Archives of General Psychiatry, 36*, 675–681.

Weiss, G., Minde, K., Werry, J., Douglas, V., & Nemeth, E. (1971). Studies on the hyperactive child. VIII. Five year follow-up. *Archives of General Psychiatry, 24*, 409–414.

Wender, P. H., Reimherr, F. W., Wood, D., & Ward, M. (1985). Controlled study of methylphenidate in treatment of attention deficit disorder, residual type, in adults. *The American Journal of Psychiatry, 142*, 547–552.

Werner, E. E., Bierman, J., & French, F. (1971). *The children of Kauai*. Honolulu: University of Hawaii Press.

Whalen, C. K. (1989). Attention deficit and hyperactivity disorders. In T. H. Ollendick & M. Hersen (Eds.), *Handbook of child psychopathology* (2nd ed., pp. 131–169). New York: Plenum Press.

Whalen, C. K., Henker, B., Collins, B. E., Fink, D., & Dotemoto, S. (1979a). A social ecology of hyperactive boys: Medication effects in structured classroom environments. *Journal of Applied Behavior Analysis, 12*, 65–81.

Whalen, C. K., Henker, B., Collins, B., McAuliffe, S., & Vaux, A. (1979b). Peer interaction in a structured communication task: Comparisons of normal and hyperactive boys and of methylphenidate (Ritalin) and placebo effects. *Child Development, 50*, 388–401.

Whalen, C. K., Henker, B., Swanson, J. M., Granger, D., Kliewer, W., & Spencer, J. (1987). Natural social behaviors in hyperactive children: Dose effects of methylphenidate. *Journal of Consulting and Clinical Psychology, 55*, 187–193.

Witt, J. C. (1986). Teachers' resistance to the use of school-based interventions. *Journal of School Psychology, 24*, 37–44.

Witt, J. C., Martens, B. K., & Elliott, S. N. (1984). Factors affecting teachers' judgments of the acceptability of behavioral interventions: Time involvement, behavior problem severity, and type of intervention. *Behavior Therapy, 15*, 204–209.

Witt, J. C., & Robbins, J. R. (1985). Acceptability of reductive interventions for the control of inappropriate child behavior. *Journal of Abnormal Child Psychology, 13*, 59–68.

Zametkin, A. J., & Rapoport, J. L. (1986). The pathophysiology of attention deficit disorder with hyperactivity: A review. In B. Lahey & A. Kazdin (Eds.), *Advances in clinical child psychology* (Vol. 9, pp. 177–216). New York: Plenum.

Zametkin, A. J., & Rapoport, J. L. (1987). Neurobiology of attention deficit disorder with hyperactivity: Where have we come in 50 years? *Journal of American Academy of Child and Adolescent Psychiatry, 26*(5), 676–686.

11

Biobehavioral Aspects of Pain in Children

Patrick J. McGrath

Professor and Co-ordinator of Clinical Psychology,
Dalhouse University
Halifax, N.S., CANADA

B. Jennifer Dunn-Geier

Psychologist
Children's Hospital of Eastern Ontario
Ottawa, Ontario, CANADA

INTRODUCTION

Relative to the extensive literature on adult pain, pain in children has only recently begun to receive the attention it deserves (Jeans, 1983).Childhood pain has been neglected because of the difficulties in measuring pain in children as well as a failure to recognize the prevalence of pain in this age group. However, within the past decade, there have been many important contributions in the area.

This chapter will review the literature on pain in children and will examine different types of childhood pain, the prevalence of pain problems, biobehavioral mechanisms of pain, measurement, management and prognosis. Of necessity, it will be limited to those types of pain that are most frequent in children. We have attempted to develop the chapter from a behavioral medicine perspective and, consequently, types of pain in which a behavioral medicine approach has been noteworthy will be emphasized. We will not discuss pain which is due to specific pathological conditions (e.g., appendicitis or trauma) except when a major contribution has been made from the behavioral sciences. The chapter will be organized into two major sections: one dealing with recurrent and chronic types of pain and the other with pain from aversive medical procedures including surgery.

RECURRENT AND CHRONIC PAIN

Differentiation Between Chronic and Recurrent Pain

Recurrent pain is pain which is intermittent and varies in intensity. There are several types of recurrent pain which occur frequently in children (i.e. migraine headache, recurrent abdominal pain, limb pain).

The differentiation between recurrent pain and chronic pain is not always clear. Recurrent pain is pain that comes and goes. However, the essential difference between chronic and recurrent pain is how well the child is coping. Individuals who have pain over an extended period of time, who are not coping well with the pain and whose lives are controlled by the pain problem regardless of whether the pain is continual or episodic can be said to have chronic intractable pain (Crue, 1985) or recurrent pain with handicap (McGrath, Mathews, & Pigeon, 1991).

Based on the above distinction, an example of recurrent pain would be a child with migraine headaches who has made a satisfactory adjustment and does not allow the headaches to interfere with his/her life. In contrast, a child with migraine headaches (a type of recurrent pain) who misses several school days each month because of pain and whose pain interferes with other daily activities, would be said to be suffering from chronic intractable pain or recurrent pain with handicap.

Prevalence

The prevalence of recurrent headache, including migraine, has been estimated to be approximately 11 percent, for children aged 7–15 years. Migraine alone has been found to occur in 4 percent of children (Bille, 1962). Other estimates of prevalence (Oster, 1972; Sillanpaa, 1983) have been higher, ranging up to 26 percent. Similarly, recurrent abdominal pain, which is severe enough to interfere with everyday activities, occurs in approximately 10–15 percent of children (Apley & Naish, 1958) and limb pain is present in 4–18 percent of children (Oster, 1972; Naish & Apley, 1951). Coleman (1984) reports that chest pain has become a major cause for referral to pediatric cardiology clinics and it accounts for 650,000 patient visits annually in patients aged 10–21 years in the United States (Brenner, Engel, & Berman, 1984). However, its actual prevalence is unknown. Therefore, the most prevalent pain problems in children are recurrent headache, abdominal, limb, and chest pain. On the other hand, back pain, while common in adults occurs infrequently in children and adolescents (King, 1984). The prevalence of chronic intractable pain or handicap due to pain in children is not known but we believe it to be rare.

Although common, recurrent limb and chest pain in children have not been extensively investigated from a behavioral medicine perspective and will be dealt with only briefly. However, contributions from a behavioral medicine perspective have been notable in recurrent headache and recurrent abdominal pain.

HEADACHE

Types of Migraine

A very wide range of organic pathology can cause headache (see Barlow, 1984, for a recent review). However, at least 99 percent of recurrent headaches are not due to any known organic pathology and are said to be benign. There are two major types of benign headache: migraine headache and muscle contraction headache. These benign headaches are the focus of this section.

The cause of migraine is not clear and both neurogenic and vascular theories are current. Typically, the pain is paroxysmal. There are a number of distinct types of migraine including: classic migraine; common migraine; complicated migraine; and cluster headache. Classic migraines are preceded by an aura which is usually visual. Common migraines which are the most frequent type of migraine in children, do not have prodromal auras and are more typically frontal and bilateral. Complicated migraine includes basilar artery migraine, hemiplegic migraine, opthalmoplegic migraine, and the "Alice in Wonderland" syndrome. They are characterized by sensory and motor defects that persist during and after the headache. Cluster headache (also known as Horton's cephalagia) are unilateral, extremely painful, brief headaches that occur in periodic clusters. More detailed descriptions of these subtypes of migraine headache are available in McGrath (1983b) and McGrath and Unruh (1987).

Factors in Migraine Headache

A number of factors have been implicated in migraine headache including genetic, operant, stress, depression, and personality factors. The following provides a brief discussion of the research related to each of these factors.

Genetic factors. A strong genetic component has been suggested in the origin of migraine. The identification of a parent who has migraine is often used as a factor in the diagnosis of migraine; however, problems often arise because diagnosis of family members is not by clinical examination. Bille (1981) reports on the only longitudinal study of the inheritance of childhood migraine. He did a 23-year follow-up on 73 persons who had been diagnosed as having severe migraine. Forty-seven individuals (19 men and 28 women) had a total of 90 children who were then 4 years of age or older. Two of the 19 fathers each had a girl with migraine and 13 of the 28 mothers had a total of 4 boys and 9 girls with migraine. Migraine seems to be inherited more frequently by way of the mother and more often by girls.

Operant factors. The notion that children usually complain about headache to avoid unpleasant events or to receive special privileges and attention appears prevalent. However, it is our clinical impression that this is usually not the case. An important diagnostic test of operant pain is the contingencies that are in effect. Operant pain occurs when it leads to special privileges or results in excuse from duties, and should disappear when the privileges or excuse from duties are not available. Operantly driven pain may be quite important in cases of chronic pain and will be discussed in greater detail in that section.

Stress. Although most researchers and clinicians agree that there is a biological disposition to migraine, many operate on the assumption that migraine is triggered by either psychological or physiological stress. However,the mechanism of action of stress has not been well investigated. Some argue that stress causes a cognitive shift which mediates autonomic arousal (Bakal, 1982) whereas others suggest a muscular or biochemical mediation.

There is a limited amount of research that has been concerned with the relationship between migraine and stress. Vahlquist (1955) found that 87 percent of a sample of 55 children reported that mental stress was a trigger for migraine attacks. Bille (1962) reports that of the 61 children who were able top identify factors that would lead to migraine, 28 mentioned school work and 7 mentioned mental stress. A recent survey of 2,181 school children in Amsterdam (Passchier & Orlebeke, 1985) found that 30 percent of the elementary school students and 40 percent of the secondary school students attributed their headaches to stress. However, both of these studies were retrospective in nature. That is, stress was not recorded before the headache and therefore, stress may just be a convenient but erroneous way to explain headache.

Depression. The role that depression may play in triggering migraine has also received some consideration. For example, Andrasik, Kabela, Quinn, Blanchard, and Rosenblum (1987) found that children with migraine were more depressed than pain-free controls. However, in our lab we have shown that the amount of pain that a child has is related to the level of depression regardless of whether the pain is migraine or musculoskeletal pain (Cunningham et al., 1987). These findings suggest that depression may be the result of, rather than the cause of, a pain disorder.

Personality. It has been suggested that children with migraine have a specific personality type that predisposes them to migraine. Migraineurs have been described as children who are delicate, shy, withdrawn, sober, polite, well-mannered, conscientious, responsible, unusually thoughtful and extremely obedient to parental wishes but obstinate, stubborn, and inflexible (Wolff, in Anderson, 1980).

There have been a number of poorly designed studies since Wolff's observations that have tended to support the image of childhood migraineurs being withdrawn, overachieving, and anxious (e.g., Koch, & Melchoir, 1969). However, the previously mentioned study (Cunningham et al., 1987) in which 20 children with migraine were compared to 20 children with musculoskeletal pain and with 20 pain-free children has suggested that the stereotyped image of the migraineur may be the result of having a longstanding pain disorder rather than a cause of migraine.

Muscle Contraction Headache

In contrast to the vascular origin of migraine, muscle contraction headaches are thought to arise from prolonged muscle tension in the head and neck. These headaches tend to be more constant in occurrence and present as a bandlike tightness. Some research (Bakal,

1982) has suggested that migraine and muscle contraction headaches are often not distinct. Many children with a serious headache disorder report both types of headaches.

In contrast to migraine, there is not thought to be a strong genetic component in muscle contraction headache. Furthermore, there are no studies on stress, personality, or depression in muscle contraction headache in children but clinical lore is similar to that of migraine.

Long-term Prognosis of Childhood Headache

Contrary to popular opinion, children often do not outgrow headache. Bille (1981), for example, found that after 23 years, approximately 60 percent of his more severe migraine headache sufferers were continuing to experience headache. Prognosis was better for males (52% remitting) than for females (30%) remitting. Similar follow-up studies on muscle contraction headaches in children have not been conducted.

Treatment of Pediatric Headache

Treatment of pediatric headache can be pharmacological, environmental, or psychological (behavioral). The pharmacological treatment of benign headache can be abortive, palliative, or prophylactic. Abortive medication which frequently consists of ergotamine preparations is not used in the treatment of muscle contraction headaches, but is occasionally appropriate for adolescents with particularly disabling migraine. However, no evaluations of abortive medications in this age group have been done. As well, abortive medication is infrequently used with younger children.

The most common type of pharmacological treatment for children with migraines is palliative medication (i.e., antiemetics, and analgesics). However, our clinical impression is that children are frequently not appropriately medicated for headache. Typically, analgesics are either not taken or are taken only after the headache becomes severe. Parents and children frequently have a strong antidrug bias that interferes with appropriate analgesic usage. No evaluations of palliative medication have been done in pediatric headache, although clinical reports indicate that early use of palliative medication reduces the severity and duration of the headaches but not the frequency.

Prophylactic medication refers to drugs which are taken daily to prevent the occurrence of migraines. Several types of prophylactic medication are used with children including propranalol, tricyclics especially amitriptyline; and antiepileptics especially dilantin; methysergide and calcium blockers. In a double-blind placebo controlled crossover study, Ludviggson (1974) found that propranalol resulted in a 70 percent reduction in frequency of attacks compared to a 9 percent reduction in response to placebo. However, a more recently published double-blind crossover study (Forsythe, Gillies, & Sills, 1984) has failed to show that propranalol is more effective than placebo. In fact, there was some indication that headaches lasted longer with propranalol. A calcium channel blocker, flunarizine, has been demonstrated effective in a randomized double-blind study with 48 children (Sorge & Marano, 1985).

The effectiveness of pharmacological treatment, although clinically widespread, has yet to be adequately empirically demonstrated in pediatric migraine.

Although pharmacological treatments are available, the most commonly researched treatment for migraine in children and adolescents follows a psychological orientation. Psychological or behavioral treatment for pediatric headache has focused on relaxation, biofeedback, or cognitive interventions. Several single-case studies have suggested the efficacy of both relaxation and biofeedback in migraine and muscle contraction headache. For a review the reader can consult McGrath and Unruh (1987). A number of controlled studies have supported the efficacy of these treatments.

Labbe and Williamson (1984) randomly assigned 28 childhood migraineurs to either a wait-list control or autogenic biofeedback. Autogenic biofeedback was superior to the control condition with 93 percent of the children in the biofeedback group reporting a reduction of 50 percent or more in headache activity. There was no improvement in the control group. Improvements were maintained at 6-month follow-up.

Richter, et al. (1986) randomly assigned 51 children with migraine to one of three groups: relaxation training, cognitive coping therapy, and a placebo treatment. The two active treatments were superior to the placebo treatment, with those children who suffered the more severe headaches doing particularly well. Gains were maintained at 16-week follow-up.

Fentress, Masek, Mehegan, and Benson (1986) randomly assigned 18 pediatric migraineurs between the ages of 8 and 12 years to one of three groups: relaxation response, relaxation-response plus biofeedback, and wait-list control group. The two active treatment groups were superior to the control condition and equivalent to each other. One-year follow-up showed that the improvements were maintained.

In a study in our lab, Davies (1987) compared group treatment, individual treatment, and a psychological placebo control in a sample of 48 adolescent female migraineurs. Individual and group treatment had the same content and consisted of relaxation and problem solving. She found that the individual treatment and the group treatment were both significantly more effective than the placebo for adolescents with moderate levels of headache. However, the individual treatment was found to be superior for adolescents with more severe headache.

Larson and Melin (1986) conducted an experimental trial of relaxation on 33 adolescent students. After a 4-week baseline, adolescents with tension and mixed tension-migraine headache were randomly assigned to either relaxation or an information-contact condition. Relaxation training resulted in a greater than 50 percent reduction in the headache activity of 9 of 11 subjects immediately posttreatment and 6 of 11 at 6-month follow-up. Only 1 of 13 information-contact subjects reported 50 percent or greater reduction after treatment and 5 of 13 reported such improvement at follow-up.

A randomized trial from our lab (McGrath et al., 1987) compared relaxation training, a psychological placebo, and an "own best efforts" therapy. All groups of patients were improved but there was no differential effect of treatment.[1]

In sum, the studies conducted to date suggest that the psychological treatment of headache in children and adolescents is promising. However, care must be taken in research in this field to include appropriate control groups.

RECURRENT ABDOMINAL PAIN

Recurrent abdominal pain can occur as a symptom of a variety of diseases or pathological conditions including appendicitis, Crohn's disease, ulcers, endometriosis, and trauma. Recently, Levine and Rappaport (1984) have summarized strategies for the differential diagnosis of these conditions. This section will not deal with issues related to pathological organic abdominal pain. Rather, it will focus on recurrent abdominal pain which, by definition, is pain which is not due to any known organic condition. Apley's criteria for recurrent abdominal pain of childhood (Apley, 1975) are universally accepted. These are: at

---

[1] Recently we (McGrath et al., 1989) reported on a reduced therapist centered treatment (referred to as the Help Yourself Treatment). Both therapist mediated and a reduced-contact treatment that relied on a manual and tapes were superior to a control condition. However, the Help Yourself treatment was far more efficient and less expensive than the therapist-based treatment. Help Yourself is now available from a commercial press (McGrath et al., 1990).

least three attacks of pain severe enough to interfere with normal activities; attacks occurring over a period of three months; and no known organic cause. Interestingly, at least 95 percent of children with recurrent abdominal pain do not develop organic etiology which could account for their pain (Barr & Feuerstein, 1983).

We have reviewed this area from the point of view of the physician (McGrath & Feldman, 1986) and this discussion borrows from that analysis.

Physiological Mechanisms in Recurrent Abdominal Pain

Physiological factors that have been implicated in recurrent abdominal pain include: autonomic instability, lactose intolerance, and constipation/gut motility. A brief discussion of the research evidence related to each of these factors follows.

Autonomic instability. Four studies are cited in the literature which have examined aspects of hypothesized autonomic defect in children with recurrent abdominal pain. Kopel, Kim, and Barbera (1967) found that following subcutaneous injection of prostigmine methyl sulphate, children with recurrent abdominal pain showed increased rectosigmoid motility in comparison to controls, suggesting an increased sensitivity to parasympathetic stimulation. Based on the results, the authors suggested that children with recurrent abdominal pain have a general autonomic imbalance. Rubin, Barbero, and Sibinga (1967) found that children with recurrent abdominal pain have an increased recovery time in pupillary response to a cold pressor stress but no differences were found in resting levels or response to stress. However, Apley, Haslam, and Tulloch (1971) failed to replicate the finding of increased recovery time but did note that children with recurrent abdominal pain were more likely to have an "unstable" recovery. Unfortunately, the authors did not precisely describe what constitutes an unstable recovery.

In a more recent comparison of children with recurrent abdominal pain and carefully matched controls using cold pressor stress, Feuerstein, Barr, Francoeur, Houle, and Rafman (1982) found no difference in physiological, behavioral, or self-report in the stress phase or in the recovery phase. Therefore, the importance of autonomic instability in recurrent abdominal pain remains unclear at this time.

Lactose intolerance. At least two studies have demonstrated the role of lactose intolerance in children with recurrent abdominal pain and their response to a lactose-free diet (Barr, Levine, & Watkins,

1979); Liebman 1979). However, a number of studies do not support these results. For example, Lebenthal, Rossi, Nord, and Branski (1981) did not find an increased prevalence of lactose intolerance in children with recurrent abdominal pain as compared to controls, nor did the lactose-intolerant children respond to a lactose-free diet more than did children who were not lactose-deficient. Similarly, Christensen (1980) and McGrath, Goodman, Shipman, Firestone, and Peters (1983) did not find any differences in lactose intolerance between children with recurrent abdominal pain and pain-free controls. Therefore, at this time the best evidence is that lactose intolerance is not a major cause of recurrent abdominal pain in children.

Constipation/gut motility. Although one well-recognized cause of abdominal pain is constipation, most children with recurrent abdominal pain are not obviously constipated. However, constipation does exist in many children without a child's awareness or without classic signs (Barr, Wilkinson, Levine, & Mulvihill, 1979). In addition, parents are unlikely to know of their children's bowel habits. In a study by Dimson (1971), 22 percent of the sample of children with recurrent abdominal pain were found to be rectally constipated and the remainder were suffering from colonic spasm. A randomized placebo-controlled trial using fiber to treat recurrent abdominal pain (Feldman, McGrath, Hodgson, Ritter, & Shipman, 1985) found that fiber supplements decreased pain at least 50 percent in half of the children studied whereas placebo was effective in about one-quarter of the children. There were no greater side effects on the fiber and the compliance to treatment was good. Although the efficacy of a treatment cannot provide definitive evidence of causation of a disorder, this study does provide suggestive evidence for the constipation/gut motility hypothesis of recurrent abdominal pain.

Research is required to determine which children are likely to benefit from an increase in dietary fiber.

Psychological/Behavioral Factors in Recurrent Abdominal Pain

Psychological factors which have been implicated in recurrent abdominal pain include: stress, modeling, depression, operant, family enmeshment, and somatization disorder. The first three of these factors will be discussed in this section. A discussion of operant factors, family enmeshment, and somatization disorder follows in the chronic pain section.

Stress factors. A number of studies have examined the relationship between stress and recurrent abdominal pain. For example, in a comparison of children and pain-free controls, McGrath et al. (1983) found no difference in the amount of life change experienced by the two groups. Similar results have been cited by Raymer, Weininger, and Hamilton (1984). In sharp contrast to these two studies are the findings of Greene, Walker, Hickson, and Thompson (1985) who were able to separate organic and nonorganic abdominal pain on the basis of negative life events in a group of adolescents attending an adolescent clinic. However, they emphasize that report of increased negative life events in patients appearing at a medical clinic with nonorganic pain does not prove causation.

Barr and Feuerstein (1983) have emphasized that stress may be a precipitant of the child not coping well with the pain even if the symptom itself is not causally related to stress. The research related to whether or not children with recurrent abdominal pain have anxious personalities that make them prone to the effects of stress is equivocal. Two surveys of children with recurrent abdominal pain which did not use standardized anxiety measures suggest that these children are more anxious (Apley & Naish, 1958; Liebman, 1978). In a controlled study using standard measures, Crossley (1982) found children with nonspecific pain to be more anxious. However, the results of two controlled studies with outpatients (McGrath et al., 1983; Raymer et al., 1984) do not support these findings. One possible explanation for these disparate results was that Crossley (1982) studied children who were hospitalized with recurrent abdominal pain, while the other studies examined out patients. Children who are hospitalized for recurrent abdominal pain are not typical and, in many hospitals, only seriously disturbed children would be hospitalized for recurrent abdominal pain (Feldman, 1986).

Modeling. The role of modeling in pain behavior is difficult to disentangle from constitutional predispositions. Oster (1972), Stone and Barbero (1970), and Apley (1975) noted that pain problems tend to run in families but the roles of physiologic tendency and psychologic modeling could not be distinguished. Christensen and Mortensen (1975) followed up 34 children who had been hospitalized for abdominal pain approximately 30 years previously. They also investigated the children of these patients and found that the children of patients with stomach pain were not more likely to have pain than were controls. However, they did find that children who had parents currently complaining of pain were much more likely to have pain. This finding suggests a modeling rather than a biological transmission of stomach pain.

Depression. There is conflicting evidence whether or not a higher percentage of children with recurrent abdominal pain are depressed than are controls and it may be that pain causes depression rather than vice versa (McGrath et al., 1983; Raymer et al., 1984). It is evident that findings of uniform depression in children with recurrent abdominal pain (Hughes, 1984) are most likely due to a sampling bias in the specific samples and not representative of the population of children with abdominal pain.

Management of Recurrent Abdominal Pain

Management of recurrent abdominal pain can be psychological or dietary. Psychological treatment consists of: reassurance that there is no major disease; teaching of strategies such as cognitive coping and relaxation to control pain; and instituting contingencies for reporting or not reporting pain. However, there are no properly conducted studies that demonstrate the degree of effectiveness of psychological treatments. Apley (1975) reported that a type of informal psychotherapy consisting of reassurance and encouragement was effective. Our own impression is that most children with recurrent abdominal pain, who are coping well, need no formal psychological contact but are well served by an understanding primary care physician. If the child is doing well, care must be taken to avoid the potential negative effects of personally invasive psychological therapy for a benign condition.

Dietary treatment consists of the addition of approximately 10 grams of fiber daily either in the form of increased consumption of high-fiber foods such as bran and vegetables or by means of a fiber supplement biscuit. The previously discussed study by Feldman et al. (1985) provides support for the use of supplementary dietary fibre in the treatment of recurrent abdominal pain.

CHEST PAIN

Chest pain is—in the lay mind—synonymous with heart problems. Fortunately, chest pain in children who do not have known cardiac pathology is rarely of cardiac origin. The more likely causes are: (a) musculoskeletal problems (31%) including costochondritis (14%), chest wall syndrome (13%), skeletal trauma (2%), or ribcage anomalies (2%); (b) hyperventilation (20%); (c) breast-related problems (5%); or (d) idiopathic (39%) (Pantell & Goodman, 1983). A number of studies have suggested that idiopathic chest pain is experienced by children and adolescents who have been subject to a high level of stressful events or who are depressed or anxious (Pantell & Goodman, 1983; Selbst, 1985). A very important related problem is that of social disability because of overprotection due to fear of heart attack in children who have innocent heart murmurs (Feldman, Rosser, & McGrath, 1987). No studies have investigated psychosocial treatment of either chest pain or social disability from cardiac nondisease.

LIMB PAIN

Limb pain can be due to trauma, orthopedic conditions, rheumatic disease, infectious disease, malignancies, benign bony tumors, endocrine disorders, nutritional abnormalities, miscellaneous disorders, or syndromes of unknown origin (Bowver & Hollister, 1984). The most common benign limb pains in children are "growing" pains and patello-femoral pain.

Growing pains usually occur in preteenage children. The pain is typically in the calf or thigh muscle, comes at night and is relieved by massage and analgesics. Growing pains are of unknown cause but are not due to growing. Patello-femoral knee pain is most common in adolescent females who are physically active. Pain is worst upon sitting for a period of time, when walking up stairs or when riding a bicycle. It is thought to be caused by a misalignment of the patella and is treated by physiotherapy.

There has been only one evaluation of psychosocial or behavioral treatments for either growing pains or patello-femoral knee pain. Baxter (1986) randomly assigned children to either a follow up or a stretching regimen. Children who did the stretching exercises became pain free more quickly than children who were only followed up.

CHRONIC INTRACTABLE PAIN SYNDROME

Any of the types of pain discussed above can become chronic intractable pain or pain with disability. As discussed previously, it is not the type or frequency of the pain which defines chronic pain, but rather it is the ability of the child to cope with the pain and the degree to which the pain interferes with daily activities. Typically, children who are missing school or other daily activities as a result of their pain are referred to as chronic pain patients. It is our impression that most children who have chronic or recurrent types of pain cope quite well; however, there is a small group of children who do not cope. Very little is known about factors which may differentiate between those children who are coping well with their pain and those who are not.

Five factors have been described in the chronic pain literature: operant factors, modeling, depression, family enmeshment, and somatization disorder. The exact role of both depression and modeling in children with chronic pain has not been detailed, although, it is our clinical impression that modeling of illness behavior by parents and childhood depression are frequently of importance.

According to the operant interpretation of chronic pain, chronic pain behaviors are the result of three basic learning processes: (a) direct, positive reinforcement of illness and pain behaviors (b) avoidance learning in which an individual's illness and pain behaviors allow him to avoid unpleasant events and (c) vicarious learning where an individual witnesses other people reinforced for illness behavior.

The major empirical support for an operant interpretation of chronic intractable pain comes from single case studies published in the behavioral psychology literature (Sank & Biglan, 1974; Miller & Kratchowill, 1979). For example, Sank & Biglan (1974) found that a token system in which nonoccurrence of severe attacks of abdominal pain and attendance at school were consequated with points that could be exchanged for money and saved for other reinforcers successfully reduced pain complaints and increased time at school.

Although reinforcement is important in the problems that some children experience, it is our opinion that the chronic intractable pain of most children cannot be explained exclusively by operant factors. Furthermore, treatment that is solely operant may reduce complaints of pain without altering the experience of pain.

Family enmeshment or overinvolvement of parents in the lives of their children, has been cited as a cause of chronic pain by clinicians (Apley, 1975; Hughes & Zimin, 1978; Stone & Barbero, 1970). Recent experimental evidence (Dunn-Geier, McGrath, Rourke, D'Astous & Latter, 1986) suggests that children who are not coping with chronic pain have mothers who intrude more in a pain-oriented situation than do mothers of children who are coping with pain. However, it is not clear if parental intrusiveness is a cause or a result of having a child who is not coping with pain. There are no other empirical studies related to the role of family enmeshment in childhood chronic pain.

Routh and Ernst (1984) found that children who have recurrent abdominal pain with no known organic cause had more symptoms of somatization disorder than children with an organic stomach pain disorder. As well, children who had experienced pain for several years had more symptoms of somatization disorder than children with recurrent abdominal pain of a more recent onset. Relatives of these children were also found to have a higher incidence of somatization disorder (Ernst, Routh, & Harper, 1984). These data can best be interpreted as evidence that the subgroup of children (approximately 17%) who have recurrent abdominal pain for more than one year may develop into adult patients with somatization disorder.

Children who have numerous widespread or changing pain symptoms without specific physical findings, who are missing school, and whose parents have similar types of problems are clearly at risk for developing a chronic pain disorder with handicap. There are no studies documenting the efficacy of interventions with these children. However, a series of guidelines has been prepared that may be of help to the clinicians faced with these most difficult patients (McGrath et al., 1986).

PAIN FROM CHRONIC DISEASE

The effectiveness of biobehavioral treatment methods to assist children in coping with pain from chronic disease has only recently been examined. For example, Varni and his associates have demonstrated that use of biobehavioral methods in helping children with chronic arthritic pain in hemophilia. In a series of properly controlled single-subject experimental studies Varni (1981a, 1981b, and Varni and Gilbert, 1982), have combined progressive muscle relaxation, meditative breathing exercises, and guided imagery. They demonstrated that these techniques were effective in reducing chronic pain without altering accurate perception of acute bleeding pain.

In an anecdotal case study, Zeltzer, Dash, and Holland (1979) report on the use of hypnosis to help two young adults to control pain due to sickle cell disease.

Additional well controlled studies examining pain in chronic illness are needed.

PAIN FROM AVERSIVE MEDICAL PROCEDURES

Two major types of painful medical procedures should be considered: postoperative pain and pain as the result of procedures such as injections, bone marrow aspirations, and lumbar punctures.

Postoperative Pain

The behavioral medicine literature that is related to postoperative pain has been very scarce and has focused on measurement. Investigation of the measurement of postoperative pain in preschool children has been limited and is a major area that behavioral medicine approaches can lead to improved medical care. Measurement of postoperative pain in the preschool child is complicated by their reduced cognitive and verbal abilities, as well as the effects of anesthesia in the immediate postoperative period. In these circumstances, self-report is of limited utility and, consequently pain behavior must be used. The most obvious pain behavior in children is crying and the presence or absence of crying is the most common way that parents and health professional judge a young child's pain. However, some type of electroacoustic analysis has been developed (Wasz-Hockert, Lind, Vuorenkoski, Partanen, & Valanne, 1968), it is not practical in the clinic. Measurement of amount and intensity of crying is also possible.

In a hospital setting, there are two practical ways to measure postoperative pain behavior in preschool children. The first method is to use a global rating by adult caregivers: the second method is to use observation of specific pain behaviors.

The most popular global rating technique is the visual analogue scale (Huskisson, 1983) which consists of a 10 cm line with an anchor point at either end. Ratings are made by making a mark on the line which is indicative of level of pain. Scoring is done by measuring the distance of the mark from the beginning of the line. Experienced adults, such as nurses, can rate the global amount of pain that they perceive that a child is suffering using Visual Analogue Scales (Martin, 1982; McGrath, et al., 1985). However, care must be taken to insure that the anchors used are clear.

In contrast to the global ratings provided by visual analogue scales, observations of specific pain behaviors permit a more detailed analysis of the pain. For example, the CHEOPS (the Children's Hospital of Eastern Ontario Pain Scale) (McGrath et al., 1985) is an observational scale that was developed following discussion with recovery room nurses, review of the literature and pretesting. The CHEOPS is a 6-item, time sampling, behavioral scale in which behaviors are sampled once every 30 seconds. A value is assigned for each behavior; "0" is assigned to a behavior that is the antithesis of pain; "1" indicates neutral behavior; "2" signifies mild or moderate pain; "3" is reserved for severe pain. The range of the CHEOPS is from 4 to 12 for every tine period sampled.

We have used both visual analogue scale and the CHEOPS to measure postoperative pain in preschoolers. Using a 10-cm visual analogue scale with anchors of "no pain and "pain as severe as possible" we had nurses make a total of 127 ratings on 30 children in the hour following surgery. Independent ratings by a research assistant demonstrated interrater reliability of 0.91. These ratings also correspond with ratings on the CHEOPS.

The CHEOPS showed interrater reliability ranging from .90 to .995. Validity was indicated by a high correlation (0.81) with nurses visual analogue scale ratings. A further indication of validity was the responsiveness of CHEOPS scores to intravenous Fentanyl. In 20 children, mean CHEOPS scores for the three minutes prior to intravenous Fentanyl were 9.9, dropping to 6.3 three minutes following the intravenous opioid.

The major advantage of using the visual analogue scale for rating pain is that it takes only a few seconds for each measure. Although the CHEOPS requires an observer dedicated to this task, the scale is easily learned with 3–4 hours of practice. The major advantage of the CHEOPS is that it gives a more fine-grained analysis of the pain behaviors. The CHEOPS may not be sensitive in some situations (Beyer et al., 1990).

Postoperative pain measurement in the school-age child should be able to make use of some of the verbal methods which are the mainstay of adult measurement. Scales that have been evaluated with children include poker chip measures (Hester, 1979), visual analogue scales (Abu-Saad, 1984, O'Hara, McGrath, D'Astous, & Vair, 1987), faces scales (LeBaron & Zeltzer, 1985), and the Oucher (Beyer, 1984).

Two groups of children that are frequently subjected to surgery are sick neonates and congenitally disabled children. The work of Grunau and Craig (1987) which is discussed below may be particularly relevant for the development of behavioral measurements of pain in neonates. The measurement of pain in congenitally disabled children such as children with cerebral palsy has not been addressed at all.

The treatment of postoperative pain in children is virtually always pharmacological.

Pain from Aversive Diagnostic Procedures

Pain from aversive procedures has been studied using behavioral medicine methodology. Two types of contributions have been made: understanding of the development of pain and treatment of painful procedures.

Research by Franck (1986) and Grunau and Craig (1987) using very different methodologies has shown that infants in their first days of life do feel pain and react in more than a simple reflex fashion. Franck (1986) used photogrammetric techniques to evaluate response to heel lance in 10 infants who were 4 hours old. She showed that even at that age the babies swipe at the affected foot with the other foot. Grunau and Craig (1987) examined facial changes measured by coding videotapes and electroacoustically analyzed cry in 140 infants who were approximately 40 hours of age. They showed differences in response due to the babies sleep/wake state, the obstetric history and to the technician taking the blood. In contrast to previous belief, it is apparent that even very young infants experience pain.

Pain from immunizations has been investigated by both Craig, McMahon, Morison, and Zaskow (1984) and by Johnson and Strada (1986). They detail the behavioral and physiological pain response to this universal medical procedure.

One group of children that undergo many very painful procedures is children who have cancer. Katz, Kellerman, and Siegel (1980) developed the Procedures Behavior Rating Scale to measure distress associated with the repeated lumbar punctures and bone marrow aspirations that children with leukemia require to guide their treatment. They found that distress could be measured and that it was at an almost uniformly high level and did not habituate over time. Subsequent research (Kellerman, Zeltzer, Ellenberg, & Dash, 1983; Zeitzer & LeBarron, 1982; Hilgard & LeBaron, 1984; Jay, Elliott, Ozolins, Olson, & Pruitt, 1985) has demonstrated that training in hypnosis can reduce the pain/distress of these procedures.

SUMMARY

Although there has been an overall lack of research in childhood pain the situation is changing. Nearly every issue of the journals devoted to pain contain at least one article on children's pain. However, there remains much work to be done on pain measurement and treatment. In particular, research is needed on medical and behavioral treatment for the common recurrent pains of childhood: headache, recurrent abdominal pain, chest pain, and limb pain. Although research in the area of measurement of postoperative pain has made major advances the treatment of postoperative pain in children has not been investigated adequately. In addition, there is a major lack of research investigating differences between children who cope well with recurrent pain and children who do not cope. A more extensive review of pain in children is provided in our text (McGrath & Unruh, 1987).

REFERENCES

Abu-Saad, H. (1984). Assessing children's responses to pain. *Pain, 19*, 163–171.

Anderson, R. W. (1980). The relation of life situations, personality features and reactions to the migraine syndrome. In D. J. Dalessio (Ed.), *Wolff's headache and other head pain* (4th ed.). New York: Oxford University Press.

Andrasik, F., Kabela, E., Quinn, S., Attanasio, V., Blanchard, E. B., & Rosenblum, E. L. (1988). Psychological functioning of children who have recurrent migraine. *Pain, 34*, 43–52.

Apley, J. (1975). *The child with abdominal pains.* London: Blackwell.

Apley, J., Haslam, D., & Tulloch, G. (1971). Pupillary reaction in children with recurrent abdominal pain. *Arch Dis Childhood, 46*, 337–340.

Apley, J., & Naish, N. (1958). Children with recurrent abdominal pains: A field survey of 1000 school children. *Arch Dis Childhood, 33*, 165–170.

Bakal, D. A. (1982). *The psychobiology of chronic headache.* New York: Springer.

Barlow, C. F. (1984). *Headaches and migraine.* Philadelphia: J. B. Lippincott.

Barr, R., & Feuerstein, M. (1983). Recurrent abdominal pain syndrome: How appropriate are our basic clinical assumptions? In P. McGrath & P. Firestone (Ed.), *Pediatric and adolescent behavioral medicine: Issues in treatment* (pp. 13–27). New York: Springer.

Barr, R., Levine, M., & Watkins, J. (1979). Recurrent abdominal pain of childhood due to lactose intolerance. *New England Journal of Medicine, 300*, 1449–1452.

Barr, R., Wilkinson, R., Levine, M., & Mulvihill, D. (1979). Chronic and occult stool retention. A clinical tool for its evaluation in school aged children. *Clinical Pediatrics, 18*, 674–685.

Baxter, M. (1986). *Growth pains and growing pains.* Paper presented at Clinical Review Day, Children's Hospital of Eastern Ontario, Canada.

Beyer, J. (1984). *The Oucher: A user's manual and technical report.* Evanston, IL: The Hospital Play Equipment Co.

Beyer, J. E., McGrath, P. J., & Berde, C. B. (1990). Discordance between self-report and behavioral pain measures in children aged 3–7 years after surgery. *Journal of Pain and Symptom Management, 5*, 350–356.

Bille, B. (1962). Migraine in schoolchildren. *Acta Pediatr Scand, 51*, (suppl 136), 1–151.

Bille, B. (1981). Migraine in childhood and its prognosis. *Cephalagia, 1*, 71–75.

Bowyer, S., & Hollister, R. (1984). Limb pain in childhood. *The Pediatric Clinics of North America, 31*(5), 1053–1081.

Brenner, J., Engel, R., & Berman, M. (1984). Cardiologic perspectives of chest pain in childhood: A referral problem? To whom? *The Pediatric Clinics of North America, 31*, 1241–1258.

Christensen, M. (1980). Prevalence of lactose intolerance in children with recurrent abdominal pain. *Arch Dis Childhood, 50*, 110–114.

Coleman, W. (1984). Recurrent chest pain in children. *The Pediatric Clinics of North America, 31*, 1007–1026.

Craig, K. D., McMahon, R. J., Morison, J. D., & Zaskow, C. (1984). Developmental changes in infant pain, expression during immunization injections. *Social Science & Medicine, 19*, 1331–1337.

Crossley, R. (1982). Hospital admissions for abdominal pain in childhood. *Journal of the Royal Society of Medicine, 75*, 772–776.

Crue, B. L. (1985). Foreword. In G. M. Aronoff (Ed.), *Evaluation and treatment of chronic pain* (pp. xv–xxi). Baltimore: Urban and Schwarzenberg.

Cunningham, S. J., McGrath, P. J., Ferguson, H. B., D'Astous, J. D., Latter, J., Goodman, J. T., & Firestone, P. (1987). Personality and behavioral characteristics in pediatric migraine. *Headache, 27*, 16–20.

Davies, K. (1987). *Group versus individual behavioral treatment in adolescent migraine.* Doctoral dissertation, University of Manitoba, Winnipeg, Canada.

Dimson, S. (1971). Transit time related to clinical findings in children with recurrent abdominal pain. *Pediatrics, 47*, 666–674.

Dunn-Geier, J., McGrath, P. J., Rourke, B., D'Astous, J., & Latter, J. (1986). Chronic pain in adolescents: The ability to cope. *Pain, 26*, 23–32.

Ernst, A., Routh, D., & Harper, D. (1984). Abdominal pain in children and symptoms of somatization disorder. *Journal of Pediatric Psychology, 91*(1), 77–86.

Feldman, W. (1986). Response to Christensen. *Am J. Dis Childhood, 140*, 739.

Feldman, W., McGrath, P., Hodgson, C., Ritter, H., & Shipman, R. (1985). The use of dietary fibre in the management of simple childhood, idiopathic, recurrent, abdominal pain: Results in a prospective, double blind, randomized, controlled trial. *American Journal of Disease of Children, 139*, 1216–1218.

Feldman, W. Rosser, W., & McGrath, P. J. (1987). *Primary medical care of children and adolescents.* New York: Oxford University Press.

Fentress, D. W., Masek, B. J., Mehegan, J. E., & Benson, H. (1986). Biofeedback and relaxation-response training in the treatment of pediatric migraine. *Develop. Med. Child Neurology, 28*, 139–146.

Feurstein, M., Barr, R., Francoeur, T., Houle, M., & Rafman, S. (1982). Potential biobehavioral mechanisms of recurrent abdominal pain in children. *Pain, 13*, 287–298.

Forsythe, W. I., Gillies, D., & Sills, M. A. (1984). Propanolol ('Inderal') in the treatment of childhood migraine. *Develop. Med. Child Neurology, 26*, 737–741.

Franck, L. S. (1986). A new method to quantitatively describe pain behavior in infants. *Nursing Research, 35*, 28–31.

Greene, J., Walker, L., Hickson, G., & Thompson, J. (1985). Stressful life events and somatic complaints in adolescents. *Pediatrics, 75*, 19–22.

Grunau, R., & Craig, K. D. (1987). Pain expression in neonates: facial action and cry. *Pain, 28*, 395–410.

Hester, N. K. O. (1979). The preoperational child's reaction to immunization. *Nursing Research, 28*, 250–255.

Hilgard, J. R., & LeBaron, S. (1984). *Hypnotherapy of pain in children with cancer.* Los Altos, CA: Kaufmann.

Hughes, M. (1984). Recurrent abdominal pain and childhood depression: Clinical observation of 23 children and their families. *American Journal of Orthography, 54*, 146–155.

Hughes, M., & Zimin, R. (1978) Children with psychogenic abdominal pain and their families: Management during hospitalization. *Clinical Pediatrics, 17*, 569–573.

Huskisson, E. C. (1983). Visual analogue scales. In R. Melzack (Ed.), *Pain Measurement and Assessment.* New York: Raven Press.

Jay, S. M., Elliot, C. H., Ozolins, M., Olson, R. A., & Pruitt, S. D. (1985). Behavioral management of children's distress during painful medical procedures. *Behavioral Research Therapy, 23*, 513–520.

Jeans, M. E. (1983). Pain in children: A neglected area. In P. Firestone, P. McGrath, & W. Feldman (Eds.), *Advances in behavioral medicine for children and adolescents* (pp. 23–37). Hillsdale, NJ: Erlbaum.

Johnston, C. C., & Strada, M. E. (1986). Acute pain response in infants: A multidimensional description. *Pain, 24*, 373–382.

King, H. (1984). Back pain in children. *The Pediatric Clinics of North America, 31*, 1083–1095.

Koch, C., & Melchoir, J. C. (1969). Headache in childhood: A five year material from a pediatric university clinic. *Dan. Medical Bulletin, 16*, 109–114.

Katz, E. R., Kellerman, J., & Siegel, S. E. (1980). Distress behavior in children with cancer undergoing medical procedures: Developmental considerations. *Journal of Cons. Clinical Psychologists, 48*, 356–365.

Kellerman, J., Zeltzer, L., Ellenberg, L., & Dash, J. (1983). Adolescents with cancer: Hypnosis for the reduction of the acute pain and anxiety associated with medical procedures. *Journal of Adolescent Health Care, 4*, 85–90.

Kopel, F., Kim, I., & Barbero, G. (1967). Comparison of rectosigmoid motility in normal children, children with recurrent abdominal pain, and children with ulcerative colitis. *Pediatrics, 39*, 539–545.

Labbe, E., & Williamson, D. (1984). Treatment of childhood migraine using autogenic feedback training. *Journal of Consulting and Clinical Psychology, 52*, 968–976.

Larsson, B., & Melin, L. (1986). Chronic headaches in adolescents: Treatment in a school setting with relaxation training as compared with information-contact and self registration. *Pain, 25*, 325–336.

LeBaron, S., & Zeltzer, L. (1985). Hypnosis for hemophiliacs: Methodlogic problems and risks. *American Journal of Hematology/Oncology, 7*, 316–319.

Lebenthal, E., Rossi, T., Nord, K., & Branski, P. (1981). Recurrent abdominal pain and lactose absorption in children. *Pediatrics, 67*, 828–832.

Levine, M., & Rappaport, L. (1984). Recurrent abdominal pain in school children: The loneliness of the long distance physician. *The Pediatric Clinics of North America, 31*, 969–991.

Liebman, W. (1978). Recurrent abdominal pain in children: A retrospective study of 119 patients. *Clinical Pediatrics, 17*, 149–153.

Liebman, W. (1979). Recurrent abdominal pain in children: Lactose and sucrose intolerance, a prospective study. *Pediatrics, 64*, 43–45.

Ludvigsson, J. (1974). Propranolol used in prophylaxis of migraine in children. *Acta Neurol. Scandinav. 20*, 109–115.

McGrath, P. J. (1983a). Psychological aspects of recurrent abdominal pain. *Canadian Family Physician, 29*, 1655–1659.

McGrath, P. J. (1983b). Migraine headaches in children and adolescents. In P. Firestone, P. J. McGrath, & W. Feldman (Eds.), *Advances in behavioral medicine for children and adolescents*. Hillsdale, NJ: Erlbaum.

McGrath, P. J., Dunn-Geier, B. J., Cunningham, S. J., Brunette, R., D'Astous, J., Humphreys, P., Latter, J., & Keene, D. (1986). Psychological guidelines for helping children cope with chronic benign intractable pain. *Clinical Journal Pain, 1*, 229–233.

McGrath, P. J., & Feldman, W. (1986). Clinical approach to recurrent abdominal pain in children. *Developmental Behavioral Pediatrics, 7*, 56–61.

McGrath, P. J., Goodman, J., Shipman, R., Firestone, P., & Peters, S. (1983). Recurrent abdominal pain: A psychogenic disorder? *Arch Dis Child, 58*, 888–890.

McGrath, P. J., Johnson, G., Goodman, J. T., Schillinger, J., Dunn, J., & Chapman, J. (1985). CHEOPS: A behavioral scale for rating pain in children. *Advances in Pain Research and Therapy, 9*, 395–402.

McGrath, P. J., Humphreys, P., Goodman, J. T., Keene, D., Firestone, P., Jacob, P., & Cunningham, S. J. (1988). Relaxation prophylaxis of childhood migraine: A randomized placebo controlled trial. *Developmental Medicine and Child Neurology, 30*, 626–631.

McGrath, P. J., & Unruh, A. (1987). *Pain in children and adolescents*. Amsterdam: Elsevier.

McGrath, P. J., Cunningham, S. J., Lascelles, M. J., & Humphreys, P. (1989). *Help Yourself: A program for treating migraine headaches*. Ottawa: University of Ottawa Press.

McGrath, P. J., Humphrey, S. P., Goodman, J. T., Keene, D., Firestone, P., Lascelles, M., Cappelli, M., & Cunningham, S. J. (1989). Evaluation of a self-administered treatment for adolescent migraine. *Journal of Pain and Symptom Management, 4*, 512.

McGrath, P.J., Mathews, J. R., & Pigeon, H. (1991). Assessment of pain in children: A systematic psychosocial model. In M. R. Bond, J. E. Charlton, & C. J. Woolf (Eds.), *Proceedings of the VIth World Congress on Pain* (pp. 509–526). Amsterdam: Elsevier.

Miller, A., & Kratchowill, T. (1979). Reduction of frequency stomach-ache complaints by time-out. *Behavioral Therapy, 10*, 211–218.

Naish, J., & Apley, J. (1951). "Growing pains." A clinical study of non-arthritic limb pains in children. *Arch Dis Child, 26*, 134–140.

O'Hara, M., McGrath, P. J., D'Astous, J., & Vair, C. A. (1987). Oral morphine versus injected meperidine (demerol) for pain relief in children after orthopedic surgery. *Journal of Pediatric Orthographic Surgery, 7*, 78–82.

Oster, J. (1972). Recurrent abdominal pain, headache and limb pain in children and adolescents. *Pediatrics, 50*, 429–436.

Pantell, R. H., & Goodman, B. W. (1983). Adolescent chest pain: A prospective study. *Pediatrics, 71*, 881–887.

Passchier, J., & Orlebeke, J. F. (1985). Headaches and stress in schoolchildren: An epidemiological study. *Cephalagia, 5*, 167–176.

Raymer, D., Weininger, O., & Hamilton, J. (1984). Psychological problems in children with abdominal pain. *Lancet, I*, 439–440.

Richter, I., McGrath, P. J., Humphreys, P., Goodman, J., Firestone, P., & Keene, D. (1986). Cognitive and relaxation treatment of pediatric migraine. *Pain, 25*, 195–203.

Routh, D., & Ernst, A. (1984). Somatization disorder in relatives of children and adolescents with functional abdominal pain. *Journal of Pediatric Psychology, 9*, 427–437.

Rubin, L., Barbero, G., & Sibinga, M. (1967). Pupillary reactivity of children with recurrent abdominal pain. *Psychosomatic Medicine, 29*, 111–120.

Selbst, S. (1985). Chest pain in children. *Pediatrics, 75*, 1068–1071.

Sillanpaa, M. (1983). Changes in the prevalence of migraine and other headache during the first seven school years. *Headache, 37*, 15–19.

Sorge, F., & Marano, E. (1985). Flunarizine v. placebo in childhood migraine: A double-blind study. *Cephalagia, Suppl 2*, 145–148.

Stone, R., & Barbero, G. (1970). Recurrent abdominal pain in childhood. *Pediatrics, 45*, 732–738.

Vahlquist, B. (1955). Migraine in children. *International Arch. Allergy, 7*, 348–355.

Varni, J. W. (1981a). Self-regulation techniques in the management of chronic arthritic pain in hemophilia. *Behavioral Therapy, 12*, 185–194.

Varni, J. W. (1981b). Behavioral medicine in hemophilia arthritic pain management: Two case studies. *Archives of Physical Medicine and Rehabilitation, 62*, 183–187.

Varni, J. W., & Gilbert, A. (1982). Self-regulation of chronic arthritic pain and long-term analgesic dependence in a hemophiliac. *Rheumatology and Rehabilitation, 22* 171–174.

Waz-Hockert, O., Lind, J., Vuorenkoski, V., Partanen, T., & Valanne, E. (1968). The infant cry: A spectrographic and auditory analysis. *Clinical Development Medicine, 29*, 9–42.

Zeltzer, L., Dash, J., & Holland, J. P. (1979). Hypnotically induced pain control in sickle cell anemia. *Pediatrics, 64*, 533–536.

Zeltzer, L., & LeBaron, S. (1982). Hypnotic and non-hypnotic techniques for the deduction of pain and anxiety during painful procedures in children and adolescents with cancer. *Journal of Pediatrics, 101*, 1032–1035.

12

Sleep Disorders and Disturbances in Children*

R. T. Pivik

University of Ottawa and Ottawa General Hospital

INTRODUCTION

Despite the fact that the new era of sleep research was ushered in over three decades ago with the discovery of rapid-eye-movement sleep (REM) in infants (Aserinksy & Kleitman, 1953), subsequent studies which have attempted to reveal the behavioral, neurophysiological, and neurochemical secrets of sleep have concentrated largely on adult subjects. To some extent this is understandable, that is, it is generally the easier task to determine generalizations and recognize laws governing relationships in mature, more stabilized systems than in those undergoing fluctuations associated with development change. Ultimately, however, it is to the developing system that attention must be turned not only to provide a more complete understanding of the fully developed behaviors, but also to deal effectively with problems peculiar to the developing organism. These statements characterize the

* Preparation of this chapter was assisted by grants from the Ontario Mental Health Foundation and the Hospital for Sick Children Foundation.

status of research knowledge regarding sleep in children. These considerations, coupled with technological advances which have made possible new or improved methodologies for investigating sleep in pediatric populations, have stimulated research into the ontogenetic characterization of sleep. It is hoped that this chapter will provide more than simply a logical recitation of facts regarding sleep in children; rather, the intention is to integrate these facts with attention given both to the historical development of the field as well as to conceptual issues relevant to sleep ontogeny.

When an ontogenetic perspective is taken with respect to early behavior and development, what is perhaps the most remarkable feature of neonatal behavior is the preeminence of sleep. Sleep is the predominant behavioral state present at birth and aspects of sleep may be in place even prior to birth. Initially it was thought that neonates slept in excess of 20 hours each day (Hellbrugge, Lange, & Rutenfranz, 1959; Kleitman & Engelmann, 1953) and although more recent studies have lowered the values to between 13 and 18 hours a day (Elias, Nicolson, Bora, & Johnston, 1986; Ellingson, 1975; Parmelee, Schultz, & Disbrow, 1961), the proportion of time that neonates spend sleeping remains prodigious. Although the prevalence of sleep at this time could simply reflect the immaturity of mechanisms essential to the maintenance of sustained wakefulness, that is, be a passive phenomenon, the differentiation and complexity of sleep mechanisms suggest that sleep is an active state which perhaps plays a critical role in the developmental process. Experimental data bearing on possible functional roles for sleep on ontogenetic development will be explored in this chapter. First, however, it is important to establish a framework within which the dynamics of sleep development and differentiation might be considered, and that framework is best provided by a description of variables and normative characteristics of sleep in the mature young adult.

Concepts regarding the nature of sleep have drastically changed in the last half-century. Prior to this time the study of sleep was based on behavioral observations which could only provide information regarding overt features of sleep behavior such as duration, body position, or respiratory patterns. With the advent in the early 1900s of the technological capability to detect and record physiological activity noninvasively over periods of time sufficient to encompass normal sleep periods, it became possible to tap into the sleeping organism and record moment-to-moment changes in physiological activity as sleep progressed. The most discriminating physiological indexes for differentiating sleep have been the measurement of electrical activity of the brain (electroencephalogram: EEG), eyes (electrooculogram: EOG) and muscles (electromyogram: EMG). This new technological window on sleep has revealed totally unexpected physiological variations which continue to challenge sleep researchers with respect to both the basis for, and significance of, these variations. One of the first revelations these recordings made possible concerned the uniformity of sleep. It had been thought that sleep was constant in its expression. However, early studies showed clearly not only that brain wave activity at sleep onset differed from that of wakefulness, but that other, even more dramatic, variations occurred as sleep progressed (Loomis, Harvey, & Hobart, 1937). For example, EEG activity at sleep onset (Stage 1 sleep, as defined in the Rechtschaffen & Kales, 1968, sleep scoring manual) is characterized by a decrease in alpha activity (8–12 Hz) in association with a background of low-voltage mixed frequency activity. As sleep progresses, the EEG becomes increasingly different from that characteristic of normal wakefulness, showing increased synchrony (12–14 Hz sinusoidal sleep spindles intermittent in Stage 2 and remarkably continuous, high amplitude .5–2 Hz delta activity in Stages 3 and 4) as well as other stage-specific waveforms (vertex sharp waves in Stage 1 and bi- or triphasic K-complexes in Stage 2).

As remarkable as the above sleep-associated EEG variations are, they did not arouse the interest or create the excitement that accompanied the reports of yet another phase of sleep which came to be called rapid eye movement or REM sleep (Aserinsky & Kleitman, 1953). In part, it was because the electrographic characteristics of this state so closely resembled those of wakefulness—that is, both show low-voltage mixed-frequency EEG in conjunction with intermittent rapid eye movements that it was not recognized earlier. When this recognition finally came it was during a study of sleep-related motility in infants. Knowing now that the amount of REM sleep is enhanced in infants relative to that of adults, we can appreciate that the probability of detecting REM sleep was enhanced in this particular subject population. However, it is instructive to note that the realization that the electroencephalographic tracings reflected a state of sleep and not active wakefulness came only after Eugene Aserinsky correlated direct visual observations of the sleeping infants with polygraphic tracings. The discovery of REM sleep and its association with the psychological experience of dreaming (Dement & Kleitman, 1957b; Foulkes, 1966) was followed by a wave of investigations that documented other features of these sleep stages, such as fluctuations in skin resistance (Broughton, Poire, & Tassinari, 1965) and growth hormone (Sassin et al., 1969) during Stages 3 and 4 (collectively termed slow-wave sleep), and marked autonomic variability (Rechtschaffen, Cornwell, & Zimmerman, 1965; Snyder, Hobson, Morrison, & Goldfrank, 1964) and inhibition of mental-submental EMG during REM sleep (Berger, 1961). These correlates, as well as stage-specific effects of behavioral (Agnew, Webb, Williams, 1967; Berger & Meier, 1966; Dement, 1960) or neurochemical (Jones, 1985; Mendelson et al., 1982; Oswald, 1974) manipulations, have validated the concept of sleep stages, demonstrating that the stage differentiations based primarily on EEG criteria are not simply arbitrary correlations of measures without empirical documentation.

Although these measures and events are basic to the identity of sleep stages, they inadequately reflect the dynamics of sleep. Additional features of sleep-wakefulness and sleep-stage interactions which are important to the understanding of normal adult sleep have been previously summarized and include:

> (a) the compartmentalization of sleep-wakefulness periods (i.e., a segregation of sleep-wakefulness episodes such that each generally occurs for an extended period of time); (b) the initiation of sleep by NREM (nonrapid eye movement) patterns, with the initial REM period occurring approximately 90 minutes after sleep onset; (c) the concentration of Stage 4 sleep in the first third of the night, particularly in the period between sleep onset and the first REM period; (d) the cyclical alternation of REM and NREM [sleep Stages 1–4] states with a period of approximately 90 minutes; and (e) the high proportion (75–80%) of total sleep time spent in NREM sleep (Dement & Kleitman, 1957a; Feinberg, 1974; Feinberg & Floyd, 1979; Williams, Agnew, & Webb, 1964, 1966). (Pivik, 1983, p. 77)

From this description of REM and NREM sleep it is obvious that each is based on the regulated occurrence of a constellation of neural and neurochemical events. While such a confluence of events may assist in reliably discriminating among stages—that is, the more state indexes, the greater the confidence in stage definition—as will become evident, it is also a major source of confusion regarding state identification when all criteria are not met, as in pathological conditions or during early development.

Sleep in the human neonate bears little resemblance to the adult sleep characteristics described above, differing in duration, distribution, and electrographic characteristics. As previously indicated, neonates sleep extensively, spending as much as 80 percent of the day asleep, as opposed to approximately 25–30 percent in mature subjects and elderly subjects (Baker, 1985). Whereas adults normally sleep in extended bouts with their sleep consolidated into a single nighttime session, the newborn's sleep is fragmented and distributed throughout the 24-hour period (Parmelee & Stern, 1972). Finally, none of the electrographic criteria applied to sleep stage differentiation in adults is present in mature form at birth. During the course of the first year of development EEG activity evolves from brief (3–10 sec) bursts of high-voltage slow waves (1–3 Hz) followed by 10–40 sec periods of inactivity present at 32–40 weeks of conceptual age, to a continuous, differentiated EEG showing both high-voltage and low-voltage fast activity (Dreyfus-Brisac, 1970). Rudimentary sleep spindles first become evident approximately 4 weeks following birth, but continue to show variation during the first 2 years of life (Lenard, 1970; Metcalf, 1970; Metcalfe & Jordon, 1972). Similarly, K-complexes, which do not make their appearance before approximately 6 months following birth, show variations in morphology and cortical distribution which may extend into adolescence (Metcalf, Mondale, & Butler, 1971). Other physiological measures which have been used as stage correlates in adults, such as eye movements and respiratory rate, exhibit developmental variations which only begin to show signs of stabilization 4–12 weeks after birth (Lynch & Aserinsky, 1986; Parmelee, 1974; Parmelee, Stern, & Harris, 1972; Petre-Quadens, deLee & Remy, 1971). Sleep-related neuroendocrine events may be even more retarded in their development, as evidenced by growth hormone secretion which typically occurs during slow wave sleep in the adult but which is reported to be absent in the infant (Finklestein, Anders, Sachar, Roffwarg, & Hellman, 1971). There is an obvious inherent difficulty in attempting to apply adult criteria for sleep stage differentiation to the infant. The differential rates at which the various physiological measures mature complicate the task of state determination and make it impractical to impose rigid criteria for state identification as in the adult (Rechtschaffen & Kales, 1968). Instead, a coding system for sleep-wakefulness state determination in infants has been developed (Anders, Emde, & Parmelee, 1971). This system allows for flexibility of state scoring, but facilitates interlaboratory comparisons since the codes are standardized.

Although these sleep-wake state determinations may be reliably determined in infants, there remain questions regarding the relationship of the determinations to adult sleep. It is notable, for example, that from among the many physiological variations used to index sleep in the infant "sustained eye closure [is] a primary criteria for defining sleep" (Anders, Emde, & Parmelee, 1971). It is recognized that although eye closure is generally a prerequisite for sleep, it clearly constitutes an insufficient index of sleep. The need for such emphasis on this index, and the indefinite information provided, warrants the caution expressed by some investigators in equating neonatal quiet sleep with NREM sleep in adults (Sterman, 1972).

Other studies documenting features of infant sleep (Delange, Castan, Cadilhac, & Passouant, 1962; Dittrichova, 1966; Dreyfus-Brisac & Monod, 1965; Roffwarg, Dement, & Fisher, 1964; Weitzman, Fishbein,

& Graziani, 1965) have noted similarities between adult and infant forms of sleep, but have also revealed dramatic differences, the more outstanding of which are listed below:

1. There are greater amounts of REM sleep in the neonate than in the adult. Reported values for REM sleep in the neonate vary between 40 percent and 60 percent of total sleep time—with the range in values reflecting the difficulty in defining REM or active sleep and depending on the specific variables used for state definition. It is generally agreed that amounts of active or REM sleep are higher in the premature than in the full-term neonate (Anders, 1975; Parmelee, Wenner, Akiyama, Schultz, & Stern, 1967; Petre-Quadens, 1968). Nevertheless, considering the extended sleep time in prematures and neonates, there is a significant enhancement of REM sleep at this time both in relative and absolute amounts.
2. Infants commonly exhibit sleep-onset REM periods. In the absence of conditions such as selective (REM) sleep deprivation (Dement, 1960; Dement & Fisher, 1963) or pathology, for example, narcolepsy (Hishikawa et al., 1968; Rechtschaffen, Wolpert, Dement, Mitchell, & Fisher, 1963) the initial REM period in the adult generally occurs approximately 90 minutes after sleep onset.
3. REM periods occur with greater frequency in infants (every 50–60 minutes) than in adults (every 90–100 minutes).
4. Primary and ancillary measures defining the REM sleep state in the adult are less coherently organized in the neonate. For example, in addition to an inconsistent reduction in mental-submental EMG activity, in the neonate there is a prominence of skin potential discharges during active sleep (Curzi-Dascalova, Pajot, & Dreyfus-Brisac, 1973), eye movements have been noted to occur in close association with spindle activity (Ornitz, 1972; Petre-Quadens, 1974), and penile erections may occur during quiet sleep periods (Korner, 1968).

The notion of excessive amounts of REM sleep early in development has recently been challenged both from an evolutionary perspective and on the basis of maturational changes in a major REM event—that is, eye movements. In a book dealing with the comparative-physiological study of sleep (Karmanova, 1982), it is suggested that true REM sleep may not emerge until the patterned sequence of slow-wave sleep and REM sleep is in place, and that what has been viewed as REM sleep before this time is a manifestation of other intermediate forms of sleep and wakefulness. This view is compatible with the idea of an ontogenetic recapitulation of phylogenetic processes with respect to the sleep-wakefulness cycle, whereas the current general consensus—in which REM sleep predates slow-wave sleep ontogenetically but not phylogenetically (Allison & Van Twyver, 1970)—is not. On the basis of a detailed examination of eye movement behavior and characteristics in full-term infants between 4 and 12 weeks following birth, Lynch and Aserinsky (1986) concluded that eye movement characteristics were determined primarily by "ocular motor developments and the mechanics of eye closure rather than by different mechanisms of neural control effected through different states of consciousness" (p. 175). These findings prompted these investigators to question whether active states present in the infant commonly identified as REM sleep might simply be a precursor to REM sleep, and to consider further the possibility that "the REM state does not develop initially in utero but further manifests itself at about 8–12 weeks of age, the time when the REM state begins to follow rather than precede non-REM sleep" (p. 182). This interpretation is not incompatible with observations made concerning development of the rest-activity and sleep-wakefulness cycles. Evidence of the rest-activity cycle is present 21 weeks postmenstrual, whereas elements of what is considered to be REM sleep do not become apparent until 28 weeks (Sterman, 1972). Consequently, the rest-activity cycle has been considered the more basic process (Kleitman, 1963, 1969) upon which sleep is superimposed, and it may well be that what has been considered or construed as the early presence of REM sleep, in fact, is a state of active wakefulness.

By the end of the first year of life many of the physiological measures used to describe sleep and the relationships among these variables have developed to the point that adult-type patterns are present. This is true for autonomic measures (such as skin potential response), the presence of more prolonged periods of quiet sleep, the initiation of sleep by quiet, rather than active, sleep and the periodic sequencing of sleep stages (Harper, Leake, Miyahara, et al., 1981; Roffwarg, Muzio, & Dement, 1966; Stern, Parmelee, Akiyama, Schultz, & Wenner, 1969). As well, by this time REM sleep has decreased to approximately 30 percent of total sleep time (Roffwarg, Muzio, & Dement, 1966) and NREM sleep has differentiated so that adult criteria can be applied (Dreyfus-Brisac, 1979). Beyond the first year of life, major developmental changes affecting sleep-wakefulness states have more to do with the temporal organization and distribution of these behavioral patterns than with variations in individual systems. Among these adjustments is the reduction in total sleep time and the segregation of sleep and wakefulness such that sleep is concentrated during the night and wakefulness during the day. Coincident with the gradual separation of extended sleep-wakefulness periods is the reorganization of sleep patterning such that slow wave sleep—Stage 4 in particular—is concentrated in the initial third of the night and the majority of REM sleep occurs in the last third of the night.

The process of diurnal state consolidation can be influenced by various factors, including habit, parental reinforcement, and nutritional demands, as well as circadian rhythms. For example, infants breastfed into the second year of life—particularly those sharing a bed with the mother—show a greater fragmentation of sleep and less total sleep time than infants weaned by the end of the first year (Elias et al., 1986). Recently, a series of studies has unmasked an influence of biological rhythms on sleep-wakefulness patterns in adults which is of relevance to the pattern with which sleep in infants becomes diurnal. It is well known that in the adjustment from a polyphasic to a biphasic sleep-wakefulness pattern, the most persistent daytime sleep period is generally the early afternoon, post-lunch nap. Persistence of this "sleepiness time zone" is evident into adulthood and across societies (as evidenced in, for example, the siesta) and has been commonly attributed to having eaten or perhaps to cultural or climatic (temperature) factors. Recent investigations, however, have revealed the presence of a biological rhythm which may be the basis for this behavior. In the sleep periods of normal individuals who have been able to extend their total sleep periods to 12 consecutive hours or more, there is evidence of the recurrence of slow-wave sleep approximately 12 hours after initial sleep onset (Broughton, 1975; Gagnon & DeKoninck, 1981, 1984; Webb, 1986). This time period coincides with the post-lunch behavioral nadir which often results in sleep. Although whether sleep occurs at this time may depend upon other factors such as the general level of arousal or motivated interest in ongoing activities, it is clear—but for reasons which remain to be determined—that the processes are in place to facilitate slow-wave sleep at this time.

Variations in the amount and patterning of sleep and sleep stages extend into adolescence (Feinberg, 1974; Karacan, Anch, Thornby, Okawa & Williams, 1975; Williams, Karacan, & Davis, 1972) and some of these variations, for example, reduction in total sleep time, may set the stage for later difficulties with waking functioning as a result of daytime sleepiness (Anders, Carskadon, & Dement, 1980; Webb, 1969; Webb & Agnew, 1975). The balanced integration and segregation of sleep-wakefulness states significantly affects our psychological and physiological functioning. This is apparent from a number of investigations examining attentive behavior and cognitive functioning in conditions in which sleep-wakefulness distinctions are blurred or disorganized (e.g., sleep deprivation, Glenville, Broughton, Wing, & Wilkinson, 1979, or in sleep disorders characterized by excessive daytime sleepiness, Guilleminault, Eldridge, Simmons, & Dement, 1976; Valley & Broughton, 1980).

With respect to sleep and sleep-wakefulness transitions, the concepts of sleep, activity, excitability, and arousal interrelate in a complicated fashion, at times coalescing to create quite unusual conditions. The very existence of a state characterized by intense physiological activation within sleep (i.e., REM sleep) flies in the face of previous considerations of sleep as a condition of repose. Even more perplexing is why this state should exist in such apparent abundance in the newborn. Studies in adults have correlated this state with the psychological experience of dreaming (Dement & Kleitman, 1957a; Foulkes, 1966), but it is difficult to imagine the nature or purpose of such extensive amounts of dreaming in neonates. The notion that neonates would spend more than half of their existence dreaming lacks intuitive appeal and, not unexpectedly, empirical support. Moreover, on the basis of a longitudinal study of REM dreams in children ranging in age from 3 to 10 years, Foulkes (1982) concluded that dreaming, as examined through dream reports, required the development of specific analytic skills which do not emerge any earlier in sleep than in wakefulness. Therefore, prior to the time that children reach an operational level of development (i.e., 5–7 years old) only rudimentary dream activity might exist, and even this would probably not begin before the age of 2 years (Foulkes, 1982).

Roffwarg, Muzio, and Dement (1966), focusing on the physiological activation present during REM sleep, suggested that in the newborn this activity provided endogenous stimulation important to central nervous system growth and differentiation. If the prevalence of REM sleep at birth is an index of its biological significance, then this theory would predict severe developmental consequences in the event of the reduction or absence of REM at this time. Although the results of earlier studies examining the effects of short-term REM sleep reduction in neonatal humans (Anders & Roffwarg, 1973) or monkeys (Berger & Meier, 1966), or long-term REM suppression in animals via pharmacologic agents (Mendelson et al., 1982), have not been remarkable, more recent investigations have shown more promise. Oksenberg et al. (1985) were able to demonstrate in kittens that REM deprivation in conjunction with monocular deprivation of visual input led to more severe visual system cell loss than monocular deprivation alone. Using neurochemical agents to suppress REM sleep in rats for a two-week period early in development, Mirmiran (1986) observed a variety of deficits and abnormalities when testing these animals once they had reached adulthood, including "hyperactivity, hyperanxiety, attentional distractibility, sleep disturbances, reduced sexual performance and reduced cerebral cortical size" (p. 283). Although unconvinced that the episodes of endogenous neural activation during sleep in the newborn animals were comparable to REM sleep in the adult, Mirmiran nonetheless concluded from his data that REM sleep serves an important role in CNS development.

If large amounts of REM sleep are required in early development to provide necessary endogenous stimulation to an immature and developing central nervous system, then it might be expected that for greater degrees of immaturity, greater amounts of REM stimulation would be required. Accordingly, relative to term infants, those born prematurely should experience increased amounts of REM sleep. There is evidence that this may be the case (Anders & Keener, 1985), but the earlier exposure to external environmental influences in conjunction with increased REM time apparently does not hasten the maturation of sleep-wakefulness states. Studies comparing premature and full-term infants on a variety of measures, such as maturation of the longest sleep period, amounts of wakefulness, and developmental patterns of diurnal and circadian organization of sleep-wake patterns (Anders & Keener, 1985) report only subtle differences between these groups. Group differences which were evident were largely restricted to state durations and transitions, suggesting less stability and greater disorganization in preterm infants (Anders & Keener, 1985; Watt & Strongman, 1985). There are indications that the stability of sleep patterns may be as important to normal development and functioning as the amounts of various sleep stages experienced (Anders & Keener, 1985; Thoman, 1975; Watt & Strongman, 1985). This inferred significance of sleep stability is underscored by the results of investigations into the reversibility of sleep.

Although there is general consensus regarding conditions which promote and disrupt sleep, the processes underlying the spontaneous initiation or termination of sleep are not clearly understood. Sleep-wakefulness transitions have been examined primarily in the context of arousal threshold studies in which the intensity of stimulation required to effect arousal from sleep is determined. Such studies agree that in the adult thresholds to arousal are greater in REM and slow-wave sleep relative to the remainder of NREM sleep, and that the threshold for arousal generally decreases across the night (Pisano, Rosadini, Rossi, & Zattoni, 1966; Rechtschaffen, Hauri, & Zeitlin, 1966). Similar investigations in neonates and infants have indicated less motor reactivity to auditory stimuli during quiet sleep at 32 weeks postmenstrual age (Monod & Garma, 1971) and reduced arousal responses in neonates and infants during both REM (Korner, 1968; Murray & Campbell, 1971; Petre-Quadens, 1974; Schmidt & Burns,

1971) and quiet sleep (Korner, 1968). Although the apparent intensity of sleep in children have not escaped notice (e.g., Dement, 1972), it has generally been considered that this sleep intensity factor was present only in very young children. Recent quantitative studies in preadolescent (8–12-year-old) children (Busby & Pivik, 1983, 1985; Pivik & Busby, 1984) have provided new insight into the intense nature of sleep maintenance processes which persist at least up to adolescence. In these studies, children were required to make behavioral responses (say "I'm awake" and press a hand-held button 3 times) whenever they became aware of brief auditory stimuli which were delivered with gradually increasing intensity via an earphone insert. There was a striking inability to arouse children to behavioral response even at intensities more than 90 dB above waking threshold values, that is, at intensities approaching levels which could cause neural damage. Although the ability to awaken children increased across the night, still only a third of the 432 arousal attempts resulted in complete awakenings. These results bring into question the capability of children to arouse from sleep and perform meaningful behavioral activities even in response to imperative stimuli, whether externally generated (e.g., signals from emergency alarm devices) or internally generated (e.g., respiratory distress). This sleep-related functional debilitation is particularly apparent during the initial cycle of sleep. With respect to arousals from sleep, it is instructive to note the consistency in the literature indicating that spontaneous awakenings from sleep occur with great frequency at the end of REM sleep periods (Schulz, Massetani, Fagioli, & Salzarulo, 1985; Weitzman, Czeisler, Zimmerman, & Ronda, 1980), a sleep stage from which it is difficult to arouse subjects experimentally. These observations suggest that it may be important to study in greater detail the physiological correlates of spontaneous awakenings in order to learn more about the basis and perhaps function of the unusually elevated thresholds to arousal present during sleep in children.

SLEEP DISTURBANCES

Since we remain ignorant of the function(s) of sleep, and since this state generally is initiated and sustained without volitional effort, our considerations regarding sleep quality emanate from presumed consequences of poor sleep for waking behavior. In this regard, concerns about sleep disruptions in infants and children often reflect inconveniences inflicted upon adults (parents and other family members), rather than any measurable negative effect of sleep disturbance on the infants and children themselves. However, it is true that many infants do have difficulty establishing regular sleep patterns (25–50 percent according to one report; Anders, Carskadon, & Dement, 1980). Furthermore, sleeplessness has been reported to be the most prevalent sleep-related problem of infancy and the toddler years (Bernal, 1973; Ferber, Boyle, & Belfer, 1981; Kohler, Coddington, & Agnew, 1968; Richman, 1981). The high incidence of sleep disturbances during development is not surprising in view of the shifting physiological and neurochemical balances which occur during normal maturation, and the need, as established from studies in adults, for these systems to be integrated not only to effect the progression and modulation of the various stages of sleep throughout the sleep period, but also to provide the most efficient relationship with wakefulness.

Parasomnias

The discrimination between normal developmentally based sleep disruptions and those which may signal a problem which will not abate with time, and which therefore warrant intervention, remains difficult and subject to marked individual variation. In his consideration of this dilemma, Ferber (1985) recommends a thorough evaluation of environmental, social, medical, and psychological factors which may be responsible for, or contributing to, the observed disruptions before dismissing the problem as a "symptom of neurologic immaturity that can be waited out" (p. 228).

There is, however, a class of sleep disturbances prevalent among children that appears to be largely related to maturation, and the symptoms of which generally disappear by midadolesence. These disturbances are termed *parasomnias*, that is, events or behaviors which, although associated with sleep, are not considered disorders of either sleep or wakefulness (Broughton, 1968; Roffwarg, 1979). Among the more common of these disturbances are sleep terrors, sleep walking, sleep talking, and sleep-related enuresis.

Sleep terrors (pavor nocturnus) are episodes characterized by marked autonomic activation (e.g., tachycardia, mydriasis, piloerection), agitation and confusion. During the event, the child is unresponsive to efforts made to placate or comfort him and may or may not come to a complete arousal when the episode subsides. When complete arousal does occur, memory for mental events preceding or coincidental with the episode, or for the event itself, is absent. This feature, and the fact that these events develop out of slow-wave sleep, distinguish sleep terrors from nightmares which occur during REM sleep and for which there is recall of a frightening dream.

Sleep walking (somnambulism) consists of motor behaviors developing out of sleep including walking as well as other perseverative motor acts and automatisms. When these episodes terminate in arousal to consciousness, there is initially confusion and disorientation. Reports of dreaming during these episodes are rare and quite fragmentary. Often, sleepwalking episodes will be ended by the child simply returning to sleep. When subjects are questioned regarding these episodes upon arising in the morning, there is generally total amnesia for the event. The observation that sleep walking can be initiated both in children who exhibit this behavior spontaneously as well as in those who do not simply by standing them on their feet in slow-wave sleep, suggests that this behavior reflects the release of motor activity which indicates or coincides with a period of incomplete arousal.

Sleep talking (somniloquy) consists of vocalizations during sleep which may take the form of speech or other psychologically meaningful sounds. These utterances are brief, often unintelligible or meaningless, and upon arousal subjects have no recall for these events.

Sleep-related enuresis or bedwetting, although generally a benign condition, may nevertheless cause considerable distress to both parents and the afflicted children (Dische, 1978; Foxman, Valdez, & Brook, 1986). A number of etiological characteristics have been variously associated with enuresis, including genetic, behavioral (late toilet training), or organic factors (urinary tract infection, outflow tract obstruction, bladder size and function). Surveys indicate that in the great majority of cases the condition generally abates by adolescence (Foxman et al., 1986, Oppel, Harber, & Rider, 1968; Rutter, Yule, & Graham, 1973).

The above discussed parasomnias have several factors in common, including: (a) occurrence in the age range of 3–15 years, (b) a positive family history, (c) a higher incidence among males than females, (d) associated occurrences in the same individuals, and (e) occurrence during the initial cycle of sleep during Stages 3 and 4—a time when arousal from sleep is extremely difficult and, when it does occur, is often incomplete, resulting in disorientation and confusion of the subject (Anders, 1982; Anders et al., 1980; Gastaut & Broughton, 1964; Hallstrom, 1972; Kales, Kales, et al., 1980; Kales, Soldatos, et al., 1980; Roffwarg, 1979; Rutter et al., 1973). Sleep talking has also been reported to occur during REM sleep (Arkin, 1966; Roffwarg, 1979), and recent studies have challenged the exclusive allocation of bedwetting episodes to slow-wave sleep (Mikkelson et al., 1980; Rapoport et al., 1980).

In general, parasomnias are amenable to treatment, but since most of these sleep-associated dysfunctions disappear by midadolescence intervention is recommended only when the disturbances endanger the child or result in excessive anxiety to either the parents or the child. These interventions take the form of pharmacological treatment [e.g., benzodiazepines, which decrease the time spent in slow-wave sleep (Fisher, Kahn, Edward, & David, 1973; Harvey, 1980) for night terrors and sleep walking; tricyclic antidepressants for enuresis (Kales, Kales, Jacobson, Humphrey, & Soldatos, 1977; Rapoport et al., 1980; Werry, Dawnick, Lampen, & Vamos, 1975)] or behavioral manipulations (preventative measures to guard the safety of the sleeping or disoriented child during night terrors or sleep walking, and a variety of training, conditioning, and arousal procedures for the treatment of enuresis; Shaffer & Ambrisoni, 1985). Although arousal procedures have been used in the treatment of enuresis, children are difficult to arouse from sleep. Furthermore, from the previous discussion indicating the presence of elevated arousal thresholds during slow-wave sleep when the majority of these disturbances occur, it is clear that this approach will meet with decided resistance. Furthermore, if the children are aroused at this time, it is likely that such arousal may enhance the disorientation, confusion, and fear which accompanies such partial awakenings.

Pharmacological treatment, although effective in many instances, is not recommended for long-term management of these sleep-associated problems because of disruptive effects (e.g., tricyclics may induce nightmares) and because the consequences of chronic pharmacologic treatment in children are unknown.

Insomnia: Developmental and Clinical Correlates

It is widely recognized that sleeplessness is among the most common problems of infants and toddlers (Anders & Keener, 1985; Ferber, 1985). Although statistics indicate that between 20 and 25 percent of children three years old or younger experience sleep difficulties which fragment sleep and shorten sleep duration (Ferber, 1985; Richman, 1981), such disruptions are not usually classified as insomnia. In fact, complaints of primary insomnia are uncommon in children (Shaffer & Ambrosini, 1985). An epidemiological study based on nearly 6,000 interviews, 12 percent of which involved children between the ages of 3 and 10 (Cirignotta, Mondini, Zucconi, Lenzi, & Lugaresi, 1985), found complaints of insomnia were rare below the age of 20 (1.6%). Another investigation which examined the prevalence of sleep disorders and sleep behaviors in children did not even include insomnia as a category of interest (Simonds & Parraga, 1982).

The above statements, that is, that sleeplessness is common yet insomnia uncommon among infants and children, appear somewhat contradictory. In part, the apparent inconsistency can be attributed to uncertainty regarding how to interpret sleep disruptions in younger populations. As one investigator put it "it is difficult to say with certainty at which point sleeplessness should be considered a problem rather than simply an annoyance; or perhaps at which point it qualifies for intervention rather than simply to be dismissed as 'developmental'." (Ferber, 1985, p. 227).

Individual differences make it difficult, if not impossible, to formulate definitive guidelines for the determination of the need and extent of intervention for sleeplessness in this subject population. There are, nevertheless, potential influences which can be readily identified and dealt with using behavioral intervention, for example, modification of feeding schedules or the conditions associated with falling asleep, or treatment of family psychological problems. If sleeplessness persists despite attempts at behavioral intervention, then pharmacological treatment is often invoked. In such instances, the admonitions previously noted regarding the development of tolerance and dependence on medications apply, and it is recommended that the need for continued pharmacotherapy be reassessed periodically (Shaffer & Ambrosini, 1985) and long-term prescriptions avoided.

Complaints of insomnia have been registered in child psychiatric patients, particularly among children falling into diagnostic categories of depression, attention deficit disorder with hyperactivity (ADDH), or conduct disorder (Dixon, Monroe, & Jakim, 1981). However, polygraphic sleep studies have not consistently found electrophysiological correlates of reported disturbances (Busby, Firestone, & Pivik, 1981; Greenhill, Puig-Antich, Goetz, Hanlon & Davies, 1983; Puig-Antich et al., 1982). For example, such studies in ADDH children have not revealed evidence of major deviations from age-matched normal controls in most sleep variables, including time to sleep onset, total sleep time, or amounts of sleep stages (Busby, Firestone, & Pivik, 1981; Feinberg, et al., 1974). There is, however, a tendency for ADDH children to exhibit more motor activity during sleep and an increased latency to onset of the initial REM period has been reported (Busby, Firestone, & Pivik, 1981; Haig, Schroeder, & Schroeder, 1974). The latter finding is consonant with a suggested maturational lag in these children.

The results of a more recent study involving learning disabled children—a population sharing some behavioral features with ADDH children—are also of relevance to the maturational lag hypothesis (Pivik, Mercier, Busby, & Butler, 1986). The children in this study were younger than the ADDH subjects (learning disabled children's mean age = 8.7 years; ADDH children's mean age = 10.9 years), and did not exhibit signs of hyperactivity. As in the ADDH group, the sleep stage patterning, amount of sleep, and latency to sleep onset of these children were normal, but—similar to the ADDH children—they demonstrated a longer latency to onset of the first REM period. Of additional interest was the observation that many children in this study, both normal control and learning-disabled, evidenced Stage 2 EEG intrusions into REM sleep and inconsistencies in the presence and extent of tonic motor inhibition during REM sleep (Figures 12.1 and 12.2). Tonic motor inhibition during REM sleep is thought to be a fundamental feature of this state and has been considered "perhaps the most essential and characteristic process of REM sleep" (Dement & Mitler, 1974, p. 283). Level of developmental organization has been related to both waking motor behaviors and motor activity in sleep (Anders, Keener, & Kraemer, 1985), and the observation of irregularities in so basic a REM-related process in these young children raises the possibility that other features of sleep might be subject to maturational influences, particularly in vulnerable populations.

The above considerations highlight the difficulties involved in differentiating normal from abnormal development of sleep processes. The significance of resolving these issues becomes apparent when it is realized that there are indications that sleep disturbances early in life may have long-term consequences. In this regard, Hauri and Olmstead (1980) reported that nearly one-third of the 73 adult insomniacs they studied had a history of insomnia with indicated onset before the age of 10. Comparisons between these subjects and others characterized as having adult-onset insomnia revealed several differences involving

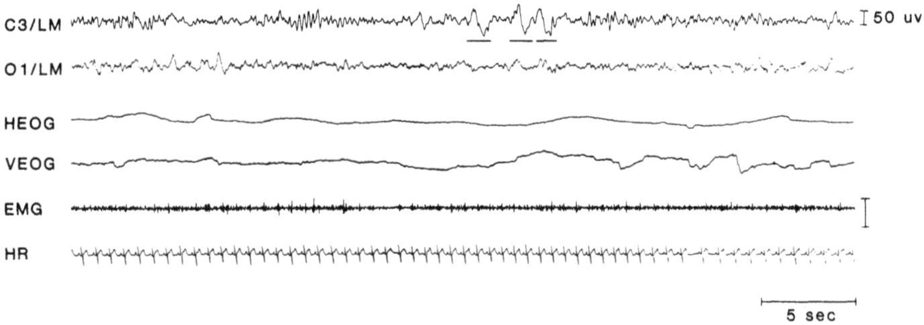

FIGURE 12.1. An illustration of a REM sleep segment in an 8-year-old normal subject which is characterized by incomplete EMG inhibition and intrusion by K-complexes (underscored, top channel). Derivations for this and subsequent figures: C3/LM and O3/LM: left central and left occipital EEG placements referenced to linked mastoid electrodes; HEOG, VEOG: bipolar horizontal and vertical electrooculograms; EMG: bipolar orbicularis oris electromyogram: HR: heart rate

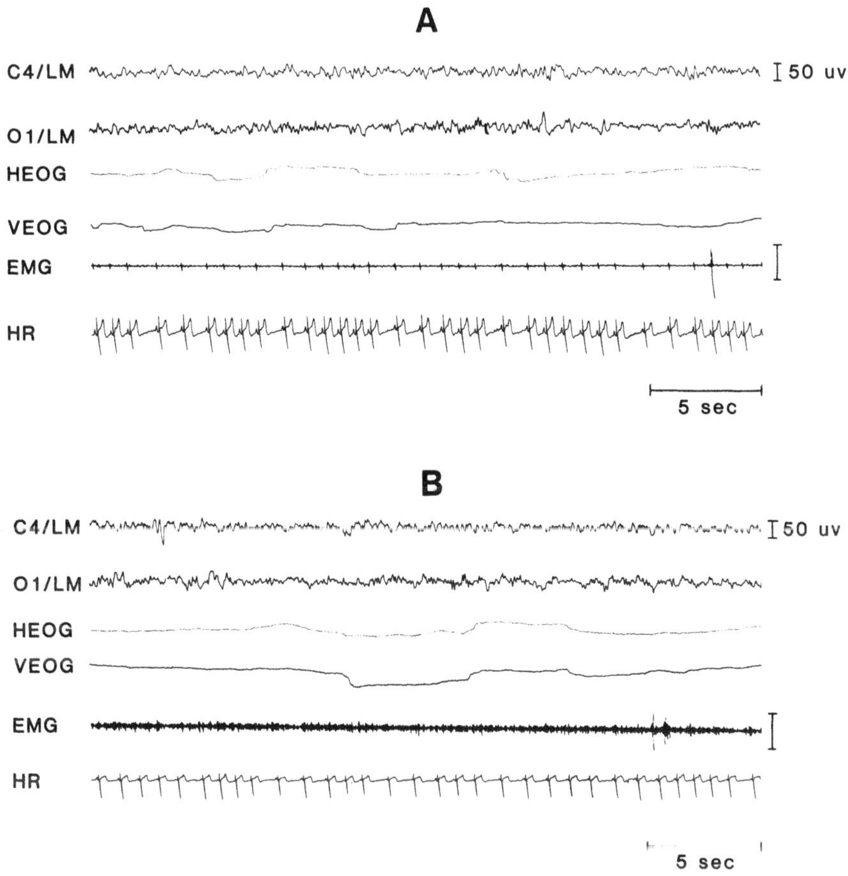

FIGURE 12.2. Polygraphic tracings from different REM episodes in the same night in an 8-year-old reading disabled subject. Note the presence of tonic EMG inhibition in panel A, but the absence of such inhibition in panel B. Irregularities in REM sleep-associated muscle tonus were common among both reading disabled and normal control children. See text for discussion.

sleep measures, neurological status and psychological parameters. Specifically, childhood-onset insomniacs experienced greater difficulty falling asleep, less sleep time, fewer eye movements in REM sleep, and more soft neurological signs. However, childhood-onset insomnia was associated with less psychological stress. The long term consequences of early sleep disruptions have not been fully appreciated, and the longitudinal studies necessary to properly evaluate this issue are yet to be conducted.

Another group of child psychiatric patients beginning to receive increased attention from the sleep research community is that exhibiting depressive symptomatology. This has come about in part because of the greater awareness of depression in children and adolescents and also because of the possibility that such studies may reveal ontogenetic processes involved in depression. In the endogenously depressed adult patient there has been an emphasis on REM-related abnormalities, including a shortened latency to onset of the first REM period and increased eye movement density during REM sleep (Kupfer, 1976; Kupfer & Foster, 1979). An initial question being addressed in studies involving depressed prepubertal and adolescent subjects is whether sleep pattern characteristics in this younger age group are similar to those of adult patients. The initial studies in this area have been quite contradictory, with some indicating the absence (Goetz et al., 1987; Puig-Antich et al., 1982; Young, Knowles, MacLean, Boag & McConville, 1982) and others the presence (Emslie, Roffwarg, Rush, Weinberg, & Parkin-Feigenbaum, 1987; Lahmeyer, Poznanski, & Bellur, 1983) of REM abnormalities in depressed children and adolescents. The basis for these opposing findings is unclear, but may reflect differences in methodology and criteria used for data selection and analysis. It is apparent, however, that these divergent outcomes could lead to quite different conclusions and applications. If sleep abnormalities in depressed prepubertal and postpubertal children are similar to those in adult depressed patients, then puberty itself has no effect on the disease process and studies in these younger depressed subjects might provide information of direct relevance to depression (Emslie et al., 1987). However, if these subjects do not display the sleep irregularities of adult depressed patients, then the later abnormalities must be subject to ontogenetic modulation and could suggest a basic difference in the prepubertal/juvenile and adult forms of depressive illness. However, Puig-Antich and colleagues (Goetz et al., 1987) view these latter results as the interaction of a disease process with maturational factors, and believe that when this age or maturational factor is taken into account, adult and childhood depression are similar in nature.

Narcolepsy

Narcolepsy is a disorder of REM sleep mechanisms which fragments both sleep and waking behaviors. It is defined by the confluence of several symptoms, including the presence of *excessive daytime sleepiness* (EDS) which leads to irresistible sleep attacks. These sleep attacks often occur in association with *cataplexy* (loss of skeletal muscle tone which is generally initiated by an emotional response such as laughter, anger, or stress), *sleep paralysis* (loss of muscle tone which occurs briefly during sleep-wakefulness or wakefulness-sleep transitions but which are not triggered by emotional affect), and *hypnagogic hallucinations* (vivid and complex dreamlike experiences occurring in the transition from wakefulness to sleep). Together these symptoms constitute the narcoleptic tetrad. Only a small percentage (11–14%) of narcoleptics experience all these symptoms in combination. Generally, excessive daytime sleepiness in association with cataplexy is considered pathognomonic of the narcoleptic syndrome (Roffwarg, 1979). This tetrad of symptoms stresses the consequences of narcolepsy for waking behavior, but there are also significant effects on sleep behavior in these patients. Prominent among these are frequent awakenings, more stage shifts, more stage 1 sleep, terrifying dreams, and a high incidence of other sleep disorders (Bixler et al., 1986; Larkin, 1984; Mosko, Shampain, & Sassin, 1984; Roth, 1978; Kellerman, 1981).

The presence of a genetic component to this disorder has been well-established (Kessler, Guilleminault, & Dement, 1974; Roth, 1978; Yoss & Daly, 1960). Recent attempts to further investigate the genetic basis for narcolepsy have examined the association between this disorder and HLA-antigen testing. The majority of these studies have indicated that an exceptionally high proportion—virtually 100 percent—of narcoleptics tested were HLV-DR2 positive (Seignalet, 1986; Honda, Juji, Matsuki, Naohara & Satake, 1985; Kramer, Dinner, Braun, Zachary, & Teresi, 1986). Despite the strength of this relationship, it may be premature to consider the absence of a positive HLV-DR2 as indicating the absence of narcolepsy since a recent report indicates exceptions to this relationship (Othman, Rundell, & Orr, 1987). The recent development of natural narcoleptic animal models presents unique opportunities for elaborating both the genetic and CNS features of this disease (Foutz, Mitler, Cavali-Sforza, & Dement, 1979; Sweeney, Hendricks, Beech, & Morrison, 1983).

With the advent of prevalence studies indicating an incidence of narcolepsy in the general population of between 0.03 percent and 0.16 percent (Bruhova & Roth, 1972; Dement et al., 1972; Dement, Carskadon & Ley, 1973; Honda & Hishikawa, 1980), it has become obvious that narcolepsy is not the rare disease it was once thought to be. Narcolepsy, in its more developed form, is not a childhood disease. The peak onset of definitive symptoms generally occurs during puberty and in the following 10 years (Billiard, 1985; Guilleminault & Anders, 1976; Roth, 1978). However, the earliest sign of this disorder—excessive daytime sleepiness—may become evident at a much earlier age. Navelet, Anders, and Guilleminault (1976) reported that 30 percent of adult narcoleptics had histories indicating excessive daytime sleepiness during their childhood or adolescent years. In another investigation involving 150 adult narcoleptics, 20 percent complained of daytime drowsiness or sleepiness before the age of 11 (Anders et al., 1980; Guilleminault & Anders, 1976). Since all narcoleptics do not report symptom onset during childhood, it becomes important to consider whether there are clinical differences between narcolepsy with and without early onset of symptomatology. In an investigation designed to address this issue, Young et al. (1987) compared groups of pediatric (mean age 11.6 years) and adult (mean age 43.4 years) narcoleptics on a variety of measures, including polygraphically recorded sleep parameters. Subsequent comparisons did not indicate major between-group differences which could not be explained by existing age differences. Both groups demonstrated disturbed sleep as indexed by number and duration of arousals and amounts of Stage 1 sleep. The presence of this disturbed sleep in pediatric populations is not a uniform finding in narcoleptic children (Guilleminault & Anders, 1976).

The full-blown expression of narcoleptic symptomatology is debilitating at any age, and studies conducted in adults have described the negative psychosocial, psychological, and behavioral effects of this disease (Kales et al., 1982; Smith, 1958; Sours, 1963). The consequences of this disorder for children are no less devastating. The early and insidious development of excessive daytime sleepiness in children results in repeated microsleep episodes which markedly disrupt attention, information acquisition and processing, and may result in total amnesia, lasting for several hours. All these effects severely retard the learning process. Guilleminault and Anders (1976) described the process and consequences of microsleep in narcoleptic children in the following way:

> EDS and daytime sleep attacks account for many of the school-related problems. The child usually fights against the sleepiness, which develops 3–4 hours after waking. Nevertheless, without overt signs of napping, recurrent micro-sleep episodes can be recorded on the polygraph . . . On the polygram, they appear either as bursts of theta activity or as typical runs of stage 1 NREM sleep, lasting 5–15 seconds. During these episodes, the child, eyes open but with a glassy look, loses perception. As the micro-sleep episodes become more repetitious . . . a typical "automatic behavior syndrome with amnesia" may appear. During this abnormal state of consciousness, the child is unaware of his actions and his performance deteriorates. The notion of time is altered and there is retrograde amnesia for the episodes. . . . Actions that do not require skill usually are performed satisfactorily in a semiautomatic way, but attempts at complex tasks fail. The ability of the patient to express himself in a coherent, appropriate manner is also impaired during these episodes. Simple answers to simple questions may not reveal the altered state of consciousness, but suddenly it becomes apparent by a string of loud, inappropriate sentences. (pp. 154–155)

Since narcolepsy is a lifelong disorder, an important part of treatment management has consisted of educating the child, family, and other relevant individuals regarding the nature and consequences of the disorder. Attempts to control narcolepsy consist of recommended frequent napping and the use of stimulant medication (e.g., methylphenidate, pemoline) to reduce the incidence of sleep attacks, and antidepressants (imipramine and chlorimipramine) to control motor inhibitory features and hypnagogic hallucinations (Billiard, 1985; Guilleminault & Anders, 1976). Considering the potential negative effects of medication on learning, it is not recommended that medication be used in children younger than 10 years of age unless the presence and interference effects on school performance of excessive daytime sleepiness are confirmed.

Sleep Apnea

Sleep constitutes an unique behavioral state which is governed by physiologic and biochemical rules and requirements in many ways distinct from those controlling wakefulness. Examples of this sleep-wakefulness distinction can be seen in the emergence during sleep of unusual patterns of EEG activity, periods of muscle inhibition, the absence of temperature control during REM sleep (Parmeggiani & Rabini, 1970), neuroendocrine regulation (Mendelson, 1982) and the reduced respiratory response to hypercapnia during REM sleep (Phillipson, 1977). Despite these state-dependent events, it is obvious that certain vital functions must be preserved, for example, pulmonary and cardiovascular functioning. It is somewhat surprising, therefore, to discover a sleep-associated respiratory dysfunction which takes the form of the momentary (≥10 sec) cessation of breathing during sleep which is terminated, and normal respiration restored, following a brief arousal. This disorder has been termed sleep apnea (Guilleminault, Eldridge, & Dement, 1973; Guilleminault, Tilkien, & Dement, 1976) and occurs in subjects in whom pulmonary functioning during wakefulness is normal. Amazingly, although individual apneic episodes may number in the hundreds each night, subjects are unaware that a cessation of breathing is responsible for their sleep disruptions. The immediate effects of these multiple sleep interruptions are insomnia and an associated excessive daytime sleepiness. In addition to these debilitating sleep-waking consequences of sleep apnea, the presence of cardiac arrhythmias has been noted in afflicted adult subjects—and this condition is by itself a common cause of sudden death (Liberthson et al., 1974). Obviously, a potentially lethal condition is created when sleep apnea and cardiovascular difficulties are combined.

Infants and children are also susceptible to sleep apnea syndromes. For these pediatric populations the clinical picture is further complicated by considerations regarding maturation of respiratory functioning as well as the deleterious effects on cognitive development and functioning resulting from the cumulative effects of intermittent hypoxia occurring throughout early stages of development. To a significant extent, the occurrence of apneic episodes in newborns and infants is related to the immaturity of mechanisms involved in respiration. Several observations support this contention, including: (a) the occurrence of apnea during wakefulness and transitional periods as well as during sleep (Spitzer & Fox, 1984); (b) the greater prevalence (>80%) of apnea among premature relative to term infants (Alden et al., 1972; Curzi-Dascalova, Christova-Gueorguieva, Lebrun, & Firtion, 1984; Daily, Klaus, & Meyer, 1969; Miller, Behrle, & Smull, 1959), particularly those of low birth weight (<1000 g; Alden et al., 1972; Thach, 1985); and, (c) the marked decrease in apneic episodes resulting from upper airway obstruction after the first few months post-delivery (Albani, Bentle, Budde, & Schulte, 1985; Curzi-Dascalova & Christova-Gueorguieva, 1983; Flores-Guevara et al., 1982; Orr et al., 1985). The relationships among several sleep variables and apneic episodes have been investigated in the search for predisposing factors or correlates of these episodes. These variables have included REM-NREM differences (Curzi-Dascalova & Christova-Gueorguieva, 1983; Hoppenbrouwers et al., 1977; Orr et al., 1985), body movement (Curzi-Dascalova & Christova-Gueorguieva, 1983), sleep position (Orr et al., 1985), and eye movements (Curzi-Dascalova & Korn, 1985; Watanabe, Inokuma, & Nigoro, 1983). Although providing new and often provocative descriptive information about apneic episodes and sleep state correlates, the results of investigations examining these variables have either been contradictory or have indicated that the variable is not systematically related to apneic events.

Children for whom apneic episodes do not resolve during the course of early development exhibit a variety of symptoms in addition to daytime sleepiness and sleep disruption. In a series of studies in 5–14 year old children with obstructive sleep apnea (Guilleminault & Anders, 1976; Guilleminault & Dement, 1978; Guilleminault et al., 1976), the following characteristics were noted: normal waking pulmonary functioning, loud snoring, reappearance of nocturnal enuresis, morning headaches, mood and personality changes, weight problems, hypertension, and poor school performance. These children averaged 345 apneic episodes during a 7-hour nocturnal sleep period. The average duration of these episodes was 20 seconds. In other words, these children spent nearly 2 hours or 27 percent of the 7 hour sleep period in apnea. In view of the scale and chronicity of the resulting hypoxia, the far-ranging effects on both sleep and waking behavior noted above are not surprising. Other apnea-associated complications and effects in children which have been reported include hemodynamic changes (Coccagna, Mantovani, Brignani, Parchi, & Lugaresi, 1972), arrhythmias (Guilleminault & Dement, 1978), cor pulmonale (Guilleminault, Souquet, Ariagno, Korobkin, & Simmons, 1984; Hunt & Brouillette, 1982), growth retardation and developmental delay (Brouillette, Fernbach, & Hunt, 1982).

A variety of treatments and interventions have been applied to infants and children afflicted with sleep apnea. These have included pharmacologic treatment (e.g., theophylline and caffeine in premature infants; Roberts, Mathew, & Thach, 1982), surgical intervention [removal of enlarged tonsils and adenoids (Guilleminault et al., 1976) or tracheostomy (Brouillette et al., 1982; Guilleminault et al., 1976)], and behavioral (weight reduction in obese patients; Simpser, Strieder, Wohl, Rosenthal, & Rockenmacker, 1977) and mechanical (positive nasal pressure; Schmidt-Nowara, 1984; Sullivan, Issa, Berthon-Jones, & Eves, 1981) procedures. Depending on the severity and type of sleep apnea syndrome involved (i.e., central—involving a cessation of breathing characterized by the termination of respiratory efforts; obstructive—impaired ventilation involving obstruction of upper airway passages; or mixed—a combination of central and obstructive types), these approaches have met with varying degrees of success. For obstructive sleep apnea, surgical procedures are generally quite effective in greatly diminishing or rapidly reversing symptomatology. Furthermore, follow-up studies in children extending 22–28 months after tracheostomy (Guilleminault et al., 1976) have not indicated complications such as those observed following this procedure in adults (Conway et al., 1981).

Sudden Infant Death Syndrome

The notion that sleep apnea may play a role in the sudden infant death syndrome (SIDS) was first advanced 65 years ago (Still, 1923). Interest in this hypothesis was reawakened by Steinschneider (1972) and the topic has been vigorously researched since that time. In one recent review dealing with sleep apnea in infancy and childhood (Thach, 1985), the relationship between sleep apnea and near-miss SIDS was considered one of 5 major apnea syndromes—major because of "their prevalence, prognostic significance or the completeness of their clinical description" (p. 1289). SIDS is reported to be the most common cause of death in infants 1 month to 1 year of age (Froggatt, Lynas, & MacKenzie, 1971; Tildon, Roeder, & Steinschnider, 1983; Valdez-Dapena, 1980). A large proportion of fatalities attributed to SIDS occurs during the winter months in infants with mild respiratory infections, and although the victims are generally discovered following periods of sleep, apneic episodes have been initiated during wakefulness or feeding (Steinschneider & Rabuzzi, 1976). The first three postnatal months have been identified as the peak risk period (Beckwith, 1973; Bergman, 1970). It is notable that this time frame is also critical to the development and stabilization of many basic physiological functions, including body temperature (Minors & Waterhouse, 1981), heart rate (Harper, Leake, Hodgman, & Hoppenbrouwers, 1982; Harper et al., 1978), and respiratory rhythm (Curzi-Dascalova, Lebrun, & Korn, 1983; Hoppenbrouwers, Jensen, Hodgman, Harper, & Sterman, 1980). Although an imminent SIDS fatality cannot be accurately identified prior to death (Avery & Frantz, 1983; Oren, Kelly, & Shannon, 1986), groups of infants designated as being "at risk" for SIDS have been described. These include subsequent siblings of SIDS victims (Irgens, Skjaerven, & Peterson, 1984; Peterson, Chinn, & Fisher, 1990)—who are reported to be a 4–5 times greater risk for SIDS than nonsiblings (Froggatt et al., 1971), premature infants (Peterson, 1966; Standfast, Jereb & Janerich, 1980; Thach, 1985), and term infants with unexplained apnea (Duffty & Bryan, 1982; Guilleminault & Korobkin, 1979). Although, like infants at risk for SIDS, normal premature and term neonates may evidence apneic episodes and associated cardiovascular and somatic changes, these events are present to a significantly greater degree in the at risk group (Guilleminault & Anders, 1976; Guilleminault, Peraita, Souquet & Dement, 1975; Harper et al., 1978; Hoppenbrouwers et al., 1978; Guilleminault et al., 1979).

The prevalence of this disorder and the large and vulnerable population which it afflicts have made the search for markers among high risk groups a top research priority. However, other than the general observations used to classify infants into the previously described "at risk" groups, significant predictive markers or factors have not been identified. Among the variables which have been examined in this regard are heart rate and respiratory pattern (Gordon et al., 1986), prolonged central apnea (Guilleminault et al., 1979: Southall et al., 1982), and frequency of upper airway obstructive episodes (Guilleminault et al., 1979). One extensive study involving monitoring of 1153 infants, of whom 76 presented with apnea during sleep, observed that infants with apneic episodes that responded only to resuscitation or who were siblings of SIDS victims had a very high risk of dying—31 percent and 25 percent, respectively (Oren et al., 1986). However, after extensive examinations which included head-computed tomographic scan, cranial ultrasound, esophageal pH probe, direct laryngoscopy, bronchoscopy, a pneumogram and recording of heart rate, the authors concluded that "physical examination, past medical history other than siblings of sudden infant death syndrome status, and laboratory evaluation on presentation were not helpful in predicting outcome in these 76 infants."

Studies of sleep organization in infants at risk for SIDS, especially those less than 12 weeks of age, have revealed a pattern of variations which suggest the presence of an arousal deficiency. These studies have indicated that these subjects exhibit: (a) fewer spontaneous awakenings (Challamel, Revol, Leszczynski, & Debilly, 1981; Coons & Guilleminault, 1984; Harper et al., 1981; Navelet, Payan, Guilhaume, & Benoit, 1984) and (b) a significant increase, relative to age-matched controls, in active sleep (Challamel, Debilly, Leszczynski, Revol, & Jouvet, 1983; Harper, Frostig, Taube, Hoppenbrouwers, & Hodgman, 1983; Navelet et al., 1984). These observations are suggestive of, or are consonant with, a relative increase in arousal threshold to wakefulness in at risk infants—a suggestion further reinforced by findings of higher arousal thresholds to hyperapnea and hypoxia tests in at risk infants (Hunt, 1981; McCulloch, Brouillette, Guzzetta, & Hunt, 1982). As Navelet et al. (1984) suggest, however, it is likely that at least two major factors are involved in these observations, namely: (a) the inability for normal homostatic regulatory mechanisms to control and reestablish normal levels of functioning without effecting arousal; and (b) the inability to effect and maintain arousal. This elevated arousal threshold hypothesis was recently tested by Kahn, Picard, and Blum (1986) who studied auditory arousal thresholds in a group of near-miss SIDS infants. These investigators confined their arousal attempts to Stage 2 sleep during the first half of the night and used 6-second, white-noise tones delivered via an earphone at intensities ranging from 40 dB to 120 dB. The index used to determine effective arousal was opening of the eyes. Under these conditions, group differences in arousal thresholds could not be demonstrated. Of interest, relative to the arousal threshold data previously presented for preadolescent subjects (Busby & Pivik, 1983, 1985; Pivik & Busby, 1984), is the observation that 28 percent of controls and 20 percent of near-miss subjects did not show signs of arousal to the highest levels of stimulus intensity. If elevated auditory arousal threshold levels are normally present from birth perhaps through adolescence, and if it is suspected that the arousal thresholds of infants at risk for SIDS exceed those of normal infants, then, given the necessary limitations on stimulus intensity, it may not be reasonable to expect group differences using this measure.

Despite the intense research focused on SIDS and SIDS-related topics, the mechanisms and effective treatment of the disorder continue to elude investigators. The dynamics of neonatal development and the various systems and processes involved in respiration and sleep have led investigators to suggest that SIDS may result from a multifactorial process (Jeffrey, Rahilly, & Read, 1983; Navelet et al., 1984; Thach, 1985). Although the present state of knowledge will not permit the prevention of SIDS, the identification of at-risk groups, and the careful monitoring of these groups are initial and very important steps in the attempted management of this disorder. Programs involving home apnea/bradycardia monitoring by parents trained in cardiovascular resuscitation techniques as well as in the operation of the home monitors have been established for infants considered at risk for SIDS (Kahn & Blum, 1982; Kelly, Shannon, & O'Connell, 1978; Korner, Guilleminault, Van den Hoed, & Baldwin, 1978; Thach, 1985; Ward et al., 1986). Despite the occurrences of infant fatalities even in the face of home monitoring (Ariagno, Guilleminault, Korobkin, Owen-Boeddiker, & Baldwin, 1983; Duffty, & Bryan, 1982), the home monitor approach has been generally well received by parents (Black, Hersher, & Steinschneider, 1978; Cain, Kelly, & Shannon, 1980; Tudehope & Cleghorn, 1984).

CONCLUSIONS

When the eminent evolutionist J. B. S. Haldane said that "the world is not only queerer than we imagine, it is queerer than we can imagine" (Forsyth, 1986), he could have been referring to sleep behavior and misbehavior (disorders), for the study of these conditions has provided us with both uncommon surprises—such as concentrations and types of EEG waveforms alien to normal wakefulness, and hallucinations and paralysis in REM sleep—as well as provocative challenges, some of which are in the form of disorders which appear to be lifelong and often life-threatening (e.g., narcolepsy, sleep apnea). The challenges are indeed formidable and continue to tax our technological, imaginative, and intuitive powers for solutions. As this review has demonstrated, the study of normal and disordered sleep in neonates, infants, and children has played a fundamental role in advancing our understanding of sleep and sleep-waking interactions. These investigations have provided a basis for evaluating maturational influences on behavior which facilitate the differentiation of normal and abnormal behaviors, have allowed us to identify sleep behaviors which are peculiar to specific developmental stages, and have further enabled us to detect emergent indications of sleep disorders which may persist beyond the developmental years into adulthood. These are important contributions to the understanding of a significant facet of human behavior, and in retrospect it seems entirely appropriate that the impetus for much of what has been accomplished in sleep research in the past third of a century was provided by a seminal sleep study in infants (Aserinsky & Kleitman, 1953).

REFERENCES

Agnew, H. W., Webb, W. B., Jr., & Williams, R. L. (1967). Comparison of stage four and REM sleep deprivation. *Perceptual and Motor Skills, 24*, 851–858.

Albani, M., Bentele, K. H. P., Budde, C., & Schulte, F. J. (1985). Infant sleep apnea profile: Preterm vs. term infants. *European Journal of Pediatrics, 143*, 261–268.

Alden, E. R., Mandelhorn, T., Woodrum, D. E., Wennberg, R. P., Parks, C. R., & Hodson, A. (1972). Morbidity and mortality of infants weighing less than 1000 grams in an intensive care nursery. *Pediatrics, 50*, 40–49.

Allison, T., & Van Twyver, H. (1970). The evolution of sleep. *Natural History, 79*, 56–66.

Anders, T. F. (1975). Maturation of sleep patterns in the newborn infant. *Advances in Sleep Research, 2*, 43–66.

Anders, T. F. (1982). Neurophysiological studies of sleep in infants and children. *Journal of Child Psychology and Psychiatry and Allied Disciplines, 23*, 75–83.

Anders, T. F., Carskadon, M. A., & Dement, W. C. (1980). Sleep and sleepiness in children and adolescents. *Pediatric Clinics of North America, 27*, 29–43.

Anders, T., Emde, R., & Parmelee, A., Jr. (Eds.). (1971). *A manual of standardized terminology, techniques and criteria for the scoring of states of sleep and wakefulness in newborn infants.* Los Angeles: Brain Information Service, School of Health Sciences, UCLA.

Anders, T. F., & Keener, M. (1985). Developmental course of nighttime sleep-wake patterns in full-term and premature infants during the first year of life. I. *Sleep, 8*, 173–192.

Anders, T. F., Keener, M. A., & Kraemer, H. (1985). Sleep-wake state organization, neonatal assessment and development in premature infants during the first year of life. II. *Sleep, 8*, 193–206.

Anders, T., & Roffwarg, H. (1973). The effects of selective interruption and deprivation of sleep in the human newborn. *Developmental Psychobiology, 6*, 77–89.

Ariagno, R. L., Guilleminault, C., Korobkin, R., Owen-Boeddiker, M., & Baldwin, R. (1983). Near-miss for sudden infant death syndrome infants: A clinical problem. *Pediatrics, 71*, 726–730.

Arkin, A. M. (1966). Sleep-talking: A review. *The Journal of Nervous and Mental Disease, 143*, 101–122.

Aserinsky, E., & Kleitman, N. (1953). Regularly occurring periods of eye motility and concomitant phenomena during sleep. *Science, 118*, 273–274.

Avery, M. E., & Frantz, I. D., III. (1983). To breathe or not to breathe, what have we learned about apneic spells and sudden infant death? *New England Journal of Medicine, 309*, 107–108.

Baker, T. L. (1985). Introduction to sleep and sleep disorders. *Medical Clinics of North America, 69*, 1123–1152.

Beckwith, J. B. (1973). The sudden infant death syndrome. *Current Problems in Pediatrics, 3*, 3.

Berger, R. J. (1961). Tonus of extrinsic laryngeal muscles during sleep and dreaming. *Science, 134*, 840.

Berger, R., & Meier, G. (1966). The effects of selective deprivation of states of sleep in the developing monkey. *Psychophysiology, 2*, 354–371.

Bergman, A. B. (1970). Sudden infant death syndrome in King County, Washington. In A. B. Bergman, J. B. Beckwith, & C. Ray (Eds.), *Sudden infant death syndrome* (pp. 47–54). Seattle, WA: University of Washington Press.

Bernal, J. (1973). Night waking in infancy during the first 14 months. *Developmental Medicine and Child Neurology, 15*, 760–769.

Billiard, M. (1985). Narcolepsy. Clinical features and aetiology. *Annals of Clinical Research, 17*, 220–226.

Bixler, E. O., Kales, A., Vela-Bueno, A., Drozdiak, R. A., Jacoby, J. A., & Manfredi, R. L. (1986). Narcolepsy/cataplexy III: Nocturnal sleep and wakefulness patterns. *International Journal of Neuroscience, 29*, 305–316.

Black, L., Hersher, L., & Steinschneider, A. (1978). Impact of the apnea monitor on family life. *Pediatrics, 62*, 681–685.

Broughton, R. (1968). Sleep disorders: Disorders of arousal? *Science, 159*, 1070–1078.

Broughton, R. (1975). Biorhythmic variations in consciousness and psychological functions. *Canadian Psychological Review, 16*, 217–239.

Broughton, R. J., Poire, R., & Tassinari, C. A. (1965). The electrodermogram (Tarchanoff effect) during sleep. *Electroencephalography and Clinical Neurophysiology, 18*, 691–708.

Brouillette, R. T., Fernbach, S. K., & Hunt, C. E. (1982). Obstructive sleep apnea in infants and children. *Journal of Pediatrics, 100*, 31–40.

Bruhova, S., & Roth, B. (1972). Heredo-familial aspects of narcolepsy and hypersomnia. *Archiv de Suisse Neurologie, Neurochirurgie, Psychiatrie, 110*, 45.

Busby, K., Firestone, P., & Pivik, R. T. (1981). Sleep patterns in hyperkinetic and normal children. *Sleep, 4*, 366–383.

Busby, K., & Pivik, R. T. (1983). Failure of high intensity auditory stimuli to effect behavioral arousal in children during the first sleep cycle. *Pediatric Research, 17*, 802–805.

Busby, K., & Pivik, R. T. (1985). Auditory arousal thresholds during sleep in hyperkinetic children. *Sleep, 8*, 332–341.

Cain, L. P., Kelly, D. H., & Shannon, D. C. (1980). Parents' perceptions of the psychological and social impact of home monitoring. *Pediatrics, 66*, 37–41.

Challamel, M. J., Debilly, G., Leszczynski, M. C., Revol, M., & Jouvet, M. (1983). A longitudinal study of sleep organization of near-miss infants during the first six months of life. In W. P. Koella (Ed.), *Sleep 1982* (pp. 304–307). Basel: Karger.

Challamel, M. J., Revol, M., Leszczynski, M. C., & Debilly, G. (1981). Organisation nycthemerale des etats de vigilance chez le nourrisson normal et le nourrisson dit "rechappe de mort subite." *Revue d'Electroencephalographie et de Neurophysiologie Clinique, 11*, 28–36.

Cirignotta, F., Mondini, S., Zucconi, M., Lenzi, P. L., & Lugaresi, E. (1985). Insomnia: An epidemiological survey. *Clinical Neuropharmacology, 8*, S49–S54.

Coccagna, G., Mantovani, M., Brignani, F., Parchi, C., & Lugaresi, E. (1972). Continuous recording of the pulmonary and systemic arterial pressure during sleep in syndromes of hypersomnia with periodic breathing. *Bulletin de Physio-Pathologie Respiratorie (Nancy), 8*, 1159–1172.

Conway, W. A., Victor, L. D., Magilligan, D. J., Jr., Fujita, S., Zorick, F. J., & Roth, T. (1981). Adverse effects of tracheostomy for sleep apnea. *Journal of the American Medical Association, 246*, 347–350.

Coons, S., & Guilleminault, C. (1984). Arousal and movement during sleep in "near miss" and normal infants. *Sleep Research, 13*, 77.

Curzi-Dascalova, L., & Christova-Gueorguieva, L. (1983). Respiratory pauses in normal prematurely born infants. A comparison with full-term newborns. *Biology of the Neonate, 44*, 325–332.

Curzi-Dascalova, L., Christova-Gueroguieva, L., Lebrun, F., & Firtion, G. (1984). Respiratory pauses in very low risk prematurely born infants reaching normal term. A comparison to full-term newborns. *Neuropediatrics, 15*, 13–17.

Curzi-Dascalova, L., & Korn, G. (1985). Respiratory pauses and REMs in sleeping premature and full-term infants. In C. T. Jones & P. T. Nathanielsz (Eds.), *The Physiological development of the fetus and newborn* (pp. 273–276). London: Academic Press.

Curzi-Dascalova, L., Lebrun, F., & Korn, G. (1983). Respiratory frequency according to sleep states and age in normal premature infants—a comparison with full-term infants. *Pediatric Research, 17*, 152–156.

Curzi-Dascalova, L., Pajot, N., & Dreyfus-Brisac, C. (1973). Spontaneous skin potential response in sleeping infants between 24 and 41 weeks of conceptional age. *Psychophysiology, 10*, 478–487.

Daily, W. J. R., Klaus, M., & Meyer, H. B. (1969). Apnea in premature infants: Monitoring, incidence, heart rate changes, and an effect of environmental temperature. *Pediatrics, 43*, 510–518.

Delange, M., Castan, P., Cadilhac, J., & Passouant, P. (1962). Les divers stades du sommeil chez le nouveau-ne et le nourisson. *Revue Neurologique, 107*, 271–276.

Dement, W. C. (1960). The effect of dream deprivation. *Science, 131*, 1705–1707.

Dement, W. C. (1972). Sleep deprivation and the organization of the behavioral states. In C. D. Clemente, D. P. Purpura, & F. E. Mayer (Eds.), *Sleep and the maturing nervous system* (pp. 319–355) New York: Academic Press.

Dement, W. C., Carskadon, M., & Ley, R. (1973). The prevalence of narcolepsy. *Sleep Research, 2*, 147.

Dement, W. C., & Fisher, C. (1963). Experimental interference with the sleep cycle. *Canadian Psychiatric Association Journal, 8*, 400–405.

Dement, W. C., & Kleitman, N. (1957a). Cyclic variations in EEG during sleep and their relation to eye movements, bodily motility and dreaming. *Electroencephalography and Clinical Neurophysiology, 9*, 673–690.

Dement, W. C., & Kleitman, N. (1957b). The relation of eye movements during sleep to dream activity: An objective method for the study of dreaming. *Journal of Experimental Psychology, 53*, 339–346.

Dement, W. C., & Mitler, M. M. (1974). An introduction to sleep. In O. Petre-Quadens & J. D. Schlag (Eds.), *Basic sleep mechanisms* (pp. 271–296). New York: Academic Press.

Dement, W. C., Zarcone, V., Varner, V., Hoddes, E., Nassau, S., Jacobs, B., Brown, J., McDonald, A., Horan, K., Glass, R., Gonzales, P., Friedman, E., & Phillips, R. (1972). The prevalence of narcolepsy. *Sleep Research, 1*, 148.

Dische, S. (1978). Childhood enuresis. *Practitioner, 221*, 323–330.

Dittrichova, J. (1966). Development of sleep in infancy. *Journal of Applied Physiology, 21*, 1243–1246.

Dixon, K. N., Monroe, L. J., & Jakim, S. (1981). Insomniac children. *Sleep, 4*, 313–318.

Dreyfus-Brisac, C. (1970). Ontogenesis of sleep in human prematures after 32 weeks of conceptual age. *Developmental Psychobiology, 3*, 91–121.

Dreyfus-Brisac, C. (1979). Ontogenesis of brain bioelectrical activity and sleep organization in neonates and infants. In F. Falkner, & J. M. Tanner (Eds.), *Human growth* (Vol. 3, pp. 157–182). New York: Plenum.

Dreyfus-Brisac, C., & Monod, N. (1965). Sleep of premature and full-term neonates—a polygraphic study. *Proceedings of the Royal Society of Medicine, 58*, 6–7.

Duffty, P., & Bryan, M. M. (1982). Home apnea monitoring in 'near-miss' sudden infant death syndrome (SIDS) and in siblings of SIDS victims. *Pediatrics, 70*, 69–74.

Elias, M. F., Nicolson, N. A., Bora, C., & Johnston, J. (1986). Sleep/wake patterns of breast-fed infants in the first 2 years of life. *Pediatrics, 77*, 322–329.

Ellingson, R. J. (1975). Ontogenesis of sleep in the human. In G. C. Lairy & P. Salzarulo (Eds.), *The experimental study of human sleep: Methodological problems* (pp. 129–146). Amsterdam: Elsevier Scientific Publishing Co.

Emslie, G. J., Roffwarg, H. P., Rush, A. J., Weinberg, W. A., & Parkin-Feigenbaum, L. (1987). Sleep EEG findings in depressed children and adolescents. *American Journal of Psychiatry, 144*, 668–670.

Feinberg, I. (1974). Changes in sleep cycle patterns with age. *Journal of Psychiatric Research, 10*, 283–306.

Feinberg, I., & Floyd, T. C. (1979). Systematic trends across the night in human sleep cycles. *Psychophysiology, 16*, 283–291.

Feinberg, I., Hibi, S., Brown, M., Cavness, C., Westerman, G., & Small, A. (1974). Sleep amphetamine effects in MBDS and normal subjects. *Archives of General Psychiatry, 31*, 723–731.

Ferber, R. (1985). Sleep, sleeplessness, and sleep disruptions in infants and young children. *Annals of Clinical Research, 17*, 227–234.

Ferber, R., Boyle, M. P., & Belfer, M. (1981). Initial experience of a pediatric sleep disorders clinic. *Sleep Research, 10*, 194.

Finklestein, J., Anders, T., Sachar, E., Roffwarg, H., & Hellman, L. (1971). Behavioral state, sleep stage and growth hormone levels in human infants. *Journal of Clinical Endocrinology and Metabolism, 32*, 368–371.

Fisher, C., Kahn, E., Edwards, A., & David, D. M. (1973). A psychophysiological study of nightmares and night terrors: The suppression of stage 4 night terrors with diazepam. *Archives of General Psychiatry, 28*, 252–259.

Flores-Guevara, R., Plouin, P., Curzi-Dascalova, L., Radvanyi, M. F., Guidasci, S., Pajot, N., & Monod, N. (1982). Sleep apnea in normal neonates and infants during the first 3 months of life. *Neuropediatrics, 13*, (Suppl.), 21–28.

Forsyth, A. (1986). *A natural history of sex*. New York: Charles Scribner's Sons.

Foulkes, D. (1966). *The psychology of sleep*. New York: Scribner.

Foulkes, D. (1982). *Children's dreams: Longitudinal studies*. New York: Wiley.

Foutz, A. S., Mitler, M. H., Cavali-Sforza, L. L., & Dement, W. C. (1979). Genetic factors in canine narcolepsy. *Sleep, 1*, 413–422.

Foxman, B., Valdez, R. B., & Brook, R. H. (1986). Childhood enuresis: Prevalence, perceived impact, and prescribed treatments. *Pediatrics, 77*, 482–487.

Froggatt, P., Lynas, M. A., & Mackenzie, G. (1971). Epidemiology of sudden unexpected death ("cot death") in northern Ireland. *British Journal of Preventive and Social Medicine, 25*, 119–134.

Gagnon, P., & DeKoninck, J. (1981). Reappearance of EEG slow waves in extended sleep. *Sleep Research, 10*, 137.

Gagnon, P., & DeKoninck, J. (1984). Reappearance of EEG slow waves in extended sleep. *Electroencephalography and Clinical Neurophysiology, 58*, 155–157.

Gastaut, H., & Broughton, R. (1964). A clinical and polygraphic study of episodic phenomena during sleep. In J. Wortis (Ed.), *Recent advances in biological psychiatry* (Vol. 7, pp. 197–221). New York: Plenum Press.

Glenville, M., Broughton, R., Wing, A. M., & Wilkinson, R. T. (1979). Effects of sleep deprivation on short-duration performance measures compared to the Wilkinson Auditory Vigilance Task. In C. MacKay & T. Cox (Eds.), *Response to stress. Occupational aspects* (pp. 169–177). England: Guilford Press.

Goetz, R. R., Puig-Antich, J., Ryan, N. Rabinovich, H. Ambrosini, P. J., Nelson, B., & Krawiec, V. (1987). Electroencephalographic sleep of adolescents with major depression and normal controls. *Archives of General Psychiatry, 44*, 61–68.

Gordon, D., Southall, D. P., Kelly, D. H., Wilson, A., Akselrod, S., Richards, J., Kenet, B., Kenet, R., Cohen, R. J., & Shannon, D. C. (1986). Analysis of heart rate and respiratory patterns in sudden infant death syndrome victims and control infants. *Pediatric Research, 20*, 680–684.

Greenhill, L., Puig-Antich, J., Goetz, R., Hanlon, C., & Davies, M. (1983). Sleep architecture and REM sleep measures in prepubertal children with attention deficit disorder with hyperactivity. *Sleep, 6*, 91–101.

Guilleminault, C., & Anders, T. F. (1976). Sleep disorders in children. Part II. *Advances in Pediatrics, 22*, 151–174.

Guilleminault, C., Ariagno, R., Korobkin, R., Nagel, L., Baldwin, R., Coons, S., & Owen, M. (1979). Mixed and obstructive sleep apnea and near miss for sudden infant death syndrome: 2. Comparisons of near miss and normal control infants by age. *Pediatrics, 64*, 882–891.

Guilleminault, C., & Dement, W. C. (1978). Sleep apnea syndromes and related sleep disorders. In R. L. Williams & I. Karacan (Eds.), *Sleep disorders: Diagnosis and treatment* (pp. 9–28). New York: Wiley.

Guilleminault, C., Eldridge, F. L., & Dement, W. C. (1973). Insomnia with sleep apnea: A new syndrome. *Science, 181*, 856–858.

Guilleminault, C., Eldridge, F. L., Simmons, F. B., & Dement, W. C. (1976). Sleep apnea in eight children. *Pediatrics, 58*, 23–30.

Guilleminault, C., & Korobkin, R. (1979). Sudden infant death: Near miss events and sleep research. Some recommendations to improve comparability of results among investigators. *Sleep, 1*, 423–433.

Guilleminault, C., Peraita, R., Souquet, M., & Dement, W. C. (1975). Apneas during sleep in infants: Possible relationship with sudden infant death syndrome. *Science, 190*, 677–679.

Guilleminault, C., Souquet, M., Ariagno, R. L., Korobkin, R., & Simmons, F. B. (1984). Five cases of near-miss sudden infant death syndrome and development of obstructive sleep apnea syndrome. *Pediatrics, 73*, 71–78.

Guilleminault, C., Tilkien, A., & Dement, W. C. (1976). The sleep apnea syndrome. *Annual Review of Medicine, 27*, 465–484.

Haig, J. R., Schroeder, C. S., & Schroeder, S. R. (1974). Effects of methylphenidate on hyperactive children's sleep. *Psychopharmacology (Berlin), 37*, 185–188.

Hallstrom, T. (1972). Night terror in adults through three generations. *Acta Psychiatrica Scandinavica, 48*, 350–352.

Harper, R. M., Frostig, Z., Taube, D., Hoppenbrouwers, T., & Hodgman, J. E. (1983). Development of sleep-waking temporal sequencing in infants at risk for the sudden infant death syndrome. *Experimental Neurology, 79*, 821–829.

Harper, R. M., Leake, B., Hodgman, J. E., & Hoppenbrouwers, T. (1982). Developmental patterns of heart rate and heart rate variability during sleep and waking in normal infants and infants at risk for the sudden infant death syndrome. *Sleep, 5*, 28–38.

Harper, R. M., Leake, B., Hoffman, H., Walter, D. L. Hoppenbrouwers, T., Hodgman, J., & Sterman, M. B. (1981). Periodicity of sleep states is altered in infants at risk for the sudden infant death syndrome. *Science, 213*, 1030.

Harper, R. M., Leake, B., Hoppenbrouwers, T., Sterman, M. B., McGinty, D. J., & Hodgman, J. (1978). Polygraphic studies of normal infants and infants at risk for the sudden infant death syndrome: Heart rate and variability as a function of state. *Pediatric Research, 12*, 778–785.

Harper, R. M., Leake, B., Miyahara, L., Mason, J., Hoppenbrouwers, T., Sterman, M. B., & Hodgman, J. (1981). Temporal sequencing in sleep and waking states during the first 6 months of life. *Experimental Neurology, 72*, 294–307.

Harvey, S. C. (1975). Hypnotics and sedatives. In A. G. Gilman, L. S. Goodman, & A. Gilman (Eds.), *The pharmacological basis of therapeutics* (pp. 102–136). New York: Macmillan.

Hauri, P., & Olmstead, E. (1980). Childhood-onset insomnia. *Sleep, 3*, 59–65.

Hellbrugge, T., Lange, J., & Rutenfranz, J. (1959). Schlafen and wachen in der Kindlichen Entwicklung. *Archiv fur Kinderheilkunde, 39*, 1–104.

Hishikawa, Y., Nan'no, H., Taclibana, M., Furuya, E., Koida, H., & Kaneko, Z. (1968). The nature of the sleep attack and other symptoms of narcolepsy. *Electroencephalography and Clinical Neurophysiology, 24*, 1–10.

Honda, Y., & Hishikawa, Y. (1980). A long term treatment of narcolepsy and excessive daytime sleepiness with pemoline (Betamin). *Current Therapeutic Research, 27*, 429–441.

Honda, Y., Juji, T., Matsuki, K., Naohara, T., & Satake, M. (1985). Positive HLA-DR2, DQ1, and DW2 in narcolepsy. *Sleep Research, 14*, 166.

Hoppenbrouwers, T., Hodgman, J. E., Arakawa, K., McGinty, D. J., Mason, J., Harper, R. M., & Sterman, M. B. (1978). Sleep apnea as part of a sequence of events: A comparison of three month old infants at low and increased risk for sudden infant death syndrome (SIDS). *Neuropadiatrie, 9*, 320–337.

Hoppenbrouwers, T., Hodgman, J. E., Harper, R. M., Hoffman, E., Sterman, M. B., & McGinty, D. J. (1977). Polygraphic studies of normal infants during the first six months of life. III. Incidence of apnea and periodic breathing. *Pediatrics, 60*, 418–425.

Hoppenbrouwers, T., Jensen, D. K., Hodgman, J., Harper, R. M., & Sterman, M. B. (1980). The emergence of a circadian pattern in respiratory rates: Comparison between control infants and subsequent siblings of SIDS. *Pediatric Research, 14*, 345–351.

Hunt, C. E. (1981). Abnormal hypercarbic and hypoxic sleep arousal responses in near-miss SIDS infants. *Pediatric Research, 15*, 1462–1464.

Hunt, C. E., & Brouillette, R. T. (1982). Abnormalities of breathing control and airway maintenance in infants and children as a cause of cor pulmonale. *Pediatric Cardiology, 3*, 249–256.

Irgens, L. M., Skjaerven, R., & Peterson, D. R. (1984). Prospective assessment of recurrence risk in sudden infant death syndrome siblings. *Journal of Pediatrics, 104*, 349–351.

Jeffrey, H. E., Rahilly, P., & Read, D. J. C. (1983). Multiple causes of asphyxia in infants at high risk for sudden infant death. *Archives of Diseases of Children, 58*, 92–100.

Jones, B. E. (1985). Neuroanatomical and neurochemical substrates of mechanisms underlying paradoxical sleep. In D. J. McGinty, R. Drucker-Colin, A. Morrison, & P. L. Parmeggiani (Eds.), *Brain mechanisms of sleep* (pp. 139–156). New York: Raven Press.

Kahn, A., & Blum, D. (1982). Home monitoring of infants at risk for the sudden infant death syndrome. *European Journal of Pediatrics, 139*, 94–100.

Kahn, A., Picard, E., & Blum, D. (1986). Auditory arousal thresholds of normal and near-miss SIDS infants. *Developmental Medicine and Child Neurology, 28*, 299–302.

Kales, A., Kales, J. D., Jacobson, A., Humphrey, F. J., & Soldatos, C. R. (1977). Effects of imipramine on enuretic frequency and sleep stages. *Pediatrics, 60*, 431–436.

Kales, J. D. Kales, A., Soldatos, C. R., Caldwell, A. B., Charney, D. S., & Martin, E. D. (1980). Night terrors. Clinical characteristics and personality patterns. *Archives of General Psychiatry, 37*, 1413–1417.

Kales, A., Soldatos, C. R., Bixler, E. O., Caldwell, A., Cadieux, R. J., Verrechio, J. M., & Kales, J. D. (1982). Narcolepsy-cataplexy. II. Psychosocial consequences and associated psychopathology. *Archives of Neurology, 39*, 169–171.

Kales, A., Soldatos, C. R., Caldwell, A. B., Kales, J. D., Humphrey, F. J. Charney, D. S., & Schweitzer, P. K. (1980). Somnambulism. Clinical characteristics and personality patterns. *Archives of General Psychiatry, 37*, 1406–1410.

Karacan, I., Anch, M., Thornby, J., Okawa, M., & Williams, R. L. (1975). Longitudinal sleep patterns during pubertal growth: Four year follow-up. *Pediatric Research, 9*, 842–846.

Karmanova, I. G. (1982). *Evolution of sleep. Stages of the formation of the "wakefulness-sleep" cycle in vertebrates*. New York: Karger.

Kellerman, H. (1981). *Sleep disorders. Insomnia and narcolepsy*. New York: Brunner Mazel.

Kelly, D. H., Shannon, D. C., & O'Connell, K. (1978). Care of infants with near miss sudden infant death syndrome. *Pediatrics, 61*, 511–514.

Kessler, S., Guilleminault, C., & Dement, W. (1974). A family study of 50 REM narcoleptics. *Acta Neurologica Scandinavica, 50*, 503–512.

Kleitman, N. (1963). *Sleep and wakefulness*. Chicago: University of Chicago Press.

Kleitman, N. (1969). Basic rest-activity cycle in relation to sleep and wakefulness. In A. Kales (Ed.), *Sleep physiology and pathology* (pp. 33–38). Philadelphia, PA: Lippincott.

Kleitman, N., & Engelmann, T. (1953). Sleep characteristics of infants. *Journal of Applied Physiology, 6*, 269–282.

Kohler, W. C., Coddington, R. D., & Agnew, H. W. (1968). Sleep patterns in 2-year-old children. *Journal of Pediatrics, 72*, 228–233.

Korner, A. F. (1968). REM organization in neonates. Theoretical implications for development and the biological function of REM. *Archives of General Psychiatry, 19*, 330–340.

Korner, A. F., Guilleminault, C., Van den Hoed, J., & Baldwin, R. B. (1978). Reduction in sleep apnea and bradycardia in preterm infants on oscillating waterbeds: A controlled polygraphic study. *Pediatrics, 61*, 528–533.

Kramer, R. E., Dinner, D. S., Braun, W. E., Zachary, A. A., & Teresi, G. A. (1986). HDA-DR2 and narcolepsy. *Sleep Research, 15*, 24.

Kupfer, D. (1976). REM latency: A psychobiological marker for primary depressive disease. *Biological Psychiatry, 11*, 159–174.

Kupfer, D. J., & Foster, F. G. (1979). EEG sleep and depression. In R. L. Williams & I. Karacan (Eds.), *Sleep disorders: Diagnosis and Treatment* (pp. 163–204). New York: John Wiley & Sons. Inc.

Lahmeyer, H. W., Poznanski, E. O., & Bellur, S. N. (1983). EEG sleep in depressed adolescents. *American Journal of Psychiatry, 140*, 1150–1153.

Larkin, K. T. (1984). The neurobiology of the narcoleptic syndrome. *International Journal of Neuroscience, 25*, 1–17.

Lenard, H. G. (1970). The development of sleep spindles in EEG during the first two years of life. *Neuropadiatrie, 1*, 264–276.

Liberthson, R. R., Nagel, E. L., Hirschman, J. C., Nussenfeld, S. R., Blackbourne, B. D., & Davis, J. H. (1974). Pathophysiologic observations in prehospital ventricular fibrillation and sudden cardiac death. *Circulation, 49*, 790–798.

Loomis, A., Harvey, E., & Hobart, G. (1937). Cerebral states during sleep as studied by human brain potentials. *Journal of Experimental Psychology, 21*, 127–144.

Lynch, J. A., & Aserinsky, E. (1986). Developmental changes of oculomotor characteristics in infants when awake and in the "active state of sleep. *Behavioural Brain Research, 20*, 175–183.

McCulloch, K., Brouillette, R. T., Guzzetta, A. J., & Hunt, C. E. (1982). Arousal responses in near miss sudden infant death syndrome and in normal infants. *Journal of Pediatrics, 101*, 911–917.

Mendelson, W. B. (1982). Studies of human growth hormone section in sleep and waking. *International Review of Neurobiology, 23*, 367–389.

Mendelson, W. B., Cohen, R. M., Campbell, I. C., Murphy, D. L., Gillin, J. C., & Wyatt, R. J. (1982). Lifetime monoamine oxidase inhibition and sleep. *Pharmacology, Biochemistry and Behavior, 16*, 429–431.

Metcalf, D. R. (1970). EEG sleep spindle ontogenesis. *Neuropadiatrie, 1*, 423–433.

Metcalf, D. B., & Jordan, K. (1972). EEG ontogenesis in normal children. In T. Smith (Ed.), *Drug, development and cerebral function* (pp. 125–144). Springfield, IL: Charles C. Thomas.

Metcalf, D. R., Mondale, J., & Butler, F. K. (1971). Ontogenesis of spontaneous K-complexes. *Psychophysiology*, 8, 340–347.

Mikkelsen, E. J., Rapoport, J. L., Nee, L., Gruenau, C., Mendelson, W., & Gillin, J. C. (1980). Childhood enuresis 1. Sleep patterns and psychopathology. *Archives of General Psychiatry, 37*, 1139–1144.

Miller, H. C., Behrle, F. C., & Smull, N. W. (1959). Severe apnea and irregular respiratory rhythms among premature infants. *Pediatrics, 23*, 676–685.

Minors, D. S., & Waterhouse, J. M. (1981). Rhythms in the infant and the aged. In D. Minors & J. M. Waterhouse (Eds.), *Circadian rhythms and the human* (pp. 166–186). Bristol: J. Wright and Sons.

Mirmiran, M. (1986). The important of fetal/neonatal REM sleep. *European Journal of Obstetrics, Gynecology, and Reproductive Biology, 21*, 283–291.

Monod, N., & Garma, L. (1971). Auditory responsivity in the human premature. *Biology of the Neonate, 17*, 292–316.

Mosko, S. S., Shampain, D. S., & Sassin, J. F. (1984). Nocturnal REM latency and sleep disturbance in narcolepsy. *Sleep, 7*, 115–125.

Murray, B., & Campbell, D. (1971). Sleep states in the newborn: Influence of sound. *Neuropadiatrie, 2*, 335–342.

Navelet, Y., Anders, T., & Guilleminault, C. (1976). Narcolepsy in children. In C. Guilleminault, W., Dement, & P. Passouant (Eds.), *Narcolepsy* (pp. 171–177). New York: Spectrum Publications.

Navelet, Y., Payan, C., Guilhaume, A., & Benoit, O. (1984). Nocturnal sleep organization in infants "at risk" for sudden infant death syndrome. *Pediatric Research, 18*, 654–657.

Oksenberg, A., Farber, J., Marks, G., Speciale, S., Malinoff, G., & Roffwarg, H. P. (1985). Testing the role of rapid eye movement (REM) sleep in the development of the CNS. *Sleep Research, 14*, 76.

Oppel, W. C., Harber, P. A., & Rider, R. V. (1968). The age of attaining bladder control. *Pediatrics, 42*, 614–626.

Oren, J., Kelly, D., & Shannon, D. C. (1986). Identification of a high-risk group for sudden infant death syndrome among infants who were resuscitated for sleep apnea. *Pediatrics, 77*, 495–499.

Ornitz, E. M. (1972). Development of sleep patterns in autistic children. In C. D. Clemente, D. P. Purpura, & F. E. Mayer (Eds.), *Sleep and the maturing nervous system* (pp. 363–381). New York: Academic Press.

Orr, W. C., Stahl, M. L., Duke, J., McCaffree, M. A., Toubas, P., Mattice, C., & Krous, H. F. (1985). Effect of sleep state and position on the incidence of obstructive and central apnea in infants. *Pediatrics, 75*, 832–835.

Oswald, I. (1974). Pharmacology of sleep. In O. Petre-Quadens & J. D. Schlag (Eds.), *Basic sleep mechanisms* (pp. 297–302). New York: Academic Press.

Othman, J., Rundell, O. H., & Orr, W. C. (1987). Not all narcoleptics are HLA-DR-2 positive. *Sleep Research, 16*, 403.

Parmeggiani, P. L., & Rabini, C. (1970). Sleep and environmental temperature. *Archives of Italian Biology, 108*, 369–387.

Parmelee, A. (1974). The ontogeny of sleep patterns and associated periodicites in infants. Prenatal and postnatal development of the human brain. *Modern Problems in Pediatrics, 13*, 298–311.

Parmelee, A., Jr., Schultz, H., & Disbrow, M. (1961). Sleep patterns of the newborn. *Journal of Pediatrics, 58*, 241–250.

Parmelee, A. H., Jr., & Stern, E. (1972). Development of states in infants. In C. D. Clemente, D. P. Purpura, & F. E. Mayer (Eds.), *Sleep and the maturing nervous system* (pp. 200–219). New York: Academic Press.

Parmelee, A. H., Stern, E., & Harris, M. A. (1972). Maturation of respiration in premature and young infants. *Neuropadiatrie, 3*, 294–304.

Parmelee, A., Jr., Wenner, W., Akiyama, Y., Schultz, M., & Stern, E. (1967). Sleep states in premature infants. *Developmental Medicine and Child Neurology, 9*, 70–77.

Peterson, D. R. (1966). Sudden unexpected death in infants: An epidemiologic study. *American Journal of Epidemiology, 84*, 478–482.

Peterson, D. R., Chinn, N. M., & Fisher, L. D. (1980). The sudden infant death syndrome: Repetitions in families. *Journal of Pediatrics, 97*, 265–267.

Petre-Quadens, O. (1968). Ontogenesis of paradoxical sleep in the human newborn. *Journal of the Neurological Sciences, 4*, 153–157.

Petre-Quadens, O. (1974). Sleep in the human newborn. In. O. Petre-Quadens & J. D. Schlag (Eds.), *Basic sleep mechanisms* (pp. 355–376). New York: Academic Press.

Petre-Quadens, O., deLee, C., & Remy, M. (1971). Eye movement density during sleep and brain maturation. *Brain Research, 26*, 49–56.

Phillipson, E. A. (1977). Regulation of breathing during sleep. *American Review of Respiratory Disease, Supplement 115*, 217–224.

Pisano, M., Rosadini, G., Rossi, G. F., & Zattoni, J. (1966). Relations between threshold of arousal and electroencephalographic patterns during sleep in man. *Physiology and Behavior, 1*, 55–58.

Pivik, R. T. (1983). Order and disorder during sleep ontogeny: A selective review. In P. Firestone, P. McGrath, & W. Feldman (Eds.), *Advances in behavioral medicine for children and adolescents* (pp. 75–102). New York: Erlbaum.

Pivik, R. T., & Busby, K. (1984). EEG response in auditory stimuli to children during the first sleep cycle as determined by power spectral analysis. *Sleep Research, 13*, 23.

Pivik, R. T., Mercier, L., Busby, K., & Butler, S. (1986, June). *Sleep patterns in reading disabled children.* Presented at the Annual Meeting of the Association of Professional Sleep Societies, Columbus, OH.

Puig-Antich, J., Goetz, R., Hanlon, C., Davies, M., Thompson, J., Chambers, W. J., Tabraizi, M. A., & Weitzman, E. D. (1892). Sleep architecture and REM sleep measures in prepubertal children with major depression. *Archives of General Psychiatry, 39*, 932–939.

Rapoport, J. L., Mikkelsen, E. J., Zavadil, A., Nee, L., Gruenau, C., Mendelson, W., & Gillin, J. C. (1980). Childhood enuresis II. Psychopathology, tricyclic concentration in plasma, and antienuretic effect. *Archives of General Psychiatry, 37*, 1146–1152.

Rechtschaffen, A., Cornwell, P., & Zimmerman, W. (1965). *Brain temperature variations with paradoxical sleep in the cat.* Unpublished manuscript.

Rechtschaffen, A., Hauri, P., & Zeitlin, M. (1966). Auditory awakening thresholds in REM and NREM sleep stages. *Perceptual and Motor Skills, 22*, 927–942.

Rechtschaffen, A., & Kales, A. (Eds.). (1968). *A manual of standardized terminology, techniques, and scoring system for sleep stages of human subjects.* Los Angeles: Los Angeles Brain Information Service/Brain Research Institute, University of California.

Rechtschaffen, A., Wolpert, E. A., Dement, W. C., Mitchell, S. A., & Fisher, C. (1963). Nocturnal sleep of narcoleptics. *Electroencephalography and Clinical Neurophysiology, 15*, 599–609.

Richman, N. (1981). A community survey of characteristics of one- to two-year-olds with sleep disruptions. *Journal of the American Academy of Child Psychiatry, 20*, 281–291.

Roberts, J. L., Mathew, O. P., & Thach, B. T. (1982). The efficacy of theophylline in premature infants with mixed and obstructive apnea and apnea associated with pulmonary and neurologic disease. *Journal of Pediatrics, 100*, 968–970.

Roffwarg, H. P. (1979). Association of sleep disorders centers. *Diagnostic Classification of Sleep and Arousal Disorders*, First Edition, prepared by the Sleep Disorders Classification Committee, H. P. Roffwarg, Chairman. *Sleep, 2*, 1–137.

Roffwarg, H. Dement, W., & Fisher, C. (1964). Preliminary observations on the sleep-dream patterns in neonates, infants, children and adults. In E. Harms (Ed.), *Problems of sleep and dreams in children* (pp. 60–72). New York: Pergamon Press.

Roffwarg, H., Muzio, J., & Dement, W. (1966). Ontogenetic development of the human sleep-dream cycle. *Science, 152*, 604–619.

Roth, B. (1978). Narcolepsy and hypersomnia. In Williams & Karacan (Eds.), *Sleep disorders: Diagnosis and treatment* (pp. 29–59). John Wiley & Sons.

Rutter, M., Yule, W., & Graham, P. (1973). Enuresis and behavioral deviance: Some epidemiological considerations. In I. Kolvin, R. Makeith, & R. Meadow (Eds.), *Bladder control and enuresis* (pp. 137–147). Philadelphia, PA: Lippincott.

Sassin, J. F., Parker, D. C., Mace, J. W., Gotlin, R. W., Johnson, L. C., & Rossman, L. G. (1969). Human growth hormone release: Relation to slow-wave sleep and sleep-waking cycles. *Science, 165*, 513–515.

Schmidt, K., & Birns, B. (1971). The behavioral arousal threshold in infant sleep as a function of time and sleep state. *Child Development, 42*, 269–277.

Schmidt-Nowara, W. W. (1984). Continuous positive airway pressure for long term treatment of sleep apnea. *American Journal of Diseases of Children, 138*, 82–84.

Schulz, H., Massetani, R., Fagioli, I., & Salzarulo, P. (1985). Spontaneous awakening from sleep in infants. *Electroencephalography and Clinical Neurophysiology, 61*, 267–271.

Seignalet, J. (1986). HLA et narcolepsie. *Pathologie Biologie (Paris), 34*, 741–746.

Shaffer, D., & Ambrosini, P. J. (1985). Enuresis and sleep disorders. In J. M. Wiener (Ed.), *Diagnosis and psychopharmacology of childhood and adolescent disorders* (pp. 305–331). New York: John Wiley & Sons.

Simonds, J. F., & Parraga, H. (1982). Prevalence of sleep disorders and sleep behaviors in children and adolescents. *Journal of the American Academy of Child Psychiatry, 21*, 383–388.

Simpser, M. D., Streider, D. J., Wohl, M. E., Rosenthal, A., & Rockenmacker, S. (1977). Sleep apnea in a child with the Pickwickian syndrome. *Pediatrics, 60*, 290–293.

Smith, C. M. (1958). Psychosomatic aspects of narcolepsy. *Journal of Mental Science, 104*, 593–607.

Snyder, F., Hobson, J., Morrison, D., & Goldfrank, F. (1964). Changes in respiration, heart rate, and systolic blood pressure in human sleep. *Journal of Applied Physiology, 19*, 417–422.

Sours, J. A. (1963). Narcolepsy and other disturbances in the sleep-waking rhythm: A study of 115 cases with review of the literature. *Journal of Nervous and Mental Diseases, 137*, 525–542.

Southall, D. P., Richards, J. M., Rhodon, K. J., Alexander, J. R., Shinebourne, E. A., Arrowsmith, W. A., Creel, S. F., Fleming, P. J., Gocalves, A., & Orme, R. L. E. (1982). Prolonged apnea and cardiac arrhythmias in infants discharged from neonatal intensive care units: Failure to predict an increased risk for sudden infant death syndrome. *Pediatrics, 70*, 844–851.

Spitzer, A. R., & Fox, W. W. (1984). Infant apnea—an approach to management. *Clinical Pediatrics, 23*, 374–380.

Standfast, S. J., Jereb, S., & Janerich, D. T. (1980). The epidemiology of sudden infant death in upstate New York: II. Birth characteristics. *American Journal of Public Health, 70*, 1061–1067.

Steinschneider, A. (1972). Prolonged apnea and the sudden infant death syndrome: Clinical and laboratory observations. *Pediatrics, 50*, 646–654.

Steinschneider, A., & Rabuzzi, D. D. (1976). Apnea and airway obstruction during feeding and sleep. *Laryngoscope, 86*, 1359–1366.

Sterman, M. B. (1972). The basic rest-activity cycle and sleep: Developmental considerations in man and cats. In C. D. Clemente, D. P. Purpura, & F. E. Mayer (Eds.), *Sleep and the maturing nervous system* (pp. 175–197). New York: Academic Press.

Stern, E., Parmelee, A. H., Akiyama, Y., Schultz, M. A., & Wenner, W. H. (1969). Sleep cycle characteristics in infants. *Pediatrics, 43*, 65–70.

Still, G. F. (1923). Attacks of arrested respiration in the newborn. *Lancet, 1*, 431–432.

Sullivan, C. E., Issa, F. G., Berthon-Jones, M., & Eves, L. (1981). Reversal of obstructive sleep apnea by continuous positive airway pressure applied through the nares. *Lancet, 1*, 862.

Sweeney, C. R., Hendricks, J. C., Beech, J., & Morrison, A. R. (1983). Narcolepsy in a horse. *Journal of the American Veterinary Medical Association, 183*, 126–128.

Thach, B. T. (1985). Sleep apnea in infancy and childhood. *Medical Clinics of North America, 69*, 1289–1315.

Thoman, E. B. (1975). Sleep and wake behaviors in neonates. Consistencies and consequences. *Merrill Palmer Quarterly, 21*, 295–314.

Tildon, J. T., Roeder, L. M., & Steinschneider, A. (1983). *Sudden infant death syndrome.* New York: Academic Press.

Tudehope, D. I., & Cleghorn, G. (1984). Home monitoring for infants at risk of sudden infant death syndrome. *Australian Paediatric Journal, 20*, 137–140.

Valdes-Dapena, M. (1980). Sudden infant death syndrome: A review of the medical literature 1974–1979. *Pediatrics, 66*, 597–614.

Valley, V., & Broughton, R. (1980). Mental impairment in relation to concomitant polygraphic recordings in patients with narcolepsy-cataplexy compared to matched controls. *Sleep Research, 9*, 228.

Ward, S. L. D., Keens, T. G., Chan, L. S., Chipps, B. E., Carson, S. H., Deming, D. D., Krishna, V., MacDonald, H. M., Martin, G. I., Meredith, K. S., Merritt, T. A., Nickerson, B. G., Stoddard, R. A., & van der Hal, A. L. (1986). Sudden infant death syndrome in infants evaluated by apnea programs in California. *Pediatrics, 77*, 451–458.

Watanabe, K. Inokuma, K., & Negoro, T. (1983). REM sleep prevents sudden infant death syndrome. *European Journal of Pediatrics, 140*, 289–292.

Watt, J. E., & Strongman, K. T. (1985). The organization and stability of sleep states in full term, preterm, and small-for-gestational-age infants: A comparative study. *Developmental Psychobiology, 18*, 151–162.

Webb, W. (1969). Twenty-four hour sleep cycling. In A. Kales (Ed.), *Sleep physiology and pathology* (pp. 53–65). Philadelphia, PA: Lippincott.

Webb, W. (1986). Enhanced slow sleep in extended sleep. *Electroencephalography and Clinical Neurophysiology, 64*, 27–30.

Webb, W., & Agnew, H. (1975). Are we chronically sleep deprived? *Bulletin of the Psychonomic Society, 6*, 47–48.

Weitzman, E. D., Czeisler, C. A., Zimmerman, J. C., & Ronda, J. (1980). The timing of REM sleep and its relation to spontaneous awakening during temporal isolation in man. *Sleep Research, 9*, 280.

Weitzman, E., Fishbein, W., & Graziani, L. (1965). Auditory evoked responses obtained from the scalp electroencephalogram of the full-term neonate during sleep. *Pediatrics, 35*, 458–462.

Werry, J., Dawnick, P., Lampen, E., & Vamos, M. J. (1975). Imipramine in enuresis: Psychological and physiological effects. *Journal of Child Psychology and Psychiatry, 16*, 289–299.

Williams, R. L., Agnew, H. W., Jr., & Webb, W. B. (1964). Sleep patterns in young adults: An EEG study. *Electroencephalography and Clinical Neurophysiology, 17*, 376–381.

Williams, R. L., Agnew, H. W., Jr., & Webb, W. B. (1966). Sleep patterns in the young adult female: An EEG study. *Electroencephalography and Clinical Neurophysiology, 20*, 264–266.

Williams, R., Karacan, I., & Davis, G. (1972). Sleep patterns of pubertal males. *Pediatric Research, 6*, 643–647.

Yoss, R. E., & Daly, D. D. (1960). Hereditary aspects of narcolepsy. *Transactions of the American Neurological Association*, pp. 239–240.

Young, W., Knowles, J., MacLean, A., Boag, L., & McConville, B. J. (1982). The sleep of childhood depressives: Comparison with age matched controls. *Biological Psychiatry, 17*, 1163–1168.

Young, D., Zorick, F., Wittig, R., Roehrs, T., Stepanski, E., & Roth, T. (1987). Narcolepsy in a pediatric population. *Sleep Research, 16*, 461.

V

ADDICTIVE BEHAVIORS

13

Minimal Interventions for Smoking Cessation: The Potentials of Self-Instructional Methods

Neville Owen

Dept. of Community Medicine
University of Adelaide, Australia

Smoking-cessation services that do not rely primarily on the face-to-face contact of individual counseling, or on the interaction and personal instruction which takes place in smoking-cessation groups, can be described as mediated programs. They involve the presentation of information, motivational messages and instruction using printed, audio, or audiovisual material. They can be distributed or sold to individual smokers who wish for assistance with their efforts at cessation, or they can be presented through the mass media, mainly television, radio, newspapers, and magazines. Information, exhortation, and advice on smoking cessation are now commonly seen and heard in the mass media, and there are familiar examples of pamphlets and kits produced for smokers.

Materials distributed or sold include self-instructional books (e.g., Danaher & Lichtenstein, 1978; Pomerleau & Pomerlau, 1977), booklets (e.g., American Lung Association, undated) quit kits (e.g., American Cancer Society, 1977; Health & Welfare Canada, 1982), and pamphlets (e.g., Anti-Cancer Council of Victoria, undated). Audiotapes marketed by commercial smoking cessation organizations, videotapes soon to be available in Australia, and combinations of audiotapes and print-media materials (e.g., Health Promotion Services, 1982a) are further examples of mediated smoking cessation materials.

Mass media interventions to promote smoking cessation include the work of the Stanford Heart Disease Prevention Program in California (e.g., Maccoby & Alexander, 1980), the North Coast "Quit for Life" program in Australia (e.g., Egger et al., 1983) and the materials for radio, television, newspapers, and magazines that are part of recent campaigns in most Australian states. In mass media campaigns, mediated smoking cessation materials include informative and motivational messages in short radio and television spots or advertisements, and television and radio segments or series on how to quit. Print media materials include informative and motivational advertisements in newspapers and magazines, and longer articles or series which deal with the health effects of smoking, the process of smoking cessation, and tips on how to quit. Mass media efforts are often coordinated around themes and carefully designed time schedules, as part of what are described as public communication campaigns (Solomon, 1981).

Mediated, as opposed to face-to-face, smoking cessation services are becoming ubiquitous, and are attracting considerable public funding, particularly for mass media campaigns. This chapter deals with mediated smoking cessation services in a critical and practical perspective, and aims to highlight some of the issues in their design and implementation. Stages of behavior change in smoking cessation are considered, along with the rationales for the use of mediated programs and the advantages and disadvantages of the social channels available to influence behavior. Guidelines for choosing appropriate mediated materials, some of the pitfalls in their use, and problems in assessing their effectiveness are discussed.

STAGES OF BEHAVIOR CHANGE AND SMOKING CESSATION

Most smokers who refrain from smoking generally only do so for a short period of time. Followup studies of participants in smoking-cessation programs have found that over 50 percent of those who quit will resume regular smoking within three months. After 12 months, over 70 percent will have resumed (Hunt, Barnett, & Branch, 1971). Maintenance of behavior change is now recognized to be a general problem, with many participants in weight loss, exercise, stuttering therapy, and other behavior change programs tending to resume the habits they have changed (Owen, 1981). Techniques for enhancing maintenance of behavior change have been given considerable attention in recent years (e.g., Goldstein & Kanfer, 1979; Karoly & Steffen, 1980; Stuart, 1982).

It should be kept in mind that any change in behavior, and particularly smoking cessation, is not a simple process, and is best understood as a series of stages. DiClemente and Prochaska (1982), for example, identify three stages: decision to change, active changing, and maintenance of the new behavior. They offer interpretations of smoking cessation programs which suggest the operation of different mechanisms at different stages of the change process, with verbal processes such as education and self-persuasion important in the first stage, and direct instruction being used in the second and third. Abrams, Elder, Lasater, and Carleton (1982) argue that behavior change should be considered in three stages: promotion of the new behavior, skill development, and maintenance. Maccoby and Alexander (1980) propose five stages: agenda setting; informing; training new behaviors; motivating and reinforcing the new behaviors; and maintenance training. This apparent variety of stages and labels appears based on similar notions of change: Behavior change requires a process of producing awareness of the problem, then motivation to change, followed by instruction on how to change, and consolidated by a final stage assisting the maintenance of the new behavior. It seems likely (e.g., Dishman, 1982) that different behavior-change techniques will be effective at different stages in the change process, and for this reason Abrams et al. (1982) recommend a multiple approach in which all stages are addressed as targets through any community intervention campaign, so that individuals at all stages of readiness to change can be influenced. This type of thinking has also been applied to self-initiated attempts at smoking cessation (Prochaska & DiClemente, 1983).

Clearly, the choice of smoking cessation materials to be used in any program or campaign, and how different materials should be introduced or combined, should take into account the stage or stages of the process of change which are being targeted. It should also be kept in mind that even following intensive, face-to-face contact programs, many smokers who succeed in quitting are likely to resume smoking.

WHY ARE SELF-INSTRUCTIONAL METHODS FAVORED?

It is well-established that most smokers who quit do so by their own efforts. Approximately 90 percent of smokers state that they simply stopped smoking, without recourse to formal assistance or to any particular aids or materials (South Australian Health Commission, 1981). From such figures, it is sometimes argued that formal programs and structured quitting aids should be given a lower priority than media campaigns designed to highlight the health hazards of smoking and to motivate smokers to quit. However, a majority of smokers have made attempts to quit, and most smokers express a wish to be able to quit. For example, in a survey in the mid-1970s in the United States, it was found that 61 percent of smokers reported at least one serious attempt at cessation. Furthermore, it was estimated that most smokers have either made a serious attempt to quit, or would do so if they believed they could succeed (United States Public Health Service, 1976).

These figures make obvious the fact that a majority of smokers probably have tried to quit without success. High priority should, and obviously is, being given to ensuring that smokers are well-informed about the health hazards of smoking. Motivating smokers to quit is also part of the widespread public education and media campaigns designed to make smoking appear undesirable, and to promote nonsmoking as an attractive alternative. However, a major challenge is to provide the large number of smokers who are motivated to quit with appropriate and effective instruction on *how* to do so. Results of a survey reported by Schwartz and Dubitzky (1967) show that less than one-third of smokers would be willing to attend a group or public health clinic for face-to-face assistance. Two-thirds of smokers expressed a preference for assistance which does not require personal contact, for example, through a television show, or by using a book or other forms of printed instruction. Similarly, McAlister (1975) reports that 70 percent of smokers surveyed would not be prepared to attend a formal smoking cessation program. Researchers working on the "Quit for Life" program in Northern N.S.W. report that when stop-smoking groups were advertised in the city of Lismore, only 1.5 percent of smokers in the population attended. When quit kits were advertised, 15 percent of smokers requested them (Egger, 1982, personal communication). Among smokers who wish to quit, there is interest in obtaining materials that they can use to aid their own efforts at cessation, rather than relying on the help of face-to-face programs.

An advantage of print-media materials such as books and quit kits is that they can be made available to large numbers of people at a relatively low cost, compared to the expense of providing facilities, trained personnel, and administrative support for groups which deal with relatively small numbers. Given that cigarette smoking is such a large-scale public health risk, with over 30 percent of the population being current, regular smokers (South Australian Health Commission, 1981; United States Public Health Service, 1979), it would be unproductive to rely on face-to-face services as the major vehicle for promoting smoking cessation. But mediated programs reaching large numbers of smokers also have disadvantages, as can be seen from the comparison of likely effects of the different social channels which may be used (see Table 13.1).

A further argument for the use of mediated materials is that they encourage individual responsibility, with smokers choosing materials which will be of use to them in their own efforts at cessation. But a problem with this approach is that it appears that there is little consistency in what smokers who quit by their own efforts actually do to achieve cessation (Baer, Foreyt, & Wright, 1977). It has also been argued that self-initiated change may result in significantly better

Table 13.1.
The relative advantages and disadvantages of mediated and face-to-face smoking cessation programs

Face-to-Face Programs	Advantages	Disadvantages
• groups • one-to-one counseling	• personalising • social support • social modeling • interactive • reliable • sequential • follow-up is easy	• expensive per unit of contact • market penetration is poor • unacceptable to many smokers • may encourage dependency
Mediated Materials	**Advantages**	**Disadvantages**
• books • pamphlets • quit kits • broadcasts radio television • newspaper and magazine advertisements and articles • combined media	• cheap per unit contact • reach large numbers • more acceptable • may stimulate self-initiated change	• unreliable • weak engagement of users • distortion and dilution of content • sequencing and follow-up are difficult

maintenance of new habits (Loro, Fisher, & Levenkron, 1979; Schachter, 1982). That is, if smokers quit by their own efforts, rather than with the assistance of structured programs, they have a greater sense of personal responsibility for this achievement, and are therefore more likely to be able to sustain the changes that they have made.

However, it should be kept in mind that smokers who ask for face-to-face assistance or who join a group may be more likely to have had a number of failures in their previous attempts at cessation. It is likely that mediated programs may appeal to smokers who are at a relatively early stage in their efforts at cessation. They may also be less physiologically addicted than are smokers who are unable to achieve cessation using mediated programs. While these suggestions are speculative, it is likely to be the case that smokers trying to quit generally desire a minimal amount of help initially, and may wish for more as they find quitting to be difficult for them.

SOCIAL CHANNELS FOR PROMOTING CESSATION: ADVANTAGES AND DISADVANTAGES

Following the preceding arguments, and observing current fashions in community antismoking campaigns, may lead to the conclusion that mediated smoking cessation services should be the prime vehicle for work in the area. However, an examination of the relative advantages and disadvantages of mediated and face-to-face methods suggests that such a conclusion oversimplifies important issues in the promotion of smoking cessation. Table 13.1 summarizes these, and may be used as a guide for decisions on the appropriateness of different intervention strategies.

While face-to-face programs have relatively low acceptability and may reach small numbers of smokers, they do have the advantages of providing: personalized information which may be selected by a well-informed expert; social support, modeling of skills, mutual exchange, and negotiation; the potential for advice and instruction to be presented reliably, with appropriate emphasis on important material; a sequence of interactions which may be tailored to each smoker's readiness to deal with each phase of the cessation process; follow-up, ongoing support, and judiciously applied social pressure.

Mediated materials do lack many of these advantages. They may not reach smokers in the form they are intended to have, and their content may be used only selectively, possibly avoiding components crucial to effective change. It is also difficult to ensure that mediated materials are used in an appropriate sequence, and it may be difficult to do follow-up assessments on people who have obtained books, kits or pamphlets (Chapman & Reynolds, 1982). In spite of these limitations, mediated materials' advantages are in areas of major importance for public health risk reduction: they can be made available to large numbers of smokers; are relatively inexpensive per unit of contact; and are more acceptable to the majority of smokers than are face-to-face methods. There is also the argument that mediated materials may be incorporated into smokers' self-directed efforts at cessation, promoting a sense of personal initiative and responsibility for change, and resulting in a greater ability on the part of those who succeed to persist with nonsmoking (Owen, 1983).

These contrasts and the material in Table 13.1 should not be taken to imply that there are mutually exclusive choices to be made between mediated and face-to-face methods, or that mediated materials are always the intervention of choice. A majority of smokers (close to two-thirds) state that they would not attend face-to-face programs (McAlister, 1975; Schwartz & Dubitzky, 1967). With such smokers, advice and follow-up from a health professional may be the most effective means for helping them to change. Given that a significant portion of the population of smokers will see a general practitioner in any one-year period, there should be efforts to provide GPs with high-quality guidelines and skill training to assist cessation among their smoking patients.

It should also be kept in mind that smoking cessation groups may provide an essential service for smokers who have experienced numerous failures in their own attempts at cessation, who have not found mediated materials or programs to be effective, or who wish for face-to-face instruction and social support. The intensive instruction, group interaction, social pressure, and social support which can be generated in group programs may be the most viable service option for many smokers.

Options for combining the advantages of mediated programs with those face-to-face programs should also be considered. For example, the correspondence course developed in Adelaide in collaboration with Health Promotion Services attracted enquiries from 310 smokers who were interested in structured assistance, but who preferred a correspondence course to participation in a group program (Owen & Ewins, 1982). Of the 208 who took part in the course; 45 percent were able to refrain from smoking for a short period; 25 percent were abstinent for at least 2 weeks, and 19 percent were abstinent for 3 months. At a 9 month follow-up, 13 percent were not smoking. Compared to the high rates of resumption following more intensive programs (Hunt, Barnett, & Branch, 1971; Lichtenstein, 1982; Owen, Ewins, Bullock, &

Lee, 1982), these apparently modest figures represent a significant effect for a totally mediated program. Correspondence courses have the advantages of being able to be made widely available, are relatively inexpensive, can elicit commitment to a definite program, can provide a sequence which participants can follow, and have the potential for being personalised using information management technology such as microcomputers and word processors (Owen, 1983; see Chapter 6). Correspondence courses for smoking cessation and for weight loss are recent developments which show considerable promise (Brengelmann, 1978; Jeffery, Danaher, Killen, Kinnear, & Farquhar, 1982; Jeffery & Gerber, 1982).

The option of combining mediated programs with face-to-face influence also has potential. An example is the "Give Up Smoking" (GUS) kits developed for general practitioners by the South Australian Health Commission (Health Promotion Services, 1982b). These are pamphlets and booklets which physicians can give to their patients, accompanied by appropriate advice and exhortation. A more structured format for such purposes has been developed, using an adaptation of the correspondence course already described. This is a program which a gastroenterologist is testing with duodenal ulcer patients in Adelaide (Owen, 1983).

In this program, the physician sees the patients for a single session of counseling in which they are shown a printed program describing the skills of preparing to quit, a technique for achieving cessation, some relaxation skills, and some means for coping with urges to smoke. The physician demonstrates aspects of the program such as diaphragm breathing and discusses any difficulties or concerns that the patient has. Four days after this session, the patients are mailed a personal letter from the physician which contains further advice on how to deal with urges to smoke, and 10 days later they are sent a further letter. The materials they are given in the face-to-face session, and the two follow-up letters, deal with the main components of the correspondence course mentioned earlier, and follow a structured sequence for achieving cessation and sustaining abstinence from cigarette smoking. There is evidence that the impact of self-instructional materials may be facilitated when combined with face-to-face instruction and counseling (Glasgow, Schafer, & O'Neill, 1981).

The correspondence course and the physicians' program are constructed of a number of elements which are common to most mediated smoking cessation materials. Like quit kits and self-instructional books, they include: protocols for recording smoking frequency and the intensity of urges to smoke; a cessation guide which often involves halving daily cigarette consumption for three days before a predetermined quit date; suggestions on how to deal with self-generated excuses to smoke; self-statements designed to support continued nonsmoking; how to recruit social support; and a relaxation protocol. Both programs follow the sequence for smoking cessation programs suggested by Best (1978). The four lessons of the correspondence course deal with: preparing for cessation; how to stop smoking; dealing with urges to smoke; and remaining a nonsmoker (maintenance). Data from the first randomized trial of the course (Owen & Ewins, 1982) have been used to guide the development of a more abbreviated three lesson course which is being tested in Adelaide as part of the South Australian Health Commission's Tobacco Awareness Campaign.

PRACTICAL ISSUES AND RESEARCH DIRECTIONS

In planning any smoking cessation program or campaign, careful attention should be given to its specific goals, to the particular target groups of concern, the audiovisual and print media materials to be used and developed, the potential roles of community services and networks, the ways in which mass media are to be used, and the funding and staff expertise that is available. Within the unique context of a particular campaign or program there will be numerous options for the judicious and creative use of mediated smoking cessation services. How these are to be used will depend on the stages of behavior change which are of concern. This should assist in making decisions about the optimal combination of material providing information, motivational content, and direct instruction on how to achieve cessation.

It is important that sound evaluation be carried out, and that long-term follow-ups of participants be conducted. However, it should be kept in mind that relatively low long-term cessation rates are to be expected following almost any stop-smoking cessation program. Generally, over 70 percent of smokers who achieve cessation will resume within twelve months (Lichtenstein, 1982; Owen, 1982, 1983).

It is always useful to consult local experts and to read the smoking cessation literature in order to gain a perspective on current issues and problems. Try to be realistic about what is likely to be achieved with the programs being used, and try to gain some sense of the current views on how such work is best conducted. Recent reviews which are worth consulting include: DiClemente and Prochaska, 1982; Health Promotion Services, 1983; Leventhal and Cleary, 1980; Marlatt and Gordon, 1980; Orleans, Shipley, Williams, and Haac, 1981a, 1981b; Pechacek and Danaher, 1979; Pechacek and McAlister, 1980; Schwartz, 1978.

Consider the advantages and disadvantages of the media, materials and social channels available (see Table 13.1). For example, if the intention is to provide services for smokers who have a long history of failed attempts at cessation, a media campaign designed to raise awareness and motivation could be combined with counseling guidelines for health professionals and the availability of intensive group programs, which may be implemented through community health services. On the other hand, if the intention is to enhance cessation among young people and new smokers, a media campaign combined with the widespread distribution of completely self-instructional materials may be most appropriate.

Keep in mind that there exists relatively little research on the effect of mediated behavior change materials such as books, kits, and pamphlets. There has been a recent evaluation in Australia (Chapman & Reynolds, 1982), but reviews of the effects of self-instructional materials (Glasgow & Rosen, 1978, 1979) make clear that their active ingredients, their effects on long-term maintenance of change, and the type of people for whom they are most effective remain to be determined.

In considering mediated smoking cessation materials, the full range of options described earlier in this chapter need to be kept in mind. Combinations of different types of materials and media can produce unique programs which may be very acceptable and effective. Current and future developments in microelectric, information-management, and broadcast technology mean that a much larger range of options for mediated programs is becoming available. Cable and satellite television will create more channels which can be used for specialized purposes such as health risk reduction. The production and marketing of audiovisual materials will become cheaper and more accessible to a wide range of health professionals and to commercial organizations. Interactive personal behavior change programs which can be used with home video systems and microcomputers will be available in the near future.

All of these developments and their commercial potential mean that low-quality, poorly conceived programs and materials may be marketed and not properly evaluated. This can lead to public disillusionment and the premature rejection of potentially effective preventive services (Agras, 1982; Owen, 1983). Priority should be given by health professionals to becoming familiar with this technology and its potentials, so that it is more likely that soundly based material is used, and that programs are well conceived, designed and evaluated. The ways in which mass media advertising can serve broad and ideological purposes at odds with the ideals of the health educator should also be a concern (Ewen, 1976; Mander, 1978).

It is important to keep in mind that any smoking cessation program faces formidable competition from expert, well-funded campaigns which promote the adoption of cigarette smoking by children and young adults (Chapman & Fitzgerald, 1982). These campaigns also provide social modeling and spuriously desirable images and aspirations which are intended to sustain the habit in established smokers (Chapman & Egger, 1980). Initiatives to counter these campaigns through lobbying, public protest, and legislative action, rather than trying only to ameliorate their effects, is necessary if rates of smoking in the community are to be reduced significantly (Chapman, 1980, 1982; Health Promotion Services, 1983).

REFERENCES

Abrams, D. B., Elder, J. P., Lasater, T. M., & Carleton, R. A. (1982). *Social learning theory principles for community health promotion: An integration across levels of intervention.* Paper presented at the 16th Annual Convention of the Association for Advancement of Behavior Therapy, Los Angeles, CA.

Agras, W. S. (1982). Behavioral medicine in the 1980s: Nonrandom connections. *Journal of Consulting and Clinical Psychology, 50* (6), 797–803.

American Cancer Society. (1977). *I quit kit* (Publication No. 2028). New York: Author.

American Lung Association. (undated). *Freedom from smoking in twenty days.* New York: Author.

Anti-Cancer Council of Victoria. (undated). *Quit kit: How to plan the five days that could save your life.* Melbourne: Author.

Baer, P. E., Foreyt, J. P., & Wright, S. (1977). Self-directed termination of excessive cigarette use among untreated smokers. *Journal of Behaviour Therapy & Experimental Psychiatry, 8,* 71–74.

Best, J. A. (1978). Targeting and self-selection of smoking modification methods. In J. L. Schwartz (Ed.), *Progress in smoking cessation.* (pp 105–118) New York: American Cancer Society.

Brengelmann, J. C. (1978). The treatment of smoking through the mail. In J. L. Schwartz (Ed.), *Progress in smoking cessation* (pp 255–265) New York: American Cancer Society.

Chapman, S. (1980). A David and Goliath story. Tobacco advertising and self-regulation in Australia. *British Medical Journal, 281*, 1187–1190.

Chapman, S. (1982). The tobacco industry: Getting our retaliation in first. *New Doctor, 25*, 27–30.

Chapman, S. & Egger, G. (1980). Forging an identity for the nonsmoker: The use of myth in health promotion. *International Journal of Health Education, Supplement 23*(3).

Chapman, S., & Reynolds, I. (1982). The mass media and smoking cessation: The ABC-TV Nationwide "I Quit" program. *Community Health Studies, 6*(3), 247–252.

Danaher, B. G. & Lichtenstein, E. (1978). *Become an ex-smoker.* Englewood Cliffs, NJ: Prentice-Hall.

DiClemente, C. C., & Prochaska, J. O. (1982). Self-change and therapy change of smoking behavior: A comparison of processes of change in cessation and maintenance. *Addictive Behaviors, 7,* 133–142.

Dishman, R. K. (1982). Compliance/adherence in health-related exercise. *Health Psychology, 1,* 237–267.

Egger, G., Fitzgerald, W., Frape, G., Monaem, A., Rubinstein, P., Tyler, C., & McKay, B. (1983). Results of large scale media antismoking campaign in Australia: North Coast "Quit for Life" program, *British Medical Journal, 287,* 1125–1128.

Ewen, S. (1976). *Captains of consciousness: Advertising and the roots of consumer culture.* New York: McGraw-Hill.

Glasgow, R. E., & Rosen, G. M. (1978). Behavioral bibliotherapy: A review of self-help behavior therapy manuals. *Psychological Bulletin, 85,* 1–23.

Glasgow, R. E. & Rosen, G. M. (1979). Self-help behavior therapy manuals: Recent developments and clinical usage. *Clinical Behavior Therapy Review, 1,* 1–20.

Glasgow, R. E., Schafer, L., & O'Neill, H. K. (1981). Self-help books and amount of therapist contact in smoking cessation programs. *Journal of Consulting and Clinical Psychology, 49*(5), 659–667.

Health and Welfare Canada. (1982). *Time to quit.* Ottawa: Health Promotion Directorate.

Health Promotion Services. (1982a). *Quit kit.* Adelaide: South Australian Health Commission.

Health Promotion Services. (1982b). *Give Up Smoking (G.U.S.) Kit.* Adelaide: South Australian Health Commission.

Health Promotion Services. (1983). *Not so much a lobby . . . more a revolution: The case for freedom from tobacco multinationals.* Adelaide: South Australian Health Commission.

Hunt, W. A., Barnett, L. W., & Branch, L. G. (1971) Relapse rates in addiction programs. *Journal of Clinical Psychology, 27,* 455–456.

Jeffery, R. W., Danaher, B. G., Killen, J., Kinnear, R., & Farquhar, J. W. (1982). Self-administered programs for health behavior change: Smoking cessation and weight reduction by mail. *Addictive Behaviors, 7,* 57–63.

Jeffery, R. W., & Gerber, W. M. (1982). Group and correspondence treatments for weight reduction used in the Multiple Risk Factor Intervention Trial. *Behavior Therapy, 13*(1), 24–30.

Karoly, P., & Steffen, J. (1980). *Improving the long-term effects of psychotherapy.* New York: Gardner Press.

Leventhal, H., & Cleary, P. D. (1980). The smoking problem: A review of the research and theory in behavioral risk modification. *Psychological Bulletin, 88*(2), 370–405.

Lichtenstein, E. (1982). The smoking problem: A behavioral perspective. *Journal of Consulting and Clinical Psychology, 50* (6), 804–819.

Loro, A. D., Fisher, E. B., Jr., & Levenkron, J. C. (1979). Comparison of established and innovative weight reduction treatment procedures. *Journal of Applied Behavior Analysis, 12,* 141–155.

Maccoby, N., & Alexander, J. (1980). Use of media in lifestyle programs. In P. Davidson (Ed.), *Behavioral medicine: Changing health lifestyles.* (pp. 351–370) New York: Brunner/Mazel.

Mander, J. (1978). *Four arguments for the elimination of television.* New York: Morrow Quill Paperback.

Marlatt, G. A., & Gordon, J. R. (1980). Determinants of relapse: Implications for the maintenance of behavior change. In P. O. Davidson & S. M. Davidson (Eds.), *Behavioral medicine: Changing health lifestyles.* (pp. 410–452) New York: Brunner/Mazel.

McAlister, A. (1975). Helping people quit smoking. In A. M. Enelow & J. B. Henderson (Eds.), *Applying behavioral science to cardiovascular risk.* (pp. 147–165) New York: American Heart Association.

Orleans, C. T., Shipley, R. H., Williams, C., & Haac, L. A. (1981a). Behavioral approaches to smoking cessation-I: A decade of research progress 1969–1979. *Journal of Behaviour Therapy and Experimental Psychiatry, 12*(2), 125–129.

Orleans, C. T., Shipley, R. H., Williams, C., & Haac, L. A. (1981b). Behavioral approaches to smoking cessation-II. Topical bibliography 1969–1979. *Journal of Behaviour Therapy and Experimental Psychiatry, 12,* 131–144.

Owen, N. (1981). Facilitating maintenance of behavior change. In E. Boberg (Ed.), *Maintenance of fluency.* New York: Elsevier.

Owen, N. (1988). Behavioural medicine: Prospects and limits. In J. L. Sheppard (Ed.), *Advances in behavioral medicine* (Vol. 5, pp. 13–30) Sydney: Cumberland College of Health Sciences.

Owen, N. & Ewins, A. (1982). Correspondence courses for quitting smoking. In T. Rogers (Chair), *Alternative delivery strategies for health behaviour change: Mass media, mail and Ma Bell. Symposium at the Association for Advancement of Behavior Therapy.* Los Angeles, CA.

Owen, N., Ewins, A., Bullock, M. & Lee, C. (1982). Adherence, relapse and health related behaviours. In J. L. Sheppard (Ed.), *Advances in behavioural medicine*, (Vol. 2, pp. 229–246) Sydney: Cumberland College of Health Sciences.

Pechacek, T. F. & Danaher, B. G. (1979). How and why people quit smoking: A cognitive-behavioral analysis. In P. C. Kendall & S. D. Hollon (Eds.), *Cognitive-behavioral interventions: Theory, research and procedures.* (pp. 162–177) New York: Academic Press.

Pechacek, T. F., & McAlister, A. L. (1980). Strategies for the modification of smoking behavior: Treatment and prevention. In J. Ferguson & C. B. Taylor (Eds.), *The comprehensive handbook of behavioral medicine* (Vol. 3, pp. 257–298) New York: Spectrum Publications.

Pomerlau, O. F., & Pomerlau, C. S. (1977). *Break the smoking habit: A behavioral program for giving up cigarettes*. Champaign, IL: Research Press.
Prochaska, J. O., & DiClemente, C. (1983). Stages and processes of self-change of smoking. Toward an integrative model of change. *Journal of Consulting and Clinical Psychology, 51*(3), 390–395.
Schachter, S. (1982). Recidivism and self-cure in smoking and obesity. *American Psychologist, 37*(4), 436–444.
Schwartz, J. L. (Ed.). (1978). *Progress in smoking cessation*. New York: American Cancer Society.
Schwartz, J. L., & Dubitzky, M. (1967). Expressed willingness of smokers to try ten smoking withdrawal methods. *Public Health Reports, 82*, 855–861.
Solomon, D. S. (1981). A social marketing perspective on campaigns. In R. E. Rice & W. J. Paisley (Eds.), *Public communication campaigns* (pp. 281–291) Beverly Hills: Sage.
South Australian Health Commission. (1981 June). *Survey of smoking in South Australia*. Adelaide: South Australian Health Commission.
Stuart, R. B. (Ed.). (1982). *Adherence, compliance and generalization in behavioral medicine*. New York: Brunner/Mazel.
United States Public Health Service. (1976). *Adult use of tobacco: 1975*. Washington DC: United States Department of Health, Education and Welfare.
United States Public Health Service. (1979). *Smoking and health. A Report of the surgeon general* (DHEW Publication No. (PHS) 79–50066). Washington, DC: United States Department of Health, Education and Welfare.

14

Eating Disorders and Their Behavioral Management

Stephen William Touyz

Head, Department of Clinical Psychology
Westmead Hospital, Westmead,
and Associate Professor,
Department of Psychiatry,
University of Sydney, New South Wales,
Australia

INTRODUCTION

In contemporary society there appears an escalating concern expressed especially by young women to maintain slimmer figures (Touyz & Ivison, 1985; Abraham, Mira, Beumont, Sowerbutts, & Llewellyn-Jones, 1983; Schwartz, Thompson, & Johnson, 1983). This concern has been associated with a rapid growth in exercise, weight control programs, and fad diets, as well as a boom in the health food industry. Schwartz, Thompson, and Johnson (1982) have even suggested that the current emphasis on diet and exercise in the United States has "shifted from a growing leisure time hobby to a national obsession" and that the pursuit of slenderness has resulted in an increased prevalence of eating disorders. Clearly, sociocultural factors have been strongly implicated with the recent increase in eating disorders.

The current obsession with dieting and slimness apparently was not shared by prehistoric women who have been described classically as having large abdomens, hips, and thighs. One of the earliest representations of human form, named the Venus of Wilendorf, dates back to the Paleolithic period of 20,000 to 30,000 B.C. (Bruch, 1973). It is a statue of an obese woman with large breasts and an extended abdomen.

In fact, as late as 1911, a French clinician, Heckel, described the frustration experienced by therapists attempting to implement weight reduction programs. These programs were actively resisted by the women of that time who wanted to remain well-rounded and plump in order to conform to cultural expectations.

As the importance attributed to maintaining a slender figure gained momentum in contemporary society, so the revulsion at being obese has begun to reach phobic proportions. Wooley, Wooley, & Dyrenforth (1979) have recently provided lucid descriptions of how obese children are ostracized by their peer group.

> The impact this hatred [of obese children by other children and by adults] has on the individual child is probably irreversible. It is not only the obese child who suffers from this hatred; anti-fat attitudes learned in childhood no doubt become the basis for self-hatred among those who become overweight at later ages, and a source of anxiety and self doubt for anyone fearful of becoming overweight.

In a noteworthy editorial, Kalucy (1983) issued a stern warning to the medical profession that it may have been overenthusiastic in promoting the notion that obesity and ill health are directly related and that this concept may have been interpreted too simplistically. He indicated that the medical profession had "contributed significantly to the prevailing weight conscious social climate and that it may now have to consider more carefully the ramifications of certain aspects of preventative health programmes. Even the best intention can sometimes have undesirable results" (p. 206).

Given the contextual issues already noted, and the fact that clinicians are now being required to treat an ever-increasing number of patients who are eating disordered, the present chapter will provide the clinician and/or research worker with recent developments in the literature concerning eating disorders (anorexia nervosa, bulimia nervosa, and obesity) and their behavioral management.

ANOREXIA NERVOSA

Characteristics of the Disorder

Anorexia nervosa is a complex, multidimensional disorder characterized by the relentless pursuit of thinness which is appropriately referred to as "magersucht" in the German literature meaning "leanness mania" (Garfinkel & Garner 1982; Beumont, 1984). It usually occurs in adolescent girls or young women and is less frequently described in prepubertal children, males, and middle-aged persons. Numerous factors contribute to the occurrence in the individual patient. Among these, sociocultural factors must be considered, as there is substantial pressure on women in our culture to diet in response to the current ideal standard for the female body shape (Bruch, 1978; Garner & Garfinkel, 1978, 1980; Garner, Garfinkel, & Schwartz, 1980; Garner, Garfield, & Olmsted, 1983; Touyz & Ivison, 1985).

Anorexia nervosa is euphemistically referred to as the "slimmers' disease" in the popular press but it is in fact a serious disorder with a mortality rate of approximately five percent (Hsu, 1980; Touyz & Beumont, 1984). It is often associated with psychological disturbances (obsessionality, depression, poor self-esteem, body image disturbance), major social effects (invalidism, regression, withdrawal), and severe physical sequelae (malnutrition, disordered body chemistry, and endocrine dysfunction) (Beumont & Touyz, 1985). Because of this complex interaction of psychological factors in the genesis of its varied symptomatology, it has been called the paradigm of psychosomatic disorders (Kaufman & Heiman, 1964).

The incidence of anorexia nervosa has increased over recent decades (Kendall, Hall, Hailey, & Babigan, 1973; Jones, Fox, Babigan, & Hutten, 1980) and it is no longer considered to be a rare illness. It is often suggested that the incidence of anorexia nervosa is reaching epidemic proportions in affluent societies but there is no scientific evidence at present to substantiate this view. Crisp, Palmer, and Kalucy (1976) reported that one out of every 100 school girls over the age of 16 years attending private schools in London is probably affected. A more recent report by Willi and Grossman (1983), who conducted a retrospective study of the incidence of anorexia nervosa in Zurich, revealed that the illness had increased significantly from .38/100,000 for 1956–1958 to .55/100,000 for 1963–1965 to 1.12/100,000 for 1973–1975. The increased occurrence of anorexia nervosa has been accompanied by a greater awareness of the disorder by medical practitioners, clinical psychologists, and school counselors and there is now a tendency to make the diagnosis earlier, before the patient has become severely emaciated (Beumont & Russell 1982).

Diagnosis

Several psychiatric illnesses such as depression, schizophrenia and anxiety states or even organic brain lesions may occasionally lead to emaciation but their presentation and optimal treatment are quite different from that of primary anorexia nervosa. For example, depressed patients usually complain of a loss of appetite and are not preoccupied with either the caloric content of their food or their body shape. Despite this, there has been an unfortunate trend in recent years to include severely undernourished patients under the generic label of "anorexia nervosa" (Hall, 1984; Garfinkel, Kaplan, Garner, & Darby, 1983). Like most psychiatric diagnoses, anorexia nervosa is a syndromal diagnosis and has a specific clinical presentation (Table 14.1). Because of this, it is generally not too difficult to differentiate anorexia nervosa patients from those with other psychiatric disorders that result in weight loss. It is a much more difficult task to distinguish anorexia nervosa from normal and even healthy lifestyles where the individual has made a commitment to diet and exercise on a regular basis (Figure 14.1) (Beumont, 1984). Behaviors found in patients with anorexia nervosa are also observed in fashion-conscious women. However, in anorexia nervosa patients, these behaviors have compulsive flavor and the patient is unable to resist them (Yates, Leehey, & Shisslak, 1983).

Eating disorders are not mutually exclusive of one another (Figure 14.1) and there is often considerable overlap. Twenty percent of patients with anorexia nervosa have been reported to develop bulimia (Hsu, Crisp, & Harding, 1979; Hall, 1984). The "night eating syndrome" characterized by nocturnal hyperplagia, insomnia, and morning anorexia was initially described in patients hospitalized with obesity (Stunkard, 1959).

The Behavioral Disorder and its Consequences

One of the earliest descriptions in the medical literature of anorexia nervosa was provided by Charles Lasegue (1873) who was intrigued by the rich phenomenology found in this disorder. He stressed the pro-

Table 14.1.
The American Psychiatric Association Diagnostic Criteria for Anorexia Nervosa (DSM III-R)

A. Refusal to maintain body weight over a minimal normal weight for age and height, e.g., weight loss leading to maintenance of body weight 15% below that expected; or failure to make expected weight gain during period of growth, leading to body weight 15% below that expected.
B. Intense fear of gaining weight or becoming fat, even though underweight.
C. Disturbance in the way in which one's body weight, size, or shape is experienced, e.g., the person claims to "feel fat" even when emaciated, believes that one area of the body is "too fat" even when obviously underweight.
D. In females, absence of at least three consecutive menstrual cycles when otherwise expected to occur (primary or secondary amenorrhea). (A woman is considered to have amenorrhea if her periods occur only following hormone, e.g., estrogen, administration.)

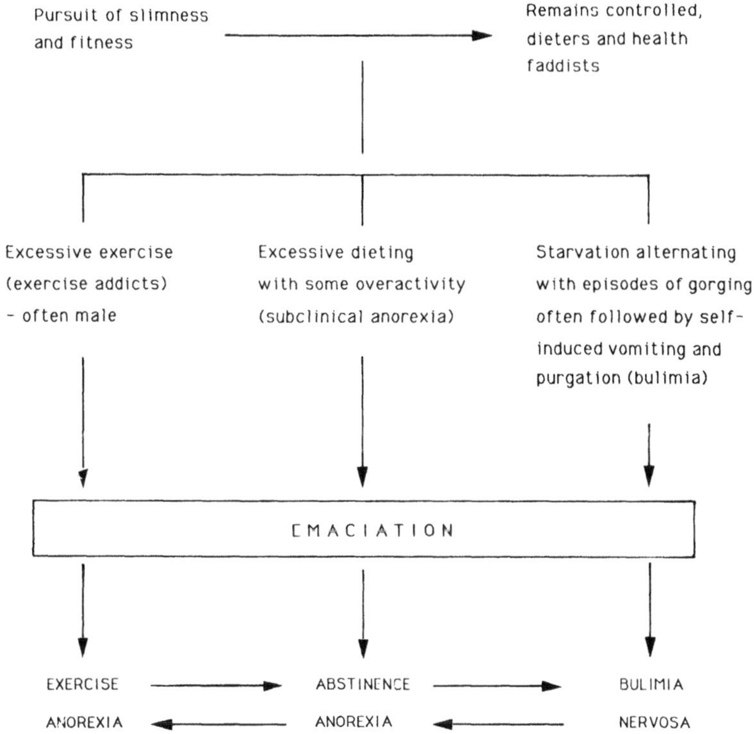

FIGURE 14.1. Anorexia nervosa and related disorders.

gressive nature of the illness and lucidly illustrated the sequential development of the numerous behavioral disturbances and the consequent physiological symptoms. Recent studies have confirmed Lasegue's earlier impressions regarding the temporal sequence of symptoms. Casper and Davis (1977) contrasted the psychological and physiological symptoms found in patients with anorexia nervosa with those of starvation reported in the medical literature (Keys et al., 1950; Schiele & Brozek 1948; Mitchell & Black 1946; Dally, 1969; and Sydenham, 1946). They were able to identify three phases of the disorder. During phase 1, which may occur months or years before the illness is diagnosed, precipitating factors are often apparent and result in a loss of self-esteem and increased self consciousness about physical appearance. In phase 2, patients develop anorexic attitudes and behaviors which include an unreasonable fear of eating and becoming fat and derive considerable satisfaction from their ability to lose weight. By phase 3, patients are forced by the severity of starvation symptoms to acknowledge that they are ill and reluctantly accept treatment.

Although many of the physical symptoms of starvation and anorexia nervosa are similar, Casper and Davis (1977) reported that patients with anorexia nervosa, in contrast to victims of starvation, showed high initiative, the ability to suppress hunger, restless hyperactivity, and body image distortion.

In a more recent study, Beumont, Booth, Abraham, Griffith, and Turney (1983) found that patients initially showed concern about their body weight and made reasonable attempts to control it. However, they became more and more preoccupied with thoughts of weight and food and used increasingly bizarre methods to control their weight such as self-induced vomiting and purgatory abuse. A notable feature of their results was the high frequency of occurrence of bulimia (76% of patients) and of self-induced vomiting (64%). However, Beumont et al. (1983) acknowledged that they did not attempt to differentiate between patients with bulimia nervosa from those with anorexia nervosa and caution that their findings may have been influenced by a high proportion of patients with bulimia nervosa.

Anorexia nervosa is primarily a behavioral disturbance and nearly all the physical and psychiatric symptoms associated with it are secondary to undernutrition. It is therefore not surprising that behaviorally oriented therapy has been found to be extremely effective in the management of this condition.

Behavioral Management of Anorexia Nervosa

Venables (1930), more than a half century ago, published practical guidelines for the treatment of anorexia nervosa. He was most optimistic about the efficacy of such treatment and his observations makes interesting reading. He reported that:

> Every patient with anorexia nervosa can be persuaded to eat normally. The condition is hysterical, and no patient should remain uncured. Full explanation should be given the patient, and the doctor should sit down with the patient and fight for every mouthful of food, which may take an hour or two per meal. The doctor must never lose his temper. With each successive meal, eating becomes easier, and the patient may eat alone in about a week. The patient must be given a full diet from the first. One must cure the anorexia before one starts on the psychology of the patient's symptoms. The author points out that he is never in favour of prolonged and deep analysis; the immediate cause is seldom hard to find. A few frank discussions, coupled with any necessary adjustments in circumstances, should be all that is necessary, and no relapses should occur. Patients should be kept in bed, and special nurses are usually needed. The patient should never be treated at home, and the parents should be excluded. (J. F. Venables, 1930, quoted in C. V. Rowland, 1970)

One of the first reports in the literature, describing the application of behavioral techniques in the management of anorexia nervosa, was provided by Bachrach and his colleagues in 1965. They treated a 37-year-old woman using social reinforcement (e.g., conversation, attention, and praise), which was made contingent upon her eating her meals. In order to maximize weight gain they placed her in a single room without the usual possessions such as a television set or books. Both staff and relatives were restricted from visiting the patient. She initially gained weight on this regime, but her weight gain tapered off after she had put on 15.84 lbs. To facilitate further increases in weight, they made rewards contingent upon weight gain rather than eating behavior. Unfortunately, the patient was discharged from hospital shortly thereafter and it is not known whether any further weight gain occurred.

Leitenberg, Agras, and Thomson (1968) replicated the work of Bachrach and his colleagues and found that conversation and attention during meals was not successful in producing weight gain. However, when they rewarded weight gain directly, a steady increase in both caloric intake and weight gain was observed.

The first experimental attempt of reinforcement in the treatment of patients with anorexia nervosa was conducted by Agras et al. (1974) using a within-subject experimental design. The authors were most interested in the unexpected findings reported in an earlier investigation (Leitenberg et al., 1968) where the removal of positive reinforcement did not result in a reduction of caloric intake. Agras et al. speculated that some other variable or variables were contributing to this therapeutic effect, for example, negative reinforcement (the patient only being allowed to leave the hospital after satisfactory weight gain). A second experiment confirmed their impression that the removal of positive reinforcement resulted in caloric intake dropping steadily and weight gain slowing down when the patient was told that weight gain would not result in discharge. Further experiments in this series indicated that informational feedback was a powerful variable in promoting weight gain.

These studies stimulated a great deal of interest in the application of principles derived from learning theory in the hospital management of patients with anorexia nervosa. Garfinkel and Garner (1982) have recently reviewed the published literature on the behavioral treatment of anorexia nervosa. Numerous techniques have been used including systematic desensitization to reduce anxiety associated with eating (Hallsten, 1965; Ollendick, 1979; Schnurer, Rubin, & Roy, 1973) and aversive counterconditioning to reduce the frequency of self-induced vomiting (Kenny & Solyom 1971). Operant conditioning has become increasingly popular in facilitating weight gain during refeeding and well over 30 studies have been cited in the literature. An extensive review of these studies is beyond the scope of this chapter but salient findings will be summarized.

Because operant techniques are known to facilitate weight gain and are relatively easy to implement on inpatient units, it is not surprising that Whyte and Kaczkowski (1983) in a recent survey found that most American psychiatrists and psychologists utilize behavioral techniques in their management of patients with anorexia nervosa. This trend was much less evident among psychiatrists in the United Kingdom (Bhanji, 1979).

Agras and Werne (1978) reported that behavioral techniques resulted in a more consistent weight gain, favorable outcome, and less use of coercive methods, for example, tube feeding and/or intravenous therapy, than nonbehavioral methods of treatment. They suggested that the less frequent use of tube feeding and/or intravenous therapy was associated with lower mortality rates and strongly advocated the use of behavior therapy in the management of the hospitalized patients with anorexia nervosa.

Bruch, on the other hand, has expressed great concern regarding the use of behavior modification in anorexia nervosa (1974, 1978). In a paper entitled "Perils of Behavior Modification in Anorexia Nervosa" she strongly criticized behavior therapists for their naive assumption that the restoration of normal body weight (the most prominent symptom) was sufficient treatment. It was her impression that most behaviorally oriented programs failed to take into account the major deficits in the personality development of these patients, namely, low self-esteem, self-doubt, lack of autonomy, and an inability to lead a self-directed life. She also indicated that behavioral programs had an adverse psychological effect on certain patients who would gain weight under the "pressure of persuasion, force or threats" and would literally "eat their way out" of the hospital. Bruch concluded by saying that "it is generally known that true benefit is derived from such weight gain only if it is part of an integrated treatment programme with correction of the underlying individual and family problems."

Garner (1986[b]) has cautioned that behavior modification can be used in a mechanical way without regard to the therapeutic relationship or individual differences among patients. It is most important that operant techniques are not used in a punitive manner to elicit the desired behaviors. Garner has drawn attention to unnecessary punitive "contingencies" such as "room isolation" (Lobb & Schaefer 1972; Schlemmer & Barnett 1977; Schmidt & Duncan, 1974), tube feeding (Newman & Gaoni, 1975; Schmidt & Duncan, 1974), and beating with a switch (Blue, 1979).

> A wooden switch was obtained from a branch and set in the parents' bedroom. Each time C threw up her food or engaged in a temper tantrum, her mother would follow these actions with five painful hits from the switch. During the punishment nothing was said. Eating continued to be followed by happy talk. (Blue, 1979, p. 707)

Garner (1986b) has stressed that "many negative contingencies may be more naturally applied upon rational parameters operating within the environment." For example, bedrest may be deemed necessary following a main meal if a patient has a history of inducing vomiting immediately after eating.

There is now a general consensus amongst clinicians that behavior modification enhances weight gain during the refeeding phase of treatment but long-term follow-up studies suggest that it may not be superior to other nontraditional treatments (Garfinkel & Garner 1982). In one of the few prospective controlled studies comparing behavioral treatment with milieu therapy alone, no significant differences were found over the 35 day period. However, this study's findings should remain tentative as patients were only rewarded every five days and rewards were not individualized.

Cognitive Therapy in Anorexia Nervosa

The use of cognitive therapy in the treatment of depression and neurotic disorders has become increasingly popular over the past decade (Beck, 1976; Beck et al., 1979). Garner and Bemis (1982, 1985) have pioneered this approach in the managment of patients with anorexia nervosa. They have modified the procedures delineated by Beck and his colleagues so as to apply to the particular distorted thinking patterns characteristic of patients with anorexia nervosa. Garner and Bemis (1985) have also incorporated ideas developed by other eminent cognitive therapists such as Ellis (1962), Goldfried (1971), Mahoney (1974), and Meichenbaum (1974), in part to deal with the deficits in self-concept that characterize patients with anorexia nervosa.

The application of cognitive procedures in the treatment of patients with anorexia nervosa is based upon the "assumption that maladaptive feelings and behaviours are mediated by distorted or maladaptive thinking and that the primary aims of clinical intervention is to alter these cognitive processes" (Garner & Bemis, 1985). Garner and Bemis (1985) stress that cognitive strategies must be adapted for the anorexic patient and should include:

1. the patient's reluctance to commence treatment, the egosyntonic nature of certain symptoms and the overall recalcitrance of the disorder
2. the interrelationship between physical and psychological elements
3. the prominence of deficits in self-concept related to the individual's lack of awareness and of confidence in the internal state
4. idiosyncratic beliefs related to weight and food. Because of these factors, the therapist must be prepared to proceed slowly so as to facilitate a more trusting therapeutic relationship and as a result, therapy may take longer than other disorders. It is also most important to recognize both the psychological and physiological sequelae of starvation and the clarification of their effects with the patient should take place early in therapy. Further the therapist needs to assist the patient in altering misperceptions without reinforcing her already inadequate trust of internal experiences.

Garner and Bemis (1985) have described some of the most common reasoning errors that occur in patients with anorexia nervosa are (a) dichotomous thinking, (b) personalization and self-reference, (c) superstitious thinkings, (d) selective abstraction, (e) overgeneralization, and (f) magnification.

Dichotomous thinking. The anorexic patient tends to think in absolute terms and usually categorizes food into "good" or "bad" categories. Their rigid attitudes and behaviors are not confined to food and weight issues and they often strive for absolute perfection in their careers, sports, and academic achievements as well. Examples of dichotomous thinking include, "If I am not in complete control, I will lose all control," "If I eat one sweet, I won't be able to stop and I will get fat."

Personalization and self-reference. Patients tend to overinterpret events relating to themselves and to make egocentric interpretations of impersonal events. Examples include "Two individuals giggled at one another as I walked by. They were probably laughing at me in that I have become so fat having recently gain 5 lbs"; "whenever I see an overweight person in the street, I immediately come to the conclusion that I will look exactly like her."

Superstitious thinking. Patients believe in the cause-effect relationship of noncontingent events. Examples include "Now that I have gained weight, I can't enjoy myself anymore"; "If I eat a doughnut, it will immediately be converted into fat inside my body."

Selective abstraction. They make assumptions on the basis of isolated information whilst ignoring contradictory and more salient evidence. Examples include "I am a terribly weak individual as I can't control my impulses. This evening I decided to eat only half my dinner and ended up eating all the food on my plate."

Overgeneralization. Patients tend to develop guidelines based upon a single event and then apply it to dissimilar situations. Examples include "When I used to eat energy dense foods such as cakes and sweets I became fat and overweight. I can never eat those foods again because if I do, I shall become overweight again."

Magnification. Patients overestimate the significance of undesirable consequent events. Examples include "Because I have gained 5 lbs, I shall never be able to go to the beach ever again as I couldn't possibly wear a bathing suit anymore!"

Thus patients with anorexia nervosa reveal a wide range of systematic distortions in both the processing and interpretation of events. It is therefore of the utmost importance to adequately document the patient cognitions when utilizing cognitive behavior therapy. Some patients may benefit from keeping a written record of their thoughts on a semi-standardized assessment form such as the Dysfunctional Thought Record (Beck et al., 1979). Psychotherapy should always be an ongoing process and the patient's cognitions should be reexamined throughout the duration of treatment to monitor change and to deal with dysfunctional thoughts not previously identified. One of the principal features of cognitive behavior therapy is to teach the patients to critically evaluate the validity of their beliefs on a moment-to-moment basis (Hollen & Beck, 1979).

Cognitive Techniques

A multitude of cognitive techniques have been recommended for treating patients with anorexia nervosa. Detailed descriptions of these procedures and their clinical applications have been previously described by Garner and Bemis (1982, 1985). Those particularly interested in this aspect of behavioral intervention are also directed to the work of Beck and his colleagues (Beck 1970, 1976; Beck et al., 1979) from which many of these techniques have been adapted. Examples of some of these techniques are presented in Table 14.2.

Many patients with anorexia nervosa have poor self-esteem, lack assertiveness, and have difficulties with both the identification and

Table 14.2.
Examples of Some of the Cognitive Techniques Recommended for Treating Patients with Anorexia Nervosa

Technique	Description of Procedure
Articulation of Beliefs	Patient should be encouraged to simplify or consolidate her beliefs in order to make the distortions more evident.
Decentering	Evaluating a belief from a different perspective in order to obtain a more objective impression.
Decatastrophizing	This technique was originally proposed by Ellis (1962) for dealing with anxiety resulting from the magnification of negative consequences of a specific event.
Challenging the "Shoulds"	Patients make excessive use of words such as "should," "must," and "ought," for example, "I must diet in order to be happy," or "I should exercise every day." This tendency has been observed in many psychological disturbances and led Horney (1950) to comment that the "tyranny of the shoulds" was the cornerstone of neurotic disturbance.

Source: Garner and Bemis, 1985.

expression of emotion. Strategies for improving self-esteem, self-awareness, and lack of assertion also should be addressed.

Cognitive therapy should not be the only focus of intervention when treating patients with anorexia nervosa but should form part of a more comprehensive treatment strategy (Touyz & Beumont, 1985). Garner and Bemis (1982) have stressed the difficulties encountered in undertaking psychotherapy in patients with anorexia nervosa. They concluded that "work with anorexic clients demands flexibility, creativity, and all the therapeutic acumen a clinician can muster." For this very reason, future research should be directed at the efficacy of this approach and as to whether it improves the longer term outcome in patients suffering from anorexia nervosa.

Behavioral Treatment: A Lenient and Flexible Approach

We recently evaluated a behavioral program that allowed patients to maintain a greater degree of control while being refed in hospital (Touyz et al. 1984b). The results were compared with data obtained using the more traditional approach where the patient is confined to bed and has all her possessions removed. She is then rewarded for gaining weight using an individualized schedule of reinforcers. Sixty-five patients with anorexia nervosa participated in the study. They were consecutive admissions to an eating disorder unit and were divided into two cohorts. The first 31 patients were treated using a strict bedrest programme with individualized schedule of reinforcers for each half pound gained. The next 34 were treated using a more lenient and flexible behavioral program. Patients were required to gain 3 lbs a week and, provided they did so, were permitted to move around the unit at their leisure. If they failed to gain the 3 lbs over a one-week period, they were placed on bedrest for a week. However, once on bedrest, they kept all their possessions such as books, radio, or television but were not permitted in visits from family or friends. The other patients in the unit were allowed to visit. While restricted to bedrest, the patients continued to attend therapeutic groups and ate their meals in the dining room.

Our most important observation was that the mean daily weight gain did not differ significantly between the two treatment programmes (0.46 lbs vs. 0.44 lbs). The mean daily weight gain for both programs also compared favorably with the best figures reported by other authors using behavioral techniques.

Furthermore, there were practical advantages in using the lenient program. It was seen as more acceptable by most of our patients, and there was a general consensus among staff members that patients on the lenient program were better motivated toward treatment and required less nursing care. It was therefore more economical and it provided less opportunity for patients to manipulate individual staff members in connection with their treatment. As a result, the staff were able to use their time more constructively in both group therapy and supportive psychotherapy with the patients. This was very much in keeping with our overall aim of providing a comprehensive integrated approach to treatment (Touyz & Beumont, 1985).

Our pragmatic multidisciplinary treatment approach consists of a series of integrated treatment approaches based upon our belief that a number of factors are involved in the causation and persistence of anorexia nervosa. Our approach has many factors in common with the one described by Anderson, Morse, and Santmyer (1983) with the notable exception being our behavioral rather than psychodynamic emphasis. Important aspects of our program are:

1. Regulated weight gain occurs in a warm supportive environment.
2. Information feedback and dietary counseling are given on a regular basis.
3. A moderate but graduated level of activity is allowed.
4. Weight gain is essential but is only part of the overall treatment program.

5. Occupational therapy, social skills, and assertiveness training groups are utilized.
6. Supportive psychotherapy with a cognitive emphasis is given on a regular basis.
7. All families are assessed and several taken into family therapy.
8. Ward outings, including visits to restaurants, are organized by the ward staff on a regular basis.
9. Patients usually return to school or work prior to discharge from the unit.

Conclusions

Despite the considerable optimism regarding the effectiveness of treatment for anorexia nervosa over the past decade, close scrutiny reveals that there have been no adequate studies of specific intervention strategies (Garner, 1986[b]). Recent attention has focused upon the methodological limitations of previous research in this area and numerous recommendations have been made for future studies aimed at identifying which components of standard treatment programs are in fact beneficial (Steinhausen & Glanville, 1983; Agras & Kraemer, 1984).

Finally, it is well worth documenting that the early recognition and effective management of anorexia nervosa has significantly reduced the mortality rate. Anderson, Morse, and Santmyer (1985) have echoed these sentiments rather well:

> While anorexia nervosa may present as a severe life-threatening disorder, it often responds well to treatment. On the positive side, many patients who have suffered from the illness may eventually become effective people as if they had never had the illness. Many of these individuals are talented people with considerable potential for growth, who can be helped by guiding them to respond in a direct rather than indirect way to life's challenges. The lack of complete response in many patients, however, reminds us that much remains to be discovered about the fundamental causes of anorexia nervosa and truly effective treatment. In the meantime the two-fold reduction in acute mortality that has occurred over the past decade, and the improvement in empirical treatment methods in many centers, suggest that there is considerable hope for the future for the truly effective treatment of anorexia nervosa.

Because of the amount of suffering experienced by the patients and their families and the huge financial cost of treatment, more effective treatment strategies need to be energetically pursued over future years.

BULIMIA NERVOSA

Bulimia nervosa occurs primarily in women and is characterized by recurrent episodes of gorging or binge eating. These episodes are usually followed by feelings of guilt and remorse at the loss of self-control and acute anxiety regarding the possibility of gaining unwanted weight (Johnson, Stuckey, Lewis, & Schwartz, 1982). Patients usually begin a stringent diet, induce vomiting or abuse purgatives to normalize their weight after an episode of binge eating.

Binge eating has been described in obese individuals (Stunkard, 1959; Wermuth, Davis, Hollister, & Stunkard, 1977) as well as in a subgroup of patients with anorexia nervosa (Beumont et al., 1976; Casper, Eckert, Halmi, Goldberg, & Davis, 1980; Garfinkel, Moldofsky, & Garner, 1980). There have been several reports in the literature suggesting that the incidence of binge eating in normally weighted young women has increased dramatically (Halmi, Falk, 1981; Hawkins & Clement 1980; Holmgren et al., 1983, Lacey, 1982; Pyle, Mitchell, & Eckert, 1981; Russell, 1979; Touyz & Ivison, 1985).

Diagnosis

As the distinctions amongst bulimia nervosa, anorexia nervosa, obesity and relatively normal eating has been difficult to make, classification has at times been controversial (Butow, Touyz, Freeman, & Beaumont, 1988). Most practitioners now accept the diagnostic criteria stated in the revised third edition of the Diagnostic and Statistical Manual of Mental Disorders of the American Psychiatric Association (DSM III-R). These criteria are listed in Table 14.3.

It will be noted that these criteria differ from earlier classificatory guidelines by the inclusion of minimum frequencies for bingeing and vomiting.

Table 14.3.
Criteria for Diagnosis of Bulimia Nervosa (DSM III-R).
(American Psychiatric Association, 1987)

A. Recurrent episodes of binge eating (rapid consumption of a large amount of food in a discrete period of time).
B. A feeling of lack of control over eating behavior during the eating binges.
C. The person regularly engages in either self-induced vomiting, use of laxatives or diuretics, strict dieting or fasting, or vigorous exercise in order to prevent weight gain.
D. A minimum average of two binge eating episodes a week for at least three months.
E. Persistent overconcern with body shape and weight.

Clinical Aspects of Bulimia Nervosa

There have been several excellent reports concerning the phenomenology of bulimia nervosa (Beumont & Abraham, 1983; Russell, 1979; Abraham & Beumont, 1982) and the data reported in this section is based largely upon their work.

Preoccupation with food. Many patients report that they are constantly preoccupied with thoughts of food to the extent that it interferes with their day-to-day functioning. They find it very difficult to concentrate for prolonged periods of time and often feel that their short-term memory is impaired. They tend to forget appointments and arrangements and become less efficient both at work and at home. Despite these subjective complaints, no evidence of cognitive deficits was found when patients with bulimia nervosa were formally assessed on tests of intellectual, neuropsychological and academic related abilities (Touyz, Beumont, & Johnstone, 1986). Their thoughts constantly revolve around food and they often spend considerable time planning which foods they will purchase to eat during the next binge episode.

Preoccupation with weight and body size. Body shape perception and its disturbance in patients with anorexia nervosa has been well documented (Bruch, 1962; Slade, 1986). We recently investigated body image perception in patients with bulimia nervosa and anorexia nervosa as well as in a control group of students using a distortion of body contours on a videomonitor (Touyz et al., 1984a; Touyz, Cowie, Collins, & Beumont, 1985). The judgments of the patients' present perceived shape and ideal shape (the shape she wanted to be) were recorded. Patients with bulimia nervosa saw themselves as being broader than they actually were and desired to be slimmer by a factor of 18.5 percent. As their mean percentage of Standard Body Weight (SBW) was 99.5 percent, the patients with bulimia nervosa could be considered as aspiring towards physiques found in patients with anorexia nervosa. It was interesting to note that the bulimia nervosa patients aspiration towards developing slimmer physiques was consistent with those of high school and college students who also desired to be slimmer by a factor of 21 percent.

Russell (1979) asked his patients with bulimia nervosa the following question: "If I advised you to put on some weight, what weight would you be willing to reach?" He found that in only 3 out of 24 patients was the desired weight equivalent to a "healthy" weight. In the remaining 21 patients, the desired weight was significantly less than the "healthy" weight and the discrepancy ranged from 2 lbs to 40 lbs (1–18 kgs) with an average of 13.64 lbs (6.2 kgs). The extreme importance attributed to being slender is therefore a significant factor in the management of patients with bulimia nervosa, and attention needs to be focused upon this during treatment.

Onset of bulimia (gorging). Prior to the onset of episodes of bulimia, there is usually an increased concern about body shape and weight and this is usually associated with an interest in the opposite sex and a desire to be attractive. Some patients report that they were teased about their weight and were determined to lose weight as rapidly as possible. In others, the onset of bulimia followed a period of successful dieting but in most instances, an initial attempt at weight loss was not sustained and this was followed by periods of abstinence alternating with periods of bulimia.

It is not uncommon for patients with anorexia nervosa to report episodes of bulimia prior to significant weight loss or during phases of emaciation. However, the episodes of bulimia tend to be less severe when patients are emaciated.

Self-induced vomiting tends to occur after the bulimic behavior has become established but can precede the first recognized episode of bulimia. The pattern of vomiting after eating is readily established as patients often recall "their delight at discovering how to induce vomiting, as they believed they would then be able to eat as much as they liked without gaining weight" (Beumont & Abraham, 1983).

The binge episode. Patients with bulimia nervosa are able to distinguish between merely eating too much and episodes of gorging which they feel they have no control over. They are initially very secretive about their episodes of bulimia and tend to choose a time and a place where their privacy is likely to be ensured and there is little possibility that they will be interrupted. However, once their behavior has been well established and social settings often in the company of family or friends. It is not infrequent that overeating and self-induced vomiting has occurred for many years without family members being aware of its presence.

Patients prefer to binge at home and many of their bulimic episodes are planned. In certain instances, the purchase of foods becomes ritualized and individuals drift from one confectionary store to the next buying small quantities of food to avoid their embarrassment at purchasing excessive quantities from a single establishment. Binge foods are often selected because they are easy to swallow or to regurgitate, for example, yogurt or ice cream. Most patients include foods they do not allow themselves to eat at other times and usually refer to these as "junk foods." It is not uncommon for individuals to dispose of food they have recently purchased to avoid eating it, despite the expense involved. Some individuals would even eat whatever food was available including pet food, frozen meat, or the contents of garbage bins!

There are large individual differences regarding the quantity of food consumed during an episode of bulimia and some patients may consume as much as 27 times the recommended daily allowance of 8.37 megajoules (Beumont & Abraham, 1983). Although it is generally accepted that patients binge predominantly on foods high in carbohydrates, an analysis of their food records reveal that a high proportion of fat and protein is consumed as well.

The duration of an episode of binge eating is often difficult to assess as there appears to be large individual differences. Some episodes may be as short as 15 minutes where individuals literally "stuff the food down their throats" whereas others may experience an almost continuous urge to binge, which persists from the time they wake up in the morning until they go to sleep at night. Binge eating usually occurs in discrete episodes at the time of the onset of the disorder and several episodes may occur on a single day.

Precipitants of individual episodes of bulimia. Numerous factors have been identified as precipitants of bulimia. These include dysphoric mood states such as anxiety and tension or boredom, preoccupation with thoughts of food, drinking alcohol, going out with members of the opposite sex, and returning home from school or work. It is worth noting that despite the fact that most patients diet between episodes, only a small proportion indicate that hunger is a precipitant of bulimia.

Methods Used to Prevent Weight Gain

Dieting. Most patients attempt to control their weight by dieting and abstaining from eating high-energy foods between bulimic episodes, whereas others attempt to starve themselves in order to lose weight. As many individuals can't fit into their clothes after episodes of binge eating, where they can gain 6–18 lbs in a day or two, there is often a considerable urgency to lose weight.

Self-induced vomiting. Approximately 50 percent regularly induce vomiting. The temptation to do so is usually the greatest in the parental home, the reason being to ensure that this behavior remains concealed from others. The most preferred method of inducing vomiting is to induce the gag reflex by inserting the fingers in the mouth and throat. Others use the handle of a toothbrush or a spoon. Some individuals are able to induce vomiting "at will" by contracting their thoracic and abdominal muscles. The use of an emetic such as Ipecac syrup is relatively rare. Some patients chew their food and spit it out afterwards.

They often continue to induce vomiting until they feel confident that they have regurgitated all the food they have consumed. It is not uncommon for "markers" such as a slice of beetroot to be eaten at the start of a binge episode to enable the patient to be reasonably confident that all the food has been regurgitated. Some patients drink large amounts of water and continue to regurgitate until there is no residue of food.

Most individuals feel relieved after they have induced vomiting. They no longer experience severe abdominal discomfort and are aware that they will not gain weight as a result of their binge.

Purgative abuse. Patients frequently take purgatives immediately after their bulimic episode but some would take them during a binge. Many individuals would consume excessive quantities of purgatives and it is not uncommon for a patient to take up to 20 times the recommended dosage.

Exercise. Individuals who have unsuccessfully attempted to induce vomiting and who are reluctant to ingest large quantities of laxatives, frequently resort to excessive exercising or starvation as a means of weight control. Exercise often becomes ritualized and individuals feel compelled to do a certain amount each day (Touyz, Beumont, & Hook, 1987). Those who jog would do so irrespective of whether it was sunny or raining. If they are unable to do so during the day because of shiftwork, they would go jogging in the middle of the night! These individuals become preoccupied with the need to exercise and often equate the amount of exercise that has to be done with the quantity of food consumed. They build up an exercise "debt." Patients will often continue to exercise despite painful injuries.

Physical symptoms and mood disturbances. Physical symptoms associated with bulimia are frequently reported. These may include abdominal pain, swollen hands and feet, fatigue, nausea, and headaches. Salivary glands may be swollen. Their teeth often require extensive dental treatment as a result of persistent self-induced vomiting. Menstrual irregularities are common and patients often report episodes of amenorrhoea. Epileptic seizures, tetany, renal complications, acute dilation of the stomach, symptoms of dehydration, and chronic hoarseness of the voice have also been noted. Patients who induce vomiting and/or abuse purgatives may have very low levels of serum potassium. Some individuals attempt to correct this deficiency by taking potassium supplements but unfortunately they often increase the dosage as their purging behavior becomes more frequent. A patient recently died from a cardiac arrest after taking an overdose of potassium supplements to restore her serum potassium level.

Most disturbances are relatively common and may occur before, during, or after a binge. These include anxiety and tension, feeling of helplessness, and failure and self-deprecatory thoughts. Relief from anxiety is often reported during a binge especially in those individuals who induce vomiting immediately thereafter. Suicidal ruminations are often present following an episode of binge eating and a survey found that 22 percent of the bulimic patients studied had made a suicide attempt at this time (Beumont & Abraham, 1983).

Behavioral Management of Bulimia Nervosa

Despite Hilde Bruch's (1974) reservations concerning the use of behavioral therapy in the management of patients with anorexia nervosa, this form of treatment has become an integral part of comprehensive inpatient programs when refeeding is a key aspect in intervention (Agras & Werne, 1978; Touyz et al., 1984b). Behavioral techniques also have gained increasing acceptance in the management of patients with bulimia nervosa.

We recently reviewed the literature concerning the behavioral management of patients with bulimia nervosa (Griffiths, Touyz, Mitchell, & Bacon, 1987). Seven behavior therapy studies have been undertaken to date (Welch, 1979; Linden, 1980; Rosen & Leitenberg, 1982; Kua, Lee, & Chee, 1982; Long & Cordle, 1982; Mizes & Lohr, 1983, Leitenberg, Gross, Peterson, & Rosen, 1984). With the exception of the study of Leitenberg et al. (1984) these have been single case studies. Most of the researchers used their own criteria for bulimia nervosa (probably as the studies were published prior to the introduction of DSM III and Russell's (1979) criteria.

Most studies treated the subjects on an out-patient basis, but no one study included a control group. Mizes and Lohr (1983) provided a better designed study than the others using a multiple baseline approach. The length of treatment used in the studies ranged from 9 weeks (Linden, 1980) to 40 weeks (Long & Cordle, 1982). A wide variety of behavioral strategies have been used, such as response prevention, assertion training, stimulus control, construction of alternative response, stimulus narrowing, self-reinforcement, self-control relaxation, contingency contracting, social reinforcement, and resocialization. Behavioral strategies have been sometimes supplemented by cognitive techniques (Long & Cordle, 1982). An important component included in the treatment program of two studies (Linden, 1980; Long & Cordle, 1982) was dietary education.

Five of the seven studies used frequency of binging as the criterion to assess outcome. Six studies used vomiting either alone or in conjunction with binging to assess outcome. All studies used other criteria for outcome such as: the number of intrusive thoughts, subjective feelings of discomfort, eating behaviors, meal size, and exercise.

The most commonly used measurement of outcome was self-monitoring of food intake and frequency of binging and vomiting. Although self-monitoring is not acknowledged as a behavioral strategy in any of the studies, it is recognized in the obesity literature (Stuart, 1967). Clearly, self-monitoring as a behavioral technique needs to be evaluated in the treatment of bulimia nervosa. The design of behavioral treatment studies could also be improved by including standardized instruments such as the EDI (Eating Disorder Inventory; Garner et al., 1983) as a measure of outcome.

In six studies (Welch 1979; Linden, 1980; Mizes & Lohr, 1983; Rosen & Leitenberg, 1982; Leitenberg et al., 1984; Long & Cordle, 1983) the patients were symptom-free at the end of the treatment and this was well maintained at follow-up. Unfortunately the follow-up periods were extremely short, ranging from 3 (Leitenberg et al., 1984) to 11 months (Welch, 1979).

The most interesting study was that of Leitenberg et al. (1984) who studied a sample of five patients. The authors used an exposure and response prevention procedure to explore the anxiety model of bulimia nervosa, which proposes that vomiting rather than binging reinforces the behavioral disorder. They postulated that purging and vomiting have a reinforcing effect as they reduce tension. They found that anxiety and the consequent urge to vomit increased while subjects ate. This stopped after eating even though subjects were not allowed to vomit. Across treatment sessions anxiety and the urge to vomit decreased as the amount of calories consumed in the treatment increased. Self-statements about eating became more positive and both binging and vomiting decreased in subjects even though the emphasis was on vomiting rather than binging. Despite the interesting speculation that either binging or vomiting might be the driving force behind bulimia nervosa, this needs to be examined with comparative groups of subjects in a much larger treatment study. In spite of this, the study by Leitenberg et al. had advantages over the other studies in that more subjects were used and a larger number of criteria to assess outcome and measurements of outcome were employed. The treatment program resulted in 60% of the patients being symptom-free at follow-up.

Cognitive Behavior Therapy

Fairburn's (1981) chapter suggested that the use of cognitive behavior therapy in treating patients with bulimia nervosa has stimulated considerable interest in the recent literature on eating disorders. Interest in the application of cognitive techniques for the treatment of bulimia nervosa can be traced to earlier programs developed for obesity (Mahoney & Mahoney, 1976). More recently Garner (1986a) has proposed a cognitive model for bulimia nervosa based upon reasoning errors, dysfunctional attitudes, and faulty assumptions which are characteristic of anorexia nervosa. This cognitive model has been derived from the principles enunciated by Beck and his colleagues (Beck, 1976; Beck et al. 1979). Despite their different historical roots, Garner (1986) has emphasized that the different origins of the cognitive models "have become less important with time since there has appeared to be a convergence in the methods advocated by various cognitive behavioural theorists treating bulimia nervosa."

One of the major limitations of the studies published thus far has been the small number of subjects who participated. In only three of six recent studies published have there been more than four subjects. However, because of the encouraging results reported thus far, it appears worthwhile to briefly summarize the findings of these investigations.

Grinc (1982) successfully treated a 26-year-old woman diagnosed as suffering from bulimia nervosa for 10 years. The treatment program involved three basic components; self-monitoring, stimulus control, and cognitive restructuring, which were instituted sequentially. However, because of inadequate experimental controls, it was not possible to determine which components of treatment were the most important.

Long and Cordle (1982) used cognitive-behavioral procedures in the successful treatment of two patients. Their treatment programme included behavioral self-control procedures, dietary restraint, cognitive restructuring, and resocialization. Because of the small sample size, their data must be regarded as tentative.

Cognitive restructuring and exposure plus vomiting prevention have been recently compared utilizing a single case methodology with a crossover design in four subjects with bulimia nervosa (Rossiter & Wilson, 1985). Binge eating and vomiting ceased in two subjects and was decreased in a third following exposure plus vomiting prevention. Improvements in attitudes towards food and weight, assertiveness and depression were also noted. They found that cognitive restructuring had little effect on any of the measures recorded, however, because of methodological limitations, these findings should be regarded as tentative.

The other three studies used larger sample sizes. Fairburn (1981) treated 11 women on an individual basis using cognitive behavior therapy. The treatment focused on increased control over eating, eliminating food avoidance, and changing maladaptive attitudes. The treatment program comprised three stages. The initial stage was designed to disrupt the habitual overeating and vomiting and then to teach cognitive strategies for self-control. During the second stage of treatment, patients were encouraged to modify abnormal attitudes to food, eating, body weight, and shape and to maintain any improvement they made. Taboo foods (usually "fattening" foods) were gradually introduced into the patient's diet in an attempt to decrease the patient's desire to binge on these foods. The patient was also taught problem-solving techniques to cope with adverse events, negative moods, and irrational thoughts. The final stage of treatment focused upon the maintenance of change. The mean duration of treatment was seven months. At the termination of treatment nine of the eleven patients had reduced their frequency of bouts of overeating and vomiting from three times daily to once per month. At one year follow-up on six of the patients, one patient had ceased to overeat or vomit, four continued to overeat and vomit (but only once every two to three months), and one patient had failed to benefit. In a more recent study (Yates & Sambrailo, 1984) compared the effectiveness of two types of intervention, that is, cognitive-behavioral group therapy vs. behavioral instruction. Of the 24 subjects who initially volunteered, only 16 completed the study. Of these, seven showed significant and positive changes in binging and purging at completion of the study. No significant differences with regard to treatment outcome were found between groups. Unfortunately, patients were recruited from a newspaper article and may not have been representative of those consulting psychiatrists or clinical psychologists in private practice or attending hospital outpatient clinics.

Ordman and Kirschenbaum (1985) assigned 20 bulimic women to either full or brief intervention programs. Results were promising in that the full intervention treatment (which included cognitive restructuring) significantly reduced the patients' binging and vomiting, improved psychological adjustment, and changed attitudes about food, dieting, and their bodies. However, the full intervention included other treatment components in addition to cognitive restructuring such as response prevention, behavioral contracting, and process-oriented psychotherapy. It is difficult to assess which of these treatment components was most effective. Other limitations of the study were that the therapists were relatively inexperienced, the patients were recruited from advertisements, and no follow-up data were available to determine the maintenance of the progress over time.

CONCLUSIONS

Despite Fairburn's (1984) cautionary note that "behavioral improvement is likely to be short lived unless it is accompanied by significant attitude changes" (Fairburn, 1984, p. 253), there have only been a few systematic studies to date which have attempted to evaluate the effectiveness of cognitive behavior therapy in the management of bulimia. Cognitive behavior therapy appears to be producing encouraging results in the treatment of bulimia nervosa but the need for further controlled trials of therapeutic intervention in the near future is urgently required. Garner (1986a) concluded his extensive review on cognitive therapy for bulimia nervosa with the following comments: "We share the opinion of others who view attitude change as a prerequisite for complete recovery for most patients with bulimia . . . Preliminary reports have been encouraging and must be followed by more systematic evaluation of the active components in treatment, predictors of outcome and durability of change."

From this review of the literature, it is apparent that no one treatment approach is more effective than another, although some have produced promising results. In fact, so many studies were comprised of multiple therapeutic components that it was difficult to ascertain which aspects of treatment made the most significant contribution to outcome.

Future studies should address the methodological limitations present in so many of the studies reviewed previously, for example, small sample sizes, failure to use standardized diagnostic criteria, inadequate outcome measures, and relatively short duration before assessing outcome.

OBESITY

Obesity is recognized as a major health problem in economically advanced countries. It is associated with many psychological and medical problems but the most serious medical hazard of obesity is its association with coronary heart disease (Kannel & Gordon, 1979). Obesity has been declared the number-one nutrition problem in the United States (Colletti & Brownell, 1982). It has been estimated that between 15 and 30 percent of all adult Americans are obese (Bray, 1976; VanItalie, 1979).

Obesity is usually considered to be present when weight is 120 percent or more of the "acceptable weight." Over the past few years considerable interest has been shown in this problem, partly because of society's perception of what constitutes an ideal body shape and its newfound concern with health and fitness, and partly because of the cost and medical consequences of overweight and obesity (Caterson, 1985).

Many possible contributing factors have been advocated to account for the problem of obesity but, despite this, many aspects of the disorder remain unclear. However, it is generally accepted that wide individual variation exists and it has even been suggested that a simple explanation may never be found (Morris & King 1986).

Obesity remains difficult to treat and it is an extremely arduous task to effect any permanent and substantial reduction in weight by dieting and exercise alone (Craddock, 1978). This fact has been rather dramatically illustrated by Craighead, Brownell, & Horan 1981, who suggested that "If a cure from obesity is defined as a reduction to ideal weight and maintenance of that weight for five years, a person is more likely to recover from cancer than from obesity" (p. 288).

Behavioral Management of Obesity

The emergence of behavioral technology was initially heralded as a landmark in the management of patients with obesity (Stuart, 1967). The enthusiasm that followed this development has been rather elegantly described by Albert Stunkard (1982):

> In 1967, a small paper on "Behavioural Control of Overeating" (Stuart) signalled, indeed provoked, the start of an explosion of interest in the use of behaviour therapy for obesity. More than a hundred papers in the professional literature placed an unprecedented interest in behaviour modification in lay publications. A concern with obesity swept departments of psychology throughout the country; the treatment of obesity

> became an increasingly common part of clinical programs, and obesity supplanted snake phobias as the largest single topic of research on treatment. (p. 535)

Unfortunately, this enthusiasm was short-lived and as early as 1977, Mahoney and his co-workers suggested that "we have begun to describe behavior procedures as more effective rather than very effective, our typical weight loss as modest rather than impressive, and our outcome as variable rather than consistent" (Mahoney 1977, p. 1). Despite this, the behavioral management of obesity has grown in popularity and more individuals are now receiving this form of treatment for their obesity than medical treatment (Stunkard, 1985).

One of the major advantages of behavioral technology is that it can be precisely specified and as a result can be easily taught and learned by others even if they lack a professional education. This has been well illustrated by Penick, Fillion, Fox, & Stunkard (1975) who found that a behavior therapy program administered by a team with little experience in the management of obesity was more effective than excellent traditional medical intervention. In this investigation the inexperienced behavior therapist obtained a twofold increase in weight reduction when compared to the traditional medical treatment.

It is beyond the scope of this report to provide an in-depth description of the behavioral treatment of obesity. Nevertheless, a brief description of some of the essential components will be documented. Those interested in a more detailed description are referred to the following texts by Mahoney and Mahoney (1976); Jordan, Levitz, and Kimbrell (1976); Stuart, (1978); and Montgomery and Harris (1985).

Behavioral Techniques

The most promising behavioral techniques commonly used in weight control programs include the following: stimulus control, response control, contingency management, assertion training, cognitive restructuring, covert sensitization, and self-monitoring (Morris & King 1986; Stunkard, 1982; Stuart, 1977).

Stimulus control. One of the most consistent features of behavioral-orientated programs for obesity is the analysis of cues that elicit and maintain eating behavior. Stimulus control of eating behavior involves multiple strategies which have become integral components of weight reduction programs. For example, an attempt is made to restrict the quantity of energy-dense foods that one usually kept in the home and to limit the availability of food kept in the home. If the individual is unable to resist eating, adequate quantities of low-calorie foods such as celery and raw carrots need to be readily available.

Further examples of stimulus control techniques include restricting the eating of all food to one room, associating no other activities with eating (it is not permissible to watch television while eating), clearing away the scraps immediately after a meal has been completed, instructing children to take their own snacks, always shopping from a list, and storing food in cupboards (out of sight).

Stimulus control techniques have thus become an integral part of weight control programs but their independent contribution to the efficacy of such programs is not known and requires further investigation (Stunkard, 1982).

Response control. Attention is also specifically focused upon eating behavior so as to assist the patient to decrease the speed of eating, to become aware of all the components of the eating process, and to gain control over these components. Exercises for reducing the speed of eating include the number of mouthfuls of food consumed during a meal, the number of chews and the number of swallows. Patients are encouraged to put down their utensils after every third mouthful until that mouthful is chewed and swallowed. They are asked to pay attention to savoring their food as they eat, enjoy the act of swallowing and to concentrate on the warmth and fullness of their stomachs. The aim of this exercise is to eat less but to derive more enjoyment from the food that is eaten. Morris and King (1986) have summarized the practical guidelines to weight control derived from a stimulus control and response control and these are presented in Table 14.4.

Contingency management. A formal system of reward and punishment is often included in weight reduction programs. Contingency contracting with patients has been used to strengthen the commitment to treatment. For example, the patient may be required to provide a monetary deposit which may be refunded either at the completion of the treatment program or during the course of treatment. This technique has been found to reduce the attrition rate (Hagan, Foreyt, & Dunham, 1976).

Stunkard (1982) has suggested that contingency management be applied to changes in eating behavior. Patients can learn points for activities they are learning, for example, record keeping, counting chews and swallows, pausing during the meal, etc. Not only do patients receive a certain number of points for each activity, but they can earn bonus points when they use their creative talents to adopt an alternative to eating in the face of strong temptation. These points are later

Table 14.4.
Practical Guidelines to Weight Control Based on Stimulus and Response Control Procedures

1. Buying food: It is important to have the correct food available for sensible eating. The client should use a shopping list, and not shop when hungry.
2. Storing food: If food is readily available many people are tempted to eat. Therefore the client is required to limit the availability and salience of food by restricting food storage to the kitchen or pantry, and by using opaque containers that require effort to open.
3. Preparing food: This is determined by the goals of a sensible eating plan and necessary nutritional guidelines. It is accomplished by the use of appropriate preparation and cooking methods, the provision of sufficient food for the meal only (hence, edible leftovers are not available), and plans to control snacking while preparing food.
4. Serving food: This involves providing a balanced and complete meal for each person. The main suggestions for accomplishing this are to avoid any serve-yourself meals and any second helpings. The strategy of serving a single balanced meal on a plate also works in smorgasbord or buffet situations.
5. Eating food: This can be controlled in two main ways. The first is to make eating a "pure" experience by using stimulus control techniques to break links between eating and any other activities (e.g., watching television). The second suggestion is to use response control techniques to slow down eating if that is a problem. Several benefits emerge from slower eating including the increased sense of control that it engenders and the biochemical benefits from a slower insulin release.
6. Cleaning up: This is an important step because any leftover food can be tempting and lead to unwise eating. The main suggestion is that clearing away should be finished as soon as possible and any surplus food should be thrown out or given to the household pet.

Source: Morris & King (1986, p. 56).

translated into tangible rewards such as going to a movie or relief from household chores.

Assertion training. Morris and King (1986) have stressed the importance of assertiveness training in the management of obese patients. They point out that unassertive behavior may result in the patient engaging in behaviors that are contrary to sensible weight management. There is often a great deal of social pressure exerted to eat unwisely and responsible assertive responses would be invaluable in such circumstances.

Cognitive restructuring. Behavioral scientists have been devoting more attention to cognitive therapy and as a result its popularity has increased dramatically over recent years. Cognitive strategies have become an important adjunct in obesity programs.

Patients are encouraged to identify negative "monologues" and to record how often they occur. Once these have been discovered, counter-arrangements against them are formulated. Thereafter, the patients are required to practice this procedure by using the more appropriate self-statements in response to negative dysfunctional thoughts. Mahoney and Mahoney (1976) have documented five kinds of negative self-statements in their description of "cleaning up the cognitive ecology." Examples of some of the common negative self-statements and counter arguments to these are presented in Table 14.5.

Covert sensitization. Covert sensitization is a procedure whereby the patient's problematic behavior is paired with an aversive stimulus in imagination (Cautela, 1972). This technique has been used with only limited success and has not gained acceptance in the behavioral management of obesity (Morris & King, 1986). Abrams (1984) has concluded that "covert sensitization does not warrant widespread use in the treatment of obesity, although its success with other compulsive behaviours (e.g., Brownell, Hayes, & Barlow 1977) makes it difficult to reject outright. If covert sensitization or aversive procedures are employed, they should be used *only* after careful consideration of less aversive alternatives" (p. 33).

Self-monitoring. Patients are asked to accurately document their food consumption in food diaries. A detailed description of a food diary can be found in Stunkard's (1985) "Behavioural Management of Obesity." On each occasion the patient eats, he or she documents precisely what has been eaten, the quantity, at what time of day, where eating occurred, who he or she was with and his or her mood at the time. Patients have found this technique extremely helpful and it has become a core component of most behavioral programs for the manage-

Table 14.5.
Some Examples of Common Negative Self-Statements and Counterarguments in Weight Control

1. Weight loss: "It's taking so long to lose weight." A counterargument is, "But I am losing it. And this time I'm going to learn how to keep if off."
2. Ability to lose weight: "I've never done it before. Why should I succeed this time?" A counterargument is, "There always has to be a first time. And this time I've got a good new program going for me."
3. Goals: "I've got to stop snacking!" A counterargument is, "That is an unrealistic goal. Just keep on trying to cut down the number of snacks."
4. Food thoughts: "I keep finding myself thinking how good chocolate tastes." A useful response is, "Stop that! It's just frustrating you. Think of lying on the beach in the sun" (or whatever activity the patient finds particularly enjoyable).
5. Excuses: "Everyone in my family has a weight problem. It's in my genes." A counterargument is, "That just makes it harder, not impossible. If I stick with this program I will succeed.

Synthesis by Morris and King (1986, p. 57) of Mahoney and Mahoney (1976), and Stunkard (1982).

ment of obesity. Should self-monitoring be used throughout the duration of weight control programmes or would it be as effective for shorter periods? Further research is needed to answer this question.

Self-Help Groups

One of the major advantages of behavioral technology is that it can be precisely specified and can be easily taught and learned by others even if they lack a professional education. This has been well illustrated by Penick et al. (1971) who found that a behavior therapy program administered by a team with little experience in the management of obesity was more effective than excellent traditional medical treatment. In this investigation, the inexperienced behavior therapists obtained a twofold increase in weight reduction when compared to the traditional medical treatment.

Self-help groups have become one of the most popular approaches to weight reduction and more obese people are receiving behavior therapy for obesity in nonmedical settings than those receiving traditional medical treatment. Stuart (1977) had recommended the use of self-help groups as an attractive, available, and cost-effective means of treating obesity. Stunkard (1985) has recently reported that, in the United States alone, half a million individuals a week receive behavior therapy for obesity under the aegis of just one commercial weight reduction program "Weight Watchers." Colletti and Brownell (1982) have expressed the possibility that the benefits of peer support in a self-help setting may outweigh the advantages of professional experience in a clinical environment. Finally, health care needs have increased so rapidly in recent years that they threaten to outstrip the supply of physicians and medical facilities and self-help groups have responded to meet this increased demand for assistance in weight reduction (Volkman, Stunkard, Woolston, & Bailey, 1981).

Behavior Therapy: A Reappraisal

Stunkard (1985) recently commented that "fifteen years of research and clinical experience have made it possible to state with some assurance what behaviour therapy can, and cannot, contribute to the treatment of obesity." There is a general consensus regarding the following six points:

1. Attrition rates: There has been a significant reduction in attrition rates. Attrition from traditional outpatient treatment programs has been as high as 25–75 percent, most behavioral programs obtain rates of 15 percent or less.

2. Side effects: Side effects such as anxiety, irritability, and depression that have plagued the routine medical office treatment of obesity are uncommon in behavioral programs.
3. Variability in weight changes during the following treatment. Wilson (1980) has indicated that the great variability found suggests that either the critical variables governing weight loss have not been identified or that current behavioral procedures are appropriate only for individuals with some as yet undetermined characteristics.
4. Prediction of outcome. As yet only a few, relatively weak predictors have been documented.
5. Weight loss. The most important criterion of successful treatment is weight loss. By this criterion, the behavioral management of obesity is only moderately effective and its results are often of little clinical significance. Ley (1985) has suggested that it is not difficult to obtain mean weight losses of 12 lbs (5.5 kg) and to maintain them for a year. The 24 lbs (10.9 kg) of weight loss in a study by Stunkard et al. (1980) probably represents an upper limit of the effectiveness of traditional behavior therapy for obesity.
6. Pharmacotherapy/diet therapy. Weight losses achieved during behavioral treatments for obesity are probably better maintained than are weight losses by either pharmacotherapy or diet therapy alone.

CONCLUSION

Stunkard (1982) has concluded that "fifteen years after its introduction, there has been no improvement on the results of the first report of the behavioural control of obesity. It appears that the limits of current behavioural technologies have been reached and that even the continuing plethora of small modifications appear unlikely to improve the situation" (p. 569).

However despite this, encouraging results are being obtained when behavioral measures have been combined with very low-calorie diets. Wadden, Stunkard, Brownell, & Day (1984) treated 17 women who averaged 87.5 percent overweight over a 6-month period with a combination of very-low-calorie diet (400–500 calories) and behavioral strategies to assist with the maintenance of weight loss. Patients lost 45 lbs (20.5 kg) and this weight loss was well maintained during the year following treatment. Patients regained no more than 4.6 lbs (2.1 kg). These results are indeed encouraging and this avenue of explanation requires further investigation.

CONCLUDING REMARKS

This chapter has reviewed the behavioral management of patients with anorexia and bulimia nervosa as well as obesity. Current therapeutic techniques have been described and avenues for further explanation alluded to.

REFERENCES

Abraham, S. F. & Beumont, P. J. V. (1982). How patients describe bulimia or binge eating. *Psychological Medicine, 12,* 625–635.

Abraham, S. F., Mira, M., Beumont, P. J. V., Sowerbutts, T. D., & Llewellyn-Jones, D. (1983). Eating behaviours among young women. *Medical Journal of Australia, 2,* 225–228.

Abrams, D. B. (1984). Current status and clinical development in the behavioural treatment of obesity. In C. M. Franks (Ed.), *New developments in behaviour therapy: From research to clinical application.* New York: Howarth Press.

Agras, W. S. Barlow, D. H., Chapin, H. N., Abel, G. G., Jackson, M., Leitenberg, H., & Burlington, V. (1974). Behaviour modification of anorexia nervosa. *Archives of General Psychiatry, 30,* 279–286.

Agras, W. S. & Kraemer, H. C. (1984). The treatment of anorexia nervosa: Do different treatments have different outcomes? In A. J. Stunkard & E. Stellar (Eds.), *Eating and its disorders.* New York: Raven Press.

Agras, W. S., & Werne, J. (1978). Behaviour therapy in anorexia nervosa: A data-based approach to the question. In J. P. Brady & H. P. Brodie (Eds.), *Controversy in psychiatry* (pp. 193–207). Philadelphia: W. B. Saunders.

American Psychiatric Association (1987). Diagnostic and Statistical Manual of Mental Disorders (3rd ed Revised) (DSM III-R). Washington, DC.

Anderson, A. E., Morse, C., & Santmyer, J. (1985). Inpatient treatment for anorexia nervosa. In D. H. Garner & P. E. Garfinkel (Eds.), *Handbook of psychotherapy for anorexia nervosa and bulimia.* New York: Guilford Press.

Bachrach, A. J., Erwin, W. J., & Mohr, J. P. (1965). The control of eating behaviour in an anorexic by operant conditioning techniques. In L. P. Ullman & L. Krasner (Eds.), *Case studies in behaviour modification* (pp. 153–163). New York: Holt, Rinehart and Winston.

Beck, A. T. (1970). Role of fantasies in psychotherapy and psychopathology. *Journal of Nervous and Mental Disease, 150,* 3–17.

Beck, A. T. (1976). *Cognitive therapy and the emotional disorders.* New York: International Universities Press.

Beck, A. T., Rush, A. J., Shaw, B. F., & Emery, G. (1979). *Cognitive therapy of depression: A treatment manual.* New York: Guilford Press.

Beumont, P. J. V. (1984). Endocrine function in Magersucht disorders. In K. M. Pirke & D. Ploog (Eds.), *The psychobiology of anorexia nervosa* (pp. 114–123). Berlin: Springer-Verlag.

Beumont, P. J. V., & Abraham, S. F. (1983). Episodes of ravenous overeating or bulimia: Their occurence in patients with anorexia nervosa and with other forms of disordered eating. In P. L. Darby, P. E. Garfinkel, D. M.

Garner, & D. V. Coscina (Eds.), *Anorexia nervosa: Recent developments in research.* New York: Alan R. Liss.

Beumont, P. J. V., Booth, A. L., Abraham, S. F., Griffiths, D. A., & Turner, T. R. (1983). A temporal sequence of symptoms in patients with anorexia nervosa: A preliminary report. In P. L. Darby, P. E. Garfinkel, D. M. Garner, & D. V. Coscina (Eds.). *Anorexia Nervosa. Recent Developments in Research* (pp. 129–136). New York: Alan R. Liss.

Beumont, P. J. V., George, G. C. W., & Smart, D. E. (1976). "Dieters" and "vomiters and purgers" in anorexia nervosa. *Psychological Medicine, 6,* 617–622.

Beumont, P. J. V., & Touyz, S. W. (1985). The syndrome of anorexia nervosa. In S. W. Touyz & P. J. V. Beumont (Eds.), *Eating disorders: Prevalence and treatment.* (pp. 1–10) Sydney: Williams and Wilkins/Adis.

Beumont, P. J. V. & Russell, J. (1982). Anorexia nervosa. In P. J. V. Beumont & G. D. Burrows (Eds.), *Handbook of psychiatry and endocrinology* (pp. 63–96). Amsterdam: Elsevier Biomedical Press.

Bhanji, S. (1979). Anorexia nervosa. Physicians' and psychiatrists, opinion and practice. *Journal of Psychosomatic Research, 23,* 7–11.

Blue, R. (1979). Use of punishment in the treatment of anorexia nervosa. *Psychological Reports, 44,* 743–746.

Bray, G. A. (1976). *The obese patient.* Philadelphia: W. B. Saunders.

Brownell, K. D., Hayes, S. & Barlow, D. (1977). Patterns of appropriate and deviant sexual arousal. The behavioural treatment of multiple sexual deviations. *Journal of Consulting and Clinical Psychology, 45,* 1144–1155.

Bruch, H. (1962). Perceptual and conceptual disturbances in anorexia nervosa. *Psychosomatic Medicine, 24,* 187–194.

Bruch, H. (1973). *Eating disorders: Obesity, anorexia nervosa and the person within.* New York: Basic Books.

Bruch, H. (1974). Perils of behaviour modification in treatment of anorexia nervosa. *Journal of the American Medical Association, 230* (10), 1419–1422.

Bruch, H. (1978). Dangers of behaviour modification in treatment of anorexia nervosa. In J. P. Brady & H. P. Brodie (Eds.), *Controversy in psychiatry.* (pp. 645–654). Philadelphia: W. B. Saunders.

Butow, P., Touyz, S. W., Freeman, R., & Beumont, P. J. V. (1988). Bulimia nervosa: Diagnosis and treatment. *Modern Medicine of Australia,* (Aug.) 64–73.

Casper, R. C., & Davis, J. M. (1977). On the course of anorexia nervosa. *American Journal of Psychiatry, 134* (9) 974–978.

Casper, R. C., Eckert, E. D., Halmi, K. A., Goldberg, S. C., & Davis, J. M. (1980). Bulimia. Its incidence and clinical importance in patients with anorexia nervosa. *Archives of General Psychiatry, 37,* 1030–1034.

Caterson, I. D. (1985). Obesity: The metabolic basis. In S. W. Touyz & P. J. V. Beumont (Eds.), *Eating disorders: Prevalence and treatment* (pp. 95–104). Sydney: Williams and Wilkins/Adis.

Cautela, J. R. (1972). The treatment of over-eating by covert conditioning. *Psychotherapy: Theory, Research, and Practice, 9,* 211–216.

Colletti, G. & Brownell, K. D. (1982). The physical and emotional benefits of social support: Application to obesity, smoking and alcoholism. *Progress in Behavior Modification, 13*, 109–178.
Craddock, D. (1978). *Obesity and its management.* London: Churchill Livingstone.
Craighead, L. W., Brownell, K. D., & Horan, J. J. (1981). Behavioural interventions for weight reduction and smoking cessation. In W. E. Craighead, A. E. Kazdin, & M. J. Mahoney (Eds.), *Behaviour modification: Principles, issues and applications* (2nd ed.). Boston: Houghton Mifflin.
Crisp, A. H., Palmer, R., & Kalucy, R. S. (1976). How common is anorexia nervosa? A prevalence study. *British Journal of Psychiatry, 128,* 549–554.
Dally, P. (1969). *General effects of starvation in anorexia nervosa.* New York: Heinneman.
Ellis, A. (1962). *Reason and emotion in psychotherapy.* New York: Lyle Stuart.
Fairburn, C. G. (1981). A cognitive behavioural approach to the management of bulimia. *Psychological Medicine, II,* 707–711.
Fairburn, C. G. (1984). Bulimia: Its epidemiology and management. In A. J. Stunkard & E. Stellar (Eds.), *Eating and its disorders* (pp. 235–258). New York: Raven Press.
Garfinkel, P. E., & Garner, D. M. (1982). *Anorexia nervosa: A multidimensional perspective.* New York: Brunner/Mazel.
Garfinkel, P. E., Kaplan, A. S., Garner, D. M., & Darby, P. L. (1983). The differentiation of vomiting/weight loss as a conversion disorder from anorexia nervosa. *American Journal of Psychiatry, 140* (8), 1019–1022.
Garfinkel, P. E., Moldofsky, H., & Garner, D. M. (1980). The heterogeneity of anorexia nervosa: Bulimia as a distinct subgroup. *Archives of General Psychiatry, 37,* 1036–1040.
Garner, D. M. (1986a). Cognitive therapy for bulimia. *Adolescent Psychiatry, 13,* 358–390.
Garner, D. M. (1986b). Iatrogenesis in anorexia nervosa and bulimia nervosa. *International Journal of Eating Disorders, 4* (4), 701–726.
Garner, D. M., & Bemis, K. M. (1982). A cognitive behavioural approach to anorexia nervosa. *Cognitive Therapy and Research, 6,* 123–150.
Garner, D. M., & Bemis, K. M. (1985). Cognitive therapy for anorexia nervosa. In D. M. Garner & P. E. Garfinkel (Eds.). (pp. 107–146). *Handbook of psychotherapy for anorexia nervosa and bulimia.* New York: Guilford Press.
Garner, D. M., & Garfinkel, P. E. (1978). Sociocultural factors in anorexia nervosa. *Lancet, 2,* 674.
Garner, D. M., & Garfinkel, P. E. (1980). Sociocultural factors in the development of anorexia nervosa. *Psychological Medicine, 10,* 647–656.
Garner, D. M., Garfinkel, P. E., & Olmstead, M. P. (1983). An overview of the socio-cultural factors in the development of anorexia nervosa. In P. L. Darby, P. E. Garfinkel, D. M. Garner, & D. V. Coscina (Eds.) *Anorexia*

Nervosa: Recent developments in research (pp. 65–82). New York: Alan R. Liss.

Garner, D. M., Garfinkel, P. E., Schwartz, D., & Thompson, M. (1980). Cultural expectations of thinness in women. *Psychological Reports, 47,* 483–491.

Garner, D. M., Olmstead, M., M. P., & Polivy, J. (1983). *Eating Disorder Inventory.* Psychological Assessment Resources, Inc.

Garner, D. M., Olmstead, M. P., Polivy, J., & Garfinkel, P. E. (1984). Comparison between weight-preoccupied women and anorexia nervosa. *Psychosomatic medicine, 46,* 255–266.

Goldfried, M. R. (1971). Systematic desensitization as training in self control. *Journal of Consulting and Clinical Psychology, 37,* 228–234.

Griffiths, R. A., Touyz, S. W., Mitchell, P. B., & Bacon, W. (1987). The treatment of bulimia nervosa: A review. *Australian and New Zealand Journal of Psychiatry, 21,* 5–15.

Grinc, G. A. (1982). A cognitive-behavioural model for the treatment of chronic vomiting. *Journal of Behavioural Medicine, 5,* 135–14.

Hagan, R. L., Foreyt, J. P., & Dunham, T. W. (1976). The drop-out problem. Reducing attrition in obesity research. *Behaviour Therapy, 7,* 462–471.

Hall, A. (1984, June). Eating disorders: Anorexia nervosa and bulimia. *Patient Management,* 105–118.

Hallsten, E. A., Jr. (1965). Adolescent anorexia nervosa treated by desensitization. *Behaviour Research and Therapy, 3,* 87–91.

Halmi, K. A., Falk, J. R., & Schwartz, E. (1981). Binge-eating and vomiting: A survey of a college population. *Psychological Medicine, 11,* 697–706.

Hawkins, R. C., & Clement, P. F. (1980). Development and construct validation of a self report measure of binge-eating tendencies. *Addictive Behaviours, 5,* 219–226.

Hollen, S. D., & Beck, A. T. (1979). Cognitive therapy for depression. In P. C. Kendell & S. D. Holton (Eds.), *Cognitive-behaviour interventions. Theory, research and procedures* (pp. 153–204). New York: Academic Press.

Holmgren, S., Humble, K., Norking, C., Roos, B., Rosmark, B., & Sohlberg, S. The anorectic bulimic conflict. *International Journal of Eating Disorders, 2* (2), 3–14.

Horney, K. (1950). *Neurosis and human growth. The struggle towards self realization.* New York: Norton.

Hsu, L. K. G. (1980). Outcome of anorexia nervosa. A review of the literature (1954–1978). *Archives of General Psychiatry, 37,* 1041–1046.

Hsu, L. K. G., Crisp, A. H., & Harding, B. (1979). Outcome of anorexia nervosa *Lancet, 1,* 61–65.

Johnson, C. L., Stuckey, M. K., Lewis, L. D., & Schwartz, D. M. (1982). Bulimia: A descriptive survey of 316 cases. *International Journal of Eating Disorders, 2* (10) 3–16.

Jones, D. J., Fox, M. M., Babigan, H. M., & Hutten, H. E. (1980). Epidemiology of anorexia nervosa in Monroe County, New York (1960–1976). *Psychosomatic Medicine, 42,* 551–558.

Jordan, H. A., Levitz, L. S., & Kimbrell, G. M. (1976). *Eating is okay.* New York: Rawson.

Kalucy, R. S. (1983). Eating disorders in young women. *Medical Journal of Australia, 2* (5), 205–206.
Kannel, W. B., & Gordon, T. (1979). Physiological and medical concomitants of obesity. The Framingham study. In G. A. Bray (Ed.), *Obesity in America.* Bethesda, MD: DHEW, NIH Publication. No. 79–359.
Kaufman, R. M., & Heiman, M. (Eds). (1964). *Evaluation of psychosomatic concepts: Anorexia nervosa: A paradigm.* New York: International Universities Press.
Kendell, R. E., Hall, D. J., Hailey, A., & Babigan, H. M. (1973). The epidemiology of anorexia nervosa. *Psychological Medicine, 3,* 200–203.
Kenny, F. T., & Solyom, L. (1971). The treatment of compulsive vomiting through faradic disruption of mental images. *Canadian Medical Association Journal, 105,* 1071.
Keys, A., Brozck, J., Henschel, A., Mickelsen, O., & Taylor, H. L. (1950). *The biology of human starvation.* Minneapolis: University of Minnesota Press.
Kua, E. H., Lee, S. L., & Chee, K. T. (1982). Bulimia Nervosa—A case report. *Singapore Medical Journal, 23,* 287–289.
Lacey, J. H. (1982). The bulimic syndrome at normal body weight: Reflections on pathogenesis and clinical features. *International Journal of Eating Disorders, 2* (1), 59–66.
Laseque, C. (1964). De l'anorexie hysterique. Arch. Gen du Med 385. In Kaufman and Heiman (Eds.), *Evolution of psychosomatic concepts: Anorexia nervosa; A paradigm.* New York: International Universities Press. (Original publication in 1873)
Leitenberg, H., Agras, W. S., & Thomson, L. E. (1968). A sequential analysis of the effects of selective positive reinforcement in modifying anorexia nervosa. *Behaviour Research and Therapy, 6,* 211–218.
Leitenberg, H., Gross, J., Peterson, J., & Rosen, J. C. (1984). Analysis of an anxiety model and the process of change during exposure plus response prevention treatment of bulimia nervosa. *Behaviour Therapy, 15,* 3–20.
Ley, P. (1985). The effectiveness of some psychological treatment for obesity. In S. W. Touyz & P. J. V. Beumont (Eds.), *Eating Disorders: Prevalence and treatment.* Sydney: Williams and Wilkins/Adis.
Linden, W. (1980). Multi-component behaviour therapy in a case of compulsive binge-eating followed by vomiting. *Journal of Behaviour Therapy and Experimental Psychiatry, II,* 297–300.
Lobb, L. G., & Shaefer, H. H. (1972). Successful treatment of anorexia nervosa through isolation. *Psychological Reports, 30,* 245–246.
Long, C. G., & Cordle, C. J. (1982). Psychological treatment of binge-eating and self-induced vomiting. *British Journal of Medical Psychology, 55,* 139–149.
Mahoney, B. K., Rogers, T., Straw, M., & Mahoney, M. J. (1977). *Results and implications of a problem solving treatment program for obesity.* Paper presented at the 11th Annual Convention of the Association for Advancement of Behaviour Therapy, Atlanta, GA.
Mahoney, M. J. (1974). *Cognitive and behaviour modification.* Cambridge, MA: Ballinger.

Mahoney, M. J., & Mahoney, K. (1976). *Permanent weight control: A total solution to the dieters dilemma.* New York: Norton.
Meichenbaum, D. (1974). *Therapist manual for cognitive behaviour modification.* Waterloo, Ontario: University of Waterloo Press.
Mitchell, J. B., & Black, J. A. (1946). Malnutrition in released prisoners-of-war and interness at Singapore. *Lancet, 2,* 855–862.
Mizes, J. S., & Lohr, J. M. (1983). The treatment of bulimia (binge-eating and self-induced vomiting). A quasi-experimental investigation of the effects of stimulus narrowing, self reinforcement and self control relaxation. *International Journal of Eating Disorders, 2,* 59–66.
Montgomery, B., & Harris, L. (1985). *You can lose weight: The new science of weight loss.* Melbourne: Thomas Nelson.
Morris, L. & King, N. J. (1986). Obesity. In N. J. King & A. Remeny (Eds.), *Health Care: A behavioural approach* (pp. 51–62). Sydney: Grune and Stratten.
Neuman, M., & Gaoni, B. (1975). Preferred food as a reinforcing agent in a case of anorexia nervosa. *Journal of Behaviour Therapy and Experimental Psychiatry, 6,* 331–333.
Ollendick, T. H. (1979). Behavioural treatment of anorexia nervosa: A five-year study. *Behaviour Modification, 3,* 124–135.
Ordman, A. M., & Kirschenbaum, D. S. (1985). Cognitive-behavioural therapy for bulimia: An initial outcome study. *Journal of Consulting and Clinical Psychology, 53* (3), 305–313.
Penick, S. B., Fillion, R., Fox, S., & Stunkard, A. J. (1971). Behaviour modification in the treatment of obesity. *Psychosomatic Medicine, 33,* 49–55.
Pyle, R. L., Mitchell, J. E., & Eckert, E. D. (1981). Bulimia: A report of 34 cases. *Journal of Clinical Psychology, 42* (2), 10–64.
Rosen, J. C., & Leitenberg, H. (1982). Bulimia nervosa: Treatment with exposure and response prevention. *Behaviour Therapy, 13,* 117–124.
Rossiter, E. M., & Wilson, G. T. (1985). Cognitive restructuring and response prevention in the treatment of bulimia nervosa. *Behaviour Research and Therapy, 23* (3), 349–359.
Rowland, C. V. (1970). Anorexia nervosa: A survey of the literature and review of 30 cases. *International Psychiatric Clinics, 7,* 37–137.
Russell, G. (1979). Bulimia nervosa: An ominous variant of anorexia nervosa. *Psychological Medicine, 9,* 429–448.
Schiele, B. C., & Brozek, J. (1948). "Experimental neurosis" resulting from semistarvation in man. *Psychosomatic Medicine, 10,* 33–50.
Schlemmer, J. K., & Barnett, P. A. (1977). Management of manipulative behaviour of anorexia nervosa patients. *Journal of Psychiatric Nursing, 15,* 35–41.
Schmidt, M. P. W., & Duncan, B. A. B. (1974). Modifying eating behaviour in anorexia nervosa. *American Journal of Nursing, 74,* 1646–1648.
Schnurer, A. T., Rubin, R. R., & Roy, A. (1973). Systematic desensitization of anorexia nervosa seen as a weight phobia. *Journal of Behaviour Therapy and Experimental Psychiatry, 4,* 149–153.
Schwartz, D. M., Thompson, M. G., & Johnson, C. L. (1983). Eating disorders and the culture. In P. L. Darby, P. E. Garfinkel, D. M. Garner, & D. V.

Coscina (Eds.), *Anorexia nervosa: Recent developments in research* (pp. 83–94). New York: Alan R. Liss.

Slade, P. (1986). A review of body-image studies in anorexia nervosa and bulimia nervosa. In G. I. Szmukler, P. D. Slade, P. Harris, D. Benton, & G. F. M. Russell (Eds.), *Anorexia nervosa and bulimic disorders* (pp. 255–266). Oxford: Pergamon.

Steinhausen, H. C., & Glanville, K. (1983). A long-term follow-up of adolescent anorexia nervosa. *Acta Psychiatrica Scandinavica, 68,* 1–10.

Stuart, R. B. (1967). Behavioural control of overeating. *Behavior, Research and Therapy, 5,* 357–365.

Stuart, R. B. (1977). Self-help group approach to self-management. In R. B. Stuart (Ed.), *Behavioral self-management.* New York: Brunner/Mazel.

Stuart, R. B. (1978). *Act thin, stay thin.* New York: Norton.

Stuart (Ed.), *Behavioural self-management.* New York: Brunner/Mazel.

Stuart, R. B. (1978). *Act thin, stay thin.* New York Norton.

Stunkard, A. J. (1959). Eating patterns and obesity. *Psychiatric Quarterly, 33,* 284–295.

Stunkard, A. J. (1982). Obesity. In A. S. Bellack, H. Herson, & A. E. Kazdin (Eds.), *International handbook of behaviour modification and therapy* (pp. 535–573). New York: Plenum.

Stunkard, A. J. (1985). Behavioural management of obesity. Special Supplement. *Medical Journal of Australia, 142,* 513–520.

Sydenham, A. (1946). Amenorrhoea at Stanley Camp, Hong Kong, during internment. *British Journal of Medicine, 159,* 249–256.

Touyz, S. W., & Beumont, P. J. V. (1984). Anorexia nervosa: A follow-up investigation. *Medical Journal of Australia, 141,* 219–222.

Touyz, S. W., & Beumont, P. J. (1985). A comprehensive, multidisciplinary approach for the management of patients with anorexia nervosa. In S. W. Touyz & P. J. V. Beumont (Eds.), *Eating disorders: Prevalence and treatment* (pp. 11–22). Sydney: Williams and Wilkins/Adis.

Touyz, S. W., Beumont, P. J. V., Collins, J. K., McCabe, M., & Jupp, J. (1984a). Body shape perception and its disturbance in anorexia nervosa. *British Journal of Psychiatry, 144,* 167–171.

Touyz, S. W., Beumont, P. J. V., Glaun, D., Philips, T., & Cowie, I. (1984b). A comparison of lenient and strict operant conditioning programmes in refeeding patients with anorexia nervosa. *British Journal of Psychiatry, 144,* 512–520.

Touyz, S. W., Beumont, P. J. V., & Hook, S., (1987). Exercise anorexia: A new dimension in anorexia nervosa? In P. J. V. Beumont, G. D. Burrows, & R. Casper (Eds.), *Handbook of eating disorders. Anorexia nervosa and bulimia* (Vol. 1, pp. 173, 189). Amsterdam: Elsevier Biomedical Press.

Touyz, S. W., Beumont, P. J. V., & Johnstone, L. C. (1986). Neuropsychological correlates of dieting disorders. *International Journal of Eating Disorders, 5* (6), 1025–1034.

Touyz, S. W., Cowie, I., Collins, J. K., & Beumont, P. J. V. (1985). Body shape perception in bulimia and anorexia nervosa. *International Journal of Eating Disorders, 4* (3), 259–266.

Touyz, S. W., & Ivison, D. J. (1985). The prevalence of bulimia in an Australia university sample. In S. W. Touyz & P. J. V. Beumont (Eds.). *Eating disorders: Prevalence and treatment* (pp. 52–61). Sydney: Williams and Wilkins/Adis.

VanItalie, T. B. (1979). Obesity: Adverse effects on health and longevity. *American Journal of Clinical Nutrition, 32*, 2723–2733.

Venables, J. F. (1930). Anorexia nervosa, study of the pathogenesis of nine cases. *Guys Hospital Report, 80*, 213.

Volkmar, F. R., Stunkard, A. J., Woolston, J., & Bailey, R. A. (1981). High attrition rates in commercial weight reduction programs. *Archives of Internal Medicine, 141*, 426–428.

Wadden, T. A., Stunkard, A. J., Brownell, K. D., & Day, S. C. (1984). Treatment of moderate obesity by behaviour therapy and very-low calorie diet: A pilot investigation. *Journal of Consulting and Clinical Psychology, 41* (3), 533–539.

Welch, G. J. (1979). The treatment of compulsive vomiting and obsessive thoughts through graduated response delay, response prevention and cognitive connection. *Journal of Behavioural Therapy and Experimental Psychiatry, 10*, 77–82.

Wermuth, B. M., Davis, K. L., Hollister, L. E., & Stunkard, A. J. (1977). Phenytoin treatment of the binge-eating syndrome. *American Journal of Psychiatry, 134*, 1249–1253.

Whyte, B. L., & Kaczkowski, H. (1983). Anorexia nervosa: A study of psychiatrists' and psychologists' opinions and practices. *International Journal of Eating Disorders, 2*, 87–92.

Willi, J. & Grossman, S. (1983). Epidemiology of anorexia nervosa in a defined region of Switzerland. *American Journal of Psychiatry, 240* (5), 564–567.

Wilson, G. T., (1980). Behaviour modification and the treatment of obesity. In A. J. Stunkard (Ed.), *Obesity* (pp. 325–344). Philadelphia: W. B. Saunders.

Wooley, O. W., Wooley, S. C., & Dyrenforth, S. R. (1979). Obesity and women II: A neglected feminist topic. *Women's Studies International Quarterly, 2*, 81–92.

Yates, A. Leehey, K., & Shisslak, C. (1983). Running an analogue of anorexia? *New England Journal of Medicine, 308*, 251–255.

Yates, A. J., & Sambrailo, F. (1984). Bulimia nervosa: A descriptive and therapeutic study. *Behaviour Research and Therapy, 5*, 503–517.

VI

THE RESPIRATORY SYSTEM

15

Pathophysiology of Breathlessness in Respiratory Disorders

Laurence A. Smolley

University of Miami School of Medicine
Chief, Pulmonary Section
Miami Veterans Administration Hospital
Miami, FL

INTRODUCTION

Difficulties in breathing comprise a variety of sensations which patients describe with an even greater variety of words (Ogilvie, 1983). Some complain of having to breathe too much, of not being able to breathe enough, of needing to take deep breaths, of gasping, suffocation, or tightness in the chest or throat. All of these expressions have in common undue awareness of a function which is normally subconscious and of discomfort which is not commensurate with the level of physical activity.

Dyspnea is the word applied clinically to these breathing difficulties. *Dyspnea,* literally: disordered breathing, is derived from the Greek, dys: abnormal or disordered, and pnoia: breath.

Table 15.3.
Studies of Conditions Related to Dyspnea

Vagal nerve blockade
Tracheobronchial irritation experiments
Chest wall blockade
Curarization
Spinal anesthesia
Breath-holding experiments
Abnormal pulmonary function tests
Detection of added respiratory loads
Carbon-dioxide stimulation experiments
Respiratory muscle dysfunction
Fatigue
Weakness
Increased central drive to breathe
Increased sense of effort
Psychopathology
Individual differences

Dyspnea is not *tachypnea,* which is rapid breathing; it is not *hyperpnea,* which is increased ventilation in proportion to increased metabolism; it is not *hyperventilation,* which is ventilation in excess of metabolic requirements. Instead, dyspnea is difficult, labored, uncomfortable breathing; it is an unpleasant type of breathing although it is not painful in the usual sense of the word. It is subjective, and like pain, it involves both perception of the sensation by the patient and his or her reaction to the sensation (Comroe, 1966). Breathlessness may indicate a different sensation, such as that felt during exercise or excitement, and may not be unpleasant. For the purposes of this chapter, the terms dyspnea and breathlessness will be used interchangeably.

Finding the cause of dyspnea in patients is frequently a diagnostic challenge. The neurophysiology of dyspnea is not agreed on and represents an exciting area of research. Possible sources of stimuli that may give rise to dyspnea include those listed in Table 15.1.

Clinically, dyspnea may be viewed in terms of the relationship between the factors that stimulate tidal breathing and the impedances that must be overcome during the act of breathing. Dyspnea may be associated with conditions that result in an abnormally increased stimulus to breathe or a requirement for greater than normal effort to breathe (Table 15.2). Conditions in which dyspnea is primarily related to the requirements for increased effort are clinically more common.

Table 15.2.
Clinical Conditions Associated with Dyspnea

Pulmonary Disorders
Increased airway resistance, e.g., asthma, emphysema, bronchitis
Intrapulmonary restrictive changes, e.g., interstitial fibrosis
Pulmonary vascular disease, e.g., emboli
Pneumothorax
Extra-pulmonary chest wall restriction
Obesity
Kyphoscoliosis
Pleural effusion
Respiratory muscle fatigue or weakness
Chemical Factors
Hypoxia
Hypercapnea, acidemia
Increased metabolic rate, e.g., fever
Cardiac Factors
Cardiac insufficiency
Valvular disease and decreased stroke volume
Myocardial disease and decreased ejection fraction
Anemia
Decreased oxygen carrying capacity
Psychogenic
Hyperventilation syndrome
Malingering (hyperventilation or hypoventilation)

STUDIES OF CONDITIONS RELATED TO DYSPNEA

In trying to comprehend the mechanism of dyspnea, experiments have been designed to block one or the other of the possibly relevant pathways. The effects of blocking these pathways on conditions known to be associated with the sensation have been examined. Other conditions apparently associated with dyspnea have also been examined (Table 15.3).

Table 15.1.
Possible Sources of Stimuli That May Induce Dyspnea

Increase or decrease in normal breathing movements
Abnormal blood chemistry (hypercapnea, hypoxia)
Stimuli arising in lung mechanoreceptors (airways, parenchyma)
Stimuli arising from mechanoreceptors in respiratory muscles
Added mechanical loads (resistive, elastic)
Cortical or psychogenic stimuli

Vagal Nerve Blockade

Afferent fibers from three intrapulmonary receptors—stretch receptors, irritant receptors, and J receptors—are carried in the vagus nerves. All have attracted interest as mediators of respiratory sensation. Transcutaneous vagal nerve anesthetic blockade using lidocaine infiltration of the base of the skull around the vagal and glossopharyngeal nerves in awake conscious subjects has been used to study respiratory sensation. Complete vagal block was assumed when aphonia from vocal cord paralysis and the development of a Horner's syndrome from a block of the sympathetic nerve fibers was noted. This experimental model permitted the intercostal muscle and diaphragmatic innervation to remain intact, while vagal-mediated afferent information from the lungs to the brain was interrupted. The effects of bilateral vagal block on breath-holding and detection of added loads are discussed in the sections below.

The results of vagal nerve blocks in patients with cardiopulmonary diseases were variable (Guz, 1970). There was no effect on dyspnea or respiratory pattern in patients with chronic airways obstruction but in patients with pulmonary vascular obstruction, left heart failure, or pulmonary parenchymal infiltration, there was a decrease in dyspnea. These effects may be due to a blockade of afferent signals from stretch receptors and J receptors stimulated by changes in lung compliance associated with these disorders.

J receptors are located close to the alveoli and pulmonary capillaries and transmit information centrally via unmyelinated fibers (Paintal, 1977). Direct examination of the role of J receptors in the mediation of dyspnea in patients with chronic airflow limitation and diffuse interstitial lung disease was attempted. A human study (Stark, 1985) was predicated on animal models in which a vagally mediated tachypnea may be induced acutely by pulmonary microembolism. This response is known to be mediated by the unmyelinated pulmonary afferent nerves in the vagus. Local anesthetic agents, administered as small particles but not as large particles, blunted the response, which suggested that the aerosol was capable of penetration to the alveolar level. The clinical study was designed to compare the effects of lignocaine or placebo both given as small-particle aerosols. Respiratory frequency, forced expiratory flow in one second, and other measurements were made. Exercise tolerance and dyspnea were measured with a six-minute walking test and visual analog scales before and after aerosol. After lignocaine, there was no clinical evidence of anesthesia of the upper airways but slight bronchoconstriction occurred as shown by changes in forced expiratory flow. Although the bronchospasm might have blunted any direct effects on afferent signals related to dyspnea, no dramatic effect of lignocaine was demonstrated and the investigators suggested that dyspnea in their study patients was not mediated by J receptors.

The role of irritant receptors in respiratory sensation is discussed in the next section.

Tracheobronchial Irritation Experiments

Studies of irritant sensations and cough response to localized electrical stimulation of the bronchial mucosa (Klassen, 1951; Morton, 1951) have shown that subjects could localize the site of the electrical stimulus on to the anterior chest wall with remarkable accuracy. Moreover, the sensations associated with cough were mediated by the vagus nerve ipsilateral to the side of irritation.

The irritating raw sensation produced in the arterior thorax by the oral inhalation of ammonia vapor was prevented by bilateral vagal blockade (Guz, 1966a). Anesthesia of the airways prevents the cough and the raw sensation in the anterior chest that results from inhalation of an aerosol of citric acid (Cross et al., 1976). When the airway of a patient with a high cervical cord transection was irritated, there was no cough response, but the irritation was still sensed in the anterior chest (Noble, 1970).

The studies outlined in this section, the one that precedes and the one that follows, suggest that the vagus nerve-mediated signals may play some role in the genesis of respiratory sensation. The exact role of the vagus in the production of breathlessness remains unclear.

Chest Wall Blockade

Studies of respiratory sensation with two types of chest wall blockade have been performed. Curarization of the respiratory muscles causes weakness or paralysis of the respiratory muscles but leaves sensation intact (Campbell, 1969). Chest wall blockade by means of spinal anesthesia (Eisele, 1968) to the sensory level of cervical seventh in awake, conscious subjects blocks both afferent and efferent signals related to the intercostal muscles while leaving intact innervation of the diaphragm via the phrenic nerve and of the lung, via the sympathetic nerves and the vagus nerves. The effects of these types of neural blockades on breath-holding and detection of added loads are discussed in the section below.

Breath-holding Experiments

The experience of breath-holding is familiar to most people and is associated with a sense of discomfort considered similar in some respects to dyspnea. The intensity of the discomfort increases with time during the breath-holding and is directly related to the arterial carbon dioxide tension and inversely related to arterial oxygen tension (Otis, 1948) and to lung volume (Mithoefer, 1959). However, with breath-holding, the thoracic sensation of discomfort coincides with the onset of diaphragmatic contractions (Agostoni, 1963). These contractions become more powerful and frequent until the subject can no longer resist the urge to inspire. The sensation is relieved during the first inspiration even if the gas mixture inhaled is hypoxic or hypercapnic (Fowler, 1954). The sensation is prevented by bilateral local anesthesia of the vagal nerves which blocks afferent nerve fibers from the lungs (Guz, 1966a). The sensation is also abolished by complete muscular paralysis with curare (Campbell, 1969). The sensation is not affected in any way by spinal anesthesia high enough to include the first thoracic segment (Eisele, 1968). These last two experiments suggest that intercostal muscle contraction is not necessary for the sensation, but that diaphragmatic muscle contraction is essential. Corroboration came from a study in which the phrenic nerves were blocked with a resultant marked alleviation of the discomfort of breath-holding and a prolonged breath-holding time (Noble, 1971). Interestingly, a study of a patient (Noble, 1971) with a nearly complete transection of the spinal cord at the third cervical segment showed that the patient could breathe and maintain normal blood gases with the use of greatly hypertrophied sternocleidomastoid muscles innervated by the spinal accessory nerve. As there was complete diaphragmatic paralysis, the breath-holding sensation was absent. The drive to breathe developed normally as shown by sternoeleidomastoid contractions whose force and rapidity increased with the duration of a breath-hold. This observation suggests that the sensation of breath-holding does not stem from a central monitoring of the drive to breathe, but that actual diaphragmatic muscular contraction is necessary.

These studies suggest that with breath-holding, a lung proprioceptive (vagal) and chemical drive to breathe develops. The sensation arises from the diaphragmatic contractions that result. Tendon receptors in the diaphragm (Agostoni, 1970) were suggested to be sources of the afferent information for the genesis of the sensation of breath-holding.

Abnormal Pulmonary Function Tests

Attempts have been made to correlate various physiologic variables, measurable in the routine clinical pulmonary function laboratory, with the sensation of dyspnea. Static lung volumes and arterial blood gases have repeatedly shown poor correlation with symptomatology (Epler, 1980; McFadden, 1973; Dudley, 1968). Early investigators suggested that dyspnea is the result of increased work of breathing due to mechanical problems in the lungs or chest wall. However, in many conditions in which dyspnea occurs, such as emphysema, the work of breathing is only slightly increased and equivalent increases in the work of breathing in normal subjects produce no symptoms (Marshall, 1954). An increased oxygen cost of breathing has also been proposed as a cause of dyspnea (Cherniak, 1959). The objection to this idea is similar to that against the theory of work of breathing. Although both the work of breathing and oxygen consumption at rest may be elevated in patients with various respiratory diseases, these parameters do not consistently correlate with the report of breathlessness. One study (Burki, 1979) of a group of patients with chronic airways obstruction showed no significant difference in oxygen uptake between the breathless compared to the nonbreathless patients.

It may be that the relationship between pulmonary dysfunction and the severity of dyspnea is close only within individual disease types. This specificity to disease is suggested by comparing the pulmonary function tests that correlate with dyspnea in obstructive and restrictive pulmonary conditions (Epler, 1980). The forced vital capacity and diffusing capacity have been found to correlate moderately with the severity of dyspnea in restrictive disease. The maximal voluntary ventilation, MVV, the largest volume of gas in liters that can be breathed per minute by voluntary effort, has the greatest reported correlation with dyspnea in obstructive diseases ($r = 0.78$). An application of the MVV more specific to the assessment of dyspnea is a dyspnea index, which expresses the minute ventilation at a given level of exercise as a percentage of the MVV. It has been found that if this index is less than 30%, dyspnea is unlikely to be experienced, but almost all subjects with an index greater than 50% are likely to report dyspnea at abnormally low levels of exercise (Morgan, 1982). However, some patients with chronic obstructive lung disease may have a dyspnea index greater than 50% at rest and therefore not complain of dyspnea.

The MVV is tiring for subjects, is dependent on maximal effort, and is difficult to reproduce. The forced expiratory volume in one second, $FEV_{1.0}$, is used more often to evaluate the degree of airway obstruction even though it has a slightly lower correlation ($r = -0.71$) with dyspnea than the MVV. In patients with obstructive pulmonary disease, flow rates such as the $FEV_{1.0}$ are used in the assessment of disability as these tests are easily performed, sensitive, and reproducible. However, the validity of these measures depends on the subject's effort and cooperation. Compatible with the subjective nature of dyspnea, in studies of pulmonary disability the relationship between $FEV_{1.0}$ and degree of reported dyspnea has been found to be influenced by the patient's reason for contacting the physician. Those patients claiming disability have been shown to have a greater degree of dyspnea for the same level of pulmonary physiologic impairment than hospitalized patients not claiming disability (Morgan, 1977).

No isolated lung function parameter has been found to predict the precise level of functional impairment or the severity of dyspnea that an individual patient will experience. These poor correlations indicate that the perception of dyspnea is influenced by factors other than the extent of pulmonary disease. In the sections that follow, the various approaches that investigators have taken to elucidate those factors that may influence the sensation of dyspnea coming to consciousness will be outlined (Table 15.3).

Detection of Added Respiratory Loads

Various studies have been carried out in which resistive or elastic loads are applied to a subject's airway. A sensation results which enables the individual to detect that the load has been added. The rationale for these studies was that the perception of added loads to respiration might be analogous to the hindered breathing of patients with obstructive or restrictive chest diseases. A threshold of detection exists in individuals for both inspiratory resistive and elastic loads, as defined by the level of the load detected 50 percent of the time (Bennett, 1962; Campbell, 1961). In normal people (Wiley, 1966) and in asthmatics (Burki, 1978) this detection threshold is a function of the individual's baseline, and intrinsic load, such as pulmonary resistance. It has been suggested that the perception of added respiratory loads is a function of a change in the relationship between respiratory muscle length and the tension developed in the muscle (Campbell, 1961). Apparently, the usual source of afferent signals responsible for the detection of these loads is the diaphragm because anesthesia of the airways (Chaudhary, 1978), chest wall blockade by spinal anesthesia (Cournand, 1954), and vagal blockade (Guz, 1970) have no effect on the detection thresholds. However, the ability to detect added loads applied to a tracheostomy has been found to be normal in patients with high cord transections up to the third cervical segment (Noble, 1972). So it is possible that sites other than the diaphragm assume a role in load perception in certain conditions. The relationship between load perception and dyspnea remains unclear.

Carbon Dioxide Inhalation Experiments

Increases in inspired carbon dioxide concentration experienced by a normal subject results in an increased depth and frequency of breathing while the subject experiences a rather typical sensation of not being able to breathe deeply enough. The sensation can be abolished by bilateral ninth and tenth nerve blocks at the base of the skull (Guz, 1966b), but the ventilatory response to carbon dioxide is markedly blunted also. Chest wall blockade has no effect on either the sensation or the ventilatory response to carbon dioxide. When carbon dioxide was added to a respirator used to provide a constant ventilation to patients completely paralyzed by poliomyelitis it was reported (Patterson, 1962; Noble, 1970) that the main sensation was "of dying away" or anesthesia. There was no apparent typical carbon-dioxide induced "air hunger." A patient with a very high cervical cord transection (Noble, 1970), who breathed using his sternocleidomastoid muscles, developed air hunger when he rebreathed from a bag containing five percent carbon dioxide at an arterial carbon-dioxide at an arterial carbon-dioxide partial pressure of 49 mmHg. However, this same patient at another time was able to tolerate an increase of arterial carbon-dioxide tension to 64 mmHg, when the carbon dioxide was added to a mechanical ventilator which maintained a steady ventilation. Subjects paralyzed with curare did not experience air hunger upon inhalation of carbon dioxide (Campbell, 1969). These data suggest that hypernea is needed for the sensation of air hunger to be experienced. Anesthesia of the airways did not prevent the sensation of air hunger or the ventilatory response to carbon dioxide (Cross et al., 1976).

An ingenious experimental approach has been attempted to overcome the challenge of dissecting out the contribution of each putative pathway of respiratory sensation alluded to in the introductory comments above. In both normal subjects and patients with obstructive and restrictive respiratory problems in whom dyspnea was induced by breathing hypoxic or hypercapnic inspirates, the investigators (Adams, 1985) made use of the fact that it is possible to stimulate the relevant anterior horn cells by the separate pathways concerned with the control of breathing, and that it is possible to dissociate the ventilatory response pattern (minute ventilation) from the arterial blood stimulus (hypoxia or hypercapnea) profile by using an oscillating stimulus and altering its frequency. In normal subjects given hypercapnic or hypoxic stimuli, the minute ventilation responses for any level of stimulus were significantly less with fast-cycle stimulation. The dyspnea ratings were also lower with fast oscillation of the stimuli. When the normal subjects were asked to voluntarily copy breathing patterns induced by reflex hypercapnic stimulation the dyspnea scores were significantly less. When the patients were asked to do voluntary copying the dyspnea was also less than during hypercapnic stimulation and interestingly, when carbon dioxide was added to their inspirate during copying, without their knowledge, both minute ventilation and dyspnea significantly increased, but dyspnea did not increase to the level experienced during carbon-dioxide oscillation stimulation, although minute ventilation was at the same level. During rapid oscillation of hypercapnic or hypoxic stimuli, the lower dyspnea ratings were associated with a reduction in either tidal volume (depth of breathing) or frequency or both. Mean inspiratory time was also reduced. During voluntary copying there were no consistent differences in the pattern of ventilation compared with reflex stimulation.

This study demonstrated that the intensity of dyspnea during both hypercapnia and hypoxia is reduced when the frequency of fixed amplitude oscillations in chemical stimuli (changes in carbon dioxide or oxygen levels) is increased. This effect reflects the reduction in the magnitude of the minute ventilation changes found when the stimulus intensity changes more rapidly. These results support the notion that breathlessness cannot result from the simple perception of afferent information from arterial chemoreceptors, and that it is the effective ventilatory response to such stimulation which is somehow involved.

For hypercapnia, the observed diminished ventilatory response to rapid-cycle oscillation probably reflects inadequate time to achieve full equilibration of carbon-dioxide partial pressure at the central chemoreceptors in the medulla. The lag relating ventilatory response to increments in arterial carbon dioxide is well known, but because it is impossible to know the stimulus level at the central site the cause of the reduction in dyspnea with rapid-cycle oscillation may be the result of reduced respiratory neuron stimulation or the reduced ventilatory response itself. For hypoxia, the site of stimulation is very clearly defined at the carotid body. The response of the human subjects in this study to hypoxic stimuli was similar to that demonstrated in animals previously. The authors concluded that the damping of the reflex ventilatory response was almost certainly occurring at the medullary respiratory complex. The fact that breathlessness is linked to the ventilatory response rather than the stimulus level is the strongest evidence that the sensation does not arise from the perception of afferent information from the chemoreceptors but rather to the efferent, motor command to the respiratory muscles or perhaps from the muscles themselves.

A remarkable finding from these studies is that voluntary activation of the ventilatory apparatus to the same level as that reached with reflex stimulation is associated with less breathlessness. This may occur because automatic (reflex) and behavioral (voluntary) "drives to breathe" follow anatomically distinct pathways such as that when descending neural information from the cortex may activate the respiratory system when unconscious medullary regulation is lost (Plum, 1981). This is in spite of a common final pathway from anterior horn cells. On this basis, the authors suggest that breathlessness may result from the perception of increased activity of respiratory-related neurons in the medulla that send efferent signals to the muscles as a consequence of effective reflex ventilatory stimulation, and that these medullary neurons may not be activated during voluntary ventilatory stimulation.

Fatigue of the Respiratory Muscles

In view of the fact that the inspiratory muscles have been shown to fatigue in various situations (Derenne, 1978), it has been suggested that fatigue plays some role in causing dyspnea. In an elegant study (Gandevia, 1981), eight normal subjects were required to sustain a maximum isometric inspiratory contraction at functional residual capacity after 20 seconds of hyperventilation while breathing pure oxygen. They had to maintain the contraction until it could no longer be tolerated. Within 30 to 60 seconds the subjects experienced a feeling of fatigue and the inspiratory pressures diminished by about 20 percent. Two minutes separated trials during which the subjects signaled subjective estimates of either inspiratory pressure or motor command. They were asked, "How big is the inspiratory pressure or tension in the (respiratory) muscles?" and "How big is your command or sense of effort?", respectively. Inspiratory loads were also applied to the airway and each subject (without knowledge of the actual magnitude of the load) was asked to select a number proportional to the size of the load. They were asked, "How big is the load?" This unrestricted magnitude scaling, using a technique described previously (Stevens, 1957), was done by each subject during several trials both after maximal contractions and after hyperventilation with oxygen and a period of breath-holding. All subjects indicated that the motor command increased monotonically during inspiratory muscle contraction, especially toward the end of the contraction when the achieved force declined. When signaling perceived inspiratory pressure, six of the subjects indicated the reduced pressure during the later part of the contraction. In one subject, the perceived pressure remained constant despite a fall in achieved pressure. In another subject, perceived pressure increased during contractions but at a rate lower than the perceived increase in motor command. Qualitatively similar performances were given by two subjects on different days. An inspiratory load seemed larger when presented at the end of a sustained maximal isometric contraction than when presented after breath-holding. For the group of subjects, an inspiratory load felt bigger when the inspiratory muscles were fatigued.

This study used fatigue as a method to disassociate the motor command (or effort) put into a maximal inspiratory contraction from the actual muscular tension (or inspiratory pressure) produced by it. Subjects were able to distinguish between their sense of motor command and their sense of achieved muscular tension. An inspiratory load was consistently overestimated when produced by fatigued muscles. Subjects preferentially used the signal of motor command, rather than achievement, when judging the size of a respiratory load. This study was consistent with the studies of limb muscles in which signals of motor command and of muscular tension were perceived, but signals of command were preferred as indicators of muscle tension (McCloskey, 1974). Experiments with anesthesia of the skin and joints combined with muscular weakness (curare induced) suggest an intramuscular origin for this signal in the limb muscles (McCloskey, 1974; Roland, 1977). The Golgi tendon organs seem most likely to be responsible for the afferent signals of tension in the muscle (Matthews, 1982). Clinical anecdotes are consistent with this study as patients frequently have dyspnea and/or an increased sense of effort associated with breathing immediately after being taken off prolonged mechanical ventilation when their respiratory muscles may be weakened by disuse.

It has been suggested that in patients with a mechanical or neuromuscular impediment to breathing, a greater motor command is needed to achieve adequate ventilation. This added command may be associated with an increased sense of effort and may result in the sensation of dyspnea in certain circumstances, just at the added command to lift a weight with fatigued limb muscles is responsible for the heavy feeling of the weight (Killian, 1985a).

Weakness of the Respiratory Muscles

In order to investigate the mechanisms involved in determining the size of a resistive load, partial curarization was used to weaken the respiratory muscles so that during neuromuscular blockade a greater motor command was required to produce the same inspiratory pressure (Campbell, 1980). This study used partial curarization as a technique to disassociate the motor command put into the efforts required to breathe against added loads from the actual muscular tensions (or pressure) generated while breathing against the loads. The perceived magnitude of resistive loads was examined over a wide range of loads using unrestricted magnitude scaling (Stevens, 1957). To determine whether curarization affects the mechanisms allowing the detection of a resistive load, thresholds for detection were determined before and during partial curarization.

Subjects estimated the size of added inspiratory resistances by assigning a number proportional to the size of the resistances before and during maintained partial curarization. By giving boluses of D-tubocurarine each minute, it was possible to maintain the maximum inspiratory pressure and inspiratory capacity at a constant low level compared to control. This reduced the possibility of selective decurarization at the neuromuscual junctions of the most frequently used muscle fibers. During partial curarization, the perceived magnitude of a particular resistance increased above control levels. Although the magnitude of each resistance was overestimated, the degree of overestimation did not increase as the size of added resistances increased. After the experiment, all subjects stated that all loads felt larger during partial curarization. There was no change in the detection threshold during curarization.

The apparent increase in the magnitude of a resistive load during partial paralysis is consistent with the hypothesis that estimation of the magnitude of the load depends in part on sensing the size of the outgoing motor command or sense of effort (McCloskey, 1974; Roland, 1977; Killian, 1985), rather than on afferent information signaling the achieved inspiratory flow and pressure developed. The failure of curarization to alter the detection threshold for resistive loads is compatible with the concept that detection depends upon sensing a disturbance in the breath-by-breath relation between inspiratory flow and pressure.

This experiment provides an interesting model because patients with airway obstruction (increased resistive loads) often are dyspneic. Moreover, these patients frequently have hyperinflated lungs and flattened diaphragms which have shortened muscle fibers which are less able to generate tension (reduced maximum inspiratory pressures)

(Sharp, 1983). It may be that the dyspnea in these patients is mediated by an increased sense of effort associated with an increased central drive to breathe (motor command).

Increased Central Drive to Breathe

Mouth occlusion pressure (P_{100}) is the pressure generated after the first 100 milliseconds of inspiration of the airway is briefly occluded at functional residual capacity or at the end of a normal expiration. P_{100} has been shown to be proportional to phrenic nerve output in cats (Eldridge, 1975) and to expired minute ventilation in normal humans. (Lederer, 1977). It is thought to reflect a central drive to breathe, and because it occurs before there is significant airflow, the measurement of P_{100} is thought to be largely independent of lung mechanics and respiratory muscle force velocity relationships (Whitelaw, 1975). Two studies of patients with respiratory muscle weakness (Aubier, 1980; Begin, 1982) observed P_{100} values much higher than anticipated on the basis of their minute ventilation levels.

The dependence of P_{100} and minute ventilation on respiratory muscle strength during carbon dioxide stimulation has been examined (Holle, 1984). Hypercapnic ventilatory response before curarization and then at several levels of respiratory muscle weakness was measured. Two to four stages of respiratory weakness were produced in each subject by partial curarization. All subjects experienced some feelings of apprehension or choking during the final stage of weakness (Schoene, 1986). At all levels of weakness, when compared to baseline, handgrip decreased more than inspiratory force, whereas inspiratory force decreased more than vital capacity, the lung volumes did not change between baseline and at the maximum level of weakness. The hypercapnic response of P_{100} with increasing weakness was greater than that of minute ventilation. The P_{100} response was significantly higher than the minute ventilation response during severe weakness at all levels of carbon dioxide and during mild and moderate weakness at a partial-pressure of carbon dioxide of 45 torr. Since there were no changes in lung volumes which might effect end-expiratory muscle length, comparison of P_{100} at different levels of weakness was felt to be valid. Prior studies had shown that curare has no direct effects of its own on a central drive to breathe (Cohen, 1959; Smith, 1951). These findings were compatible with the hypothesis that weakened respiratory muscles should require greater neural input to maintain ventilation. Unfortunately, the investigators did not formally examine respiratory sensation during this study. A correlation between muscle weakness, central drive to breathe, and dyspnea still awaits confirmation.

The relationship between dyspnea and P_{100} has been reported by Burki (1979). A group of 24 patients with chronic airways obstructions was divided into two groups on the basis of the presence or absence of dyspnea at rest. Assignment of individual patients to the breathless or nonbreathless group was made before pulmonary function or other measurements were done. The breathless group had a greater degree of airway obstruction. Lung volumes were similar in the two groups as were the carbon dioxide levels in arterial blood. The breathless group had a slightly (perhaps clinically insignificant) but statistically significant lower arterial blood level of oxygen. There were no differences in resting minute ventilation or breathing frequency between the groups. In both groups of patients, resting P_{100} was significantly above the normal range, however, the P_{100} was significantly greater in the breathless group compared to the nonbreathless patients. This study suggests a correlation between dyspnea and central drive to breathe which may be related to the motor command and sense of effort.

Recently, a study was done examining the mechanisms responsible for the relief of dyspnea in patients with chronic obstructive lung disease after participation in a comprehensive pulmonary rehabilitation program (Smolley, 1986a). The patients strengthened their inspiratory muscles by using a resistive inspiratory muscle training device in which the resistive loads could gradually be increased as the patients improved. The patients also did walking exercises. In this controlled study, the patients in the treatment group experienced a significant decrease in their dyspneic symptoms during their activities of daily living in conjunction with increases in inspiratory muscle strength, distance walked during a 12-minute walk test, and in oxygen consumption at rest. Interestingly, the P_{100} decreased significantly from baseline in this group of patients. This study also suggests that a decreased central drive to breathe and a decrease in breathlessness are related to respiratory muscle function.

Also, in a study of patients with large pleural effusions who were dyspneic (Smolley, 1986b) it was found that after removal of some of the fluid the patients felt better. Their dyspnea was significantly improved as measured by a category scale of respiratory sensation which described sense of effort during breathing. Moreover, there was a significant decrease in the P_{100}. There was no change in muscle strength or in minute ventilation. It was suggested that the decrease in dyspnea and decrease in the central drive to breathe were related to improvement in respiratory muscle function. After removal of fluid, it was presumed that the size of the thorax decreased with concomitant stretching of the inspiratory muscles, thus allowing them to function on a more advantageous portion of their length-tension curve (Estenne, 1983). With such enhancement of respiratory muscle contractibility less neural input was needed for a given muscle tension. The decrease in respiratory center output or central motor command may reach conscious awareness as less dyspnea through a decreased sense of effort.

The sense of effort alluded to in the previous sections discussing respiratory muscle fatigue and weakness will be further elucidated in terms of its relationship to dyspnea in the section that follows.

Increased Sense of Effort

When breathing is hindered by the addition of obstructive or restrictive loads, the perceived magnitude of the load is directly related to the peak inspiratory pressure, the duration of inspiration, and the frequency of breathing (Killian, 1982, 1985b). The sensory magnitude is related to the magnitude of the muscular response and is only indirectly related to the magnitude of the load. However, the neurophysiology of the sensory mechanism which permits perception of the size of a load is unclear. The close relationship with inspiratory pressure suggests that the sense of achieved muscular tension (mediated by muscle mechanoreceptors) or the sense of effort (mediated in part by an awareness of the efferent, motor command) are the most likely mechanisms. It has been demonstrated that the perceived magnitude of an added load or a static inspiratory pressure is not increased by shortening the operating length of the respiratory muscle (Altose, 1982; Stubbing, 1983).

A study was done to determine whether the sensation of tension and effort were affected differently by changing lung volume and associated length of the inspiratory muscles and if so, with which sensation the sensation of breathlessness was more closely associated (Killian, 1984). The technique of increasing lung volume to shorten and weaken the inspiratory muscles was used. This was meant to be a model for patients with obstructive lung disease and hyperinflation. Five normal subjects were asked to scale the magnitude of sensory experiences while breathing on an apparatus which allowed the investigators to apply varying elastic loads. They were told that while breathing with the added load they might require an increased effort to breathe and that the force or tension required by the inspiratory muscles would also increase. These loads would make it more difficult to breathe and possibly make them experience breathlessness and discomfort while breathing. The magnitude of the specific sensations while breathing on an added load was estimated using a category scale in which numbers from 0 to 10 are anchored to descriptions of increasing magnitudes of sensation, for example, nothing at all, to weak, to very, very strong (Borg, 1982). During each study period, the initial load and lung volume was randomized, as were all subsequent loads. The volume, duration, and frequency of breathing were held constant. Lung volumes were controlled by having the subjects in the recumbent position completely enclosed in a modified Drinker respirator. Only one sensation (breathlessness, effort, or tension) was studied during a single session. In another part of the study, targeted inspiratory pressures were the stimuli. The magnitude of the pressure and lung volumes were randomized. In the latter part of the study, the open-scale magnitude estimation and sensory matching (magnitude production) techniques were used to assess sense of effort.

The magnitude of breathlessness and perceived effort as estimated by the subjects using the category scale increased significantly with the inspiratory airway pressure and the lung volume. The magnitude of perceived tension as estimated by the subject using the category scale increased significantly with the inspiratory airway pressure, but was unaffected by the increase in lung volume. At baseline lung volumes, there was no significant difference between target pressures and the pressures reproduced to match the same effort. To reproduce the same effort at baseline lung volume to match the target pressures generated at increased lung volumes, the subjects produced significantly greater pressures.

The magnitude of perceived breathlessness, effort, and tension increase as the tension developed by the inspiratory muscle increases; whereas breathlessness and effort increase proportionately more when the inspiratory muscle is weakened by shortening the resting length. These results suggest that breathlessness and effort are closely related and may be mediated by the same pathway. Breathlessness occurs when ventilation is increased, when the impedance to the action of the inspiratory muscle is increased, and when the respiratory muscle is weakened. In all these situations, the sense of effort may intensify along with the drive to breathe. In patients with chronic obstructive lung disease in acute exacerbation and respiratory failure, the central drive to breathe is increased (Aubier, 1980), and in patients with muscle weakness due to myotonic dystrophy the central drive is also increased (Begin, 1982). In subjects with respiratory muscle fatigue the sense of effort is also increased (Gandevia, 1981).

Psychopathology

It is frequently noted that people experiencing intense emotion, especially anxiety, may become dyspneic. It is true that in individual cases of asthma acute bronchospasm may be triggered by emotional distress and dyspnea ensues. Some behaviors that may result in bronchospasm in asthmatics are crying, laughing, yelling, hyperventilating, coughing, or choking. These actions may stimulate afferent receptors in the airways, resulting in bronchospasm and therefore dyspnea, by a reflex mechanism. Anger, anxiety, and frustration are emotions that have been observed to occur during asthma attacks. Similar observations have been made for the changes in respiration that occur with intense emotion in patients with other pulmonary diseases as well as in normal subjects (Dudley, 1968). However, patients with asthma and those with exacerbations or complications of underlying lung disease have acute episodic attacks of dyspnea, and findings from studies of these patients cannot be generalized to patients with chronic unremitting dyspnea at rest or at a moderate level of physical exertion.

In the introduction to this chapter it was emphasized that dyspnea is subjective and involves both perception of the sensation by the patient and his or her reaction to the sensation (Comroe, 1966). Unlike many measures related to metabolism, there is a wide variation between persons, and between occasions in the same individual, with regard to a response to a threatening situation. The nature and degree of the response, both psychic and physical, is dependent upon personality traits, and is influenced by previous experience, even remote in time. Exactly how higher cerebral function or psychologic substrate impacts on the sensation of dyspnea is not clear.

A syndrome of disproportionately severe breathlessness has been described in chronic bronchitis (Burns, 1969). Two groups, each of 31 subjects, were studied. Members of the patient group were selected because they were much more breathless than would be expected from their lung disease. The $FEV_{1.0}$ in each case was better than one liter. The control group was considered to have proportionate breathlessness and the $FEV_{1.0}$ in each case was less than one liter. Comparisons of the two groups in terms of medical and psychiatric history and state were made by physicians and psychiatrists. The patient group differed from the control group in that the symptom of breathlessness had a shorter duration, the mean age of the group was younger, and the patients were more socially isolated. The patient group was also subject to more recent stress including bereavement, had more previous psychiatric illnesses, and had more current psychiatric symptoms. All of the patients were found to be psychiatrically ill, whereas few of the control group had formal psychiatric illnesses. Breathlessness in the patient group was characterized by a cluster of symptoms including difficulty in inspiration rather than expiration, poor relationship of dyspnea to exercise, aggravation by social stress, and relief by alcohol and tranquilizers. The patient group underwent psychiatric treatment, and in 26 of these cases, this included benzodiazepines. The other five cases received other psychotropic drugs. The authors reported that in all cases who improved psychiatrically, a marked alleviation of dyspnea occurred.

Such factors as mood and general psychiatric disorder along with beliefs and attitudes concerning their illness has been examined with regard to exercise performance in patients with chronic bronchitis (Morgan, 1983). The 12-minute walk test was used as a measure of functional impairment. In this test, patients were asked to walk as fast as they could for 12 minutes, resting only if dyspnea limited their ability to proceed. Routine measures of pulmonary function were made. Psychological assessments were of several types. Mood disturbance was assessed with a multiple affect adjective checklist which used words to describe their feelings of anxiety, depression, or hostility. General psychiatric disorder was assessed with a general health questionnaire. Attitudes and beliefs were measured by means of a semantic differential using concept and adjective scales. A significant correlation was found between ventilatory capacity and the 12-minute walking distance. A score greater than 4 out of 30 on the general health questionnaire was taken to indicate the presence of a general psychiatric disorder. Thirty-nine of the 50 patients studied had scores greater than this. Despite this evidence of psychiatric morbidity, the individual scores did not correlate significantly with the distance walked. In contrast, scores for disturbances of mood assessed with the multiple-affect adjective checklist in 49 patients had significant negative correlations with anxiety, hostility, and depression. When beliefs and attitudes were analyzed many beliefs held by the patients, particularly fear of exercise and negative attitudes towards treatment, correlated negatively with walking distance. Positive attitudes correlated positively with exercise tolerance. Subjective perception of exertion was the factor that accounted for the largest proportion of the variance in distance walked. Relatively speaking, ventilatory capacity was a poor predictor of exercise tolerance in chronic bronchitis patients. The impairment of everyday physical performance was more closely related to mood, especially depression, than to the nonspecific disturbances estimated by the general health questionnaire. Attitudes and beliefs in turn appeared to be of even greater importance than disturbances of mood or measurements of ventilatory capacity in predicting exercise tolerance.

Interestingly, another study (Light, 1985) could find no significant relationships between the 12-minute walking test and depression or anxiety scores in patients with chronic obstructive pulmonary disease. Differences between studies might be explained on the basis of different patient populations or different psychological instruments used to assess the various parameters.

Individual Differences

In view of the common clinical and experimental evidence that the severity of breathlessness reported by patients often correlates poorly with the degree of functional impairment that can be measured, some investigators (Adams, 1986) speculated that there might be consistent differences between individuals in the degree to which they quantify the sensation of breathlessness before they become ill.

Breathlessness was induced in normal subjects by hypercapnic or hypoxic stimulation or by progressive exercise. Subjective assessment of breathlessness was done using a visual analog scale and a magnitude estimation technique. Subjects consistently stated that they were able to discriminate breathlessness from other sensations, such as fatigue or awareness of increased breathing, and in general were confident that they could scale this sensation adequately with the techniques provided. During progressive ventilatory stimulation there were marked individual differences in the level of ventilation threshold at which breathlessness was first noted for each of the three stimulus types, and these differences were consistent on repeat testing. Visual analogue scores showed wide individual variability for a standard level of ventilation.

With the chemical stimulation, those reporting initial breathlessness at a high minute ventilation were generally less breathless at the higher standard ventilation. Inspection of the distribution of subjects' sex, height, $FEV_{1.0}$, or forced vital capacity, in terms of their relative order of threshold minute ventilation and visual analog scales, suggested that these were not important factors for any stimulus type. To test the hypothesis that the observed variability in subjective breathlessness would be related to differences in ventilatory sensitivity to hypercapnea or hypoxia, linear correlation coefficients were computed between the indices of objective and subjective measures. These correlations did not reach statistical significance.

There was no consistent evidence that the pattern of breathing adopted during stimulation was a major factor in determining the intensity of breathlessness. There was a weak association between the differing intensities of breathlessness and one objective index of physical fitness during exercise. This was compatible with the common observation that sedentary individuals experience more breathlessness when undergoing physical exertion than those who are accustomed to regular activity. This association was maintained when ventilation was increased by the chemical stimuli. This might suggest several mechanisms by which physical conditioning could modulate the perception of breathlessness. It could alter the nature of afferent information arising from the respiratory apparatus for a given level of activity, or it could cause changes in the way such information is processed centrally, or it could be associated with decreased central drive to a more efficient respiratory system.

It is interesting that similar individual variability has been reported in the ratio scaling of another sensory modality for which associated neurophysiological information was available. Magnitude estimation exponents were obtained from carefully controlled indentations of slowly adopting mechanoreceptors in the palms of the hands of normal subjects. Simultaneously was recorded the different activity in neurons supplying these receptors (Knibestol, 1980). Relatively little between-subject variability was noted for the relationship between applied pressure and resultant afferent neural impulse frequency, but marked and reproducible individual differences in the sensory perception of this stimulus, which did not correlate with the small differences in the nature of the afferent information, were demonstrated. The interpretation of these data is that differences in the perception of sensory stimuli could result from characteristic individual differences in the central processing of afferent information.

SUMMARY

In this chapter, the possible sources of stimuli that may induce dyspnea in patients with respiratory diseases have been reviewed (Table 15.1). Various studies of conditions related to the sensation of breathlessness (Table 15.3) have suggested that the genesis of the sensation may be within a complex interaction of afferent signals from the lungs themselves, but especially from the respiratory muscles and the central processing of these signals with a resultant conscious awareness of the motor command to breathe. This further is associated with the sense of effort which is modulated by some personality characteristics of the individual patients experiencing the symptom.

REFERENCES

Adams, L., Lane, R., Shea, S. A., Cockroft, A., & Guz, A. (1985). Breathlessness during different forms of ventilatory stimulation: A study of mechanisms in normal subjects and respiratory patients. *Clinical Science, 69,* 663–672.

Adams, L., Chronos, N., Lane, R., & Guz, A. (1986). The measurement of breathlessness induced in normal subjects: Individual differences. *Clinical Science, 70,* 131–140.

Agostoni, E. (1963). Diaphragm activity during breath-holding: Factors related to its onset. *Journal of Applied Physiology, 18,* 30–36.

Agostoni, E., & Sant'Ambrogio, G. (1970). The diaphragm. In E. J. M. Campbell, E. Agostoni, & J. Newson-Davis (Eds.), *The respiratory muscles* (pp. 145–160). Philadelphia: W. B. Saunders.

Altose, M. D., DiMarco, A. F., & Strohl, K. P. (1982). The sensation of respiratory muscle force. *American Review of Respiratory Disease, 126,* 807–816.

Altose, M. D., Cherniack, N., & Fishman, A. P. (1985). Respiratory sensations and dyspnea. *Journal of Applied Physiology, 58,* 1051–1054.

Aubier, N. D., Murciano, D., Milic-Emili, J., Pariente, R., & Derenne, P. H. (1980). Central respiratory drive in acute respiratory failure in patients with COPD. *American Review of Respiratory Disease, 122,* 191–199.

Begin, R., Bureau, M. A., Lupieu, L., Bernier, J. P., & Lemieux, B. (1982). Pathogenesis of respiratory insufficiency in myotonic dystrophy. *American Review of Respiratory Disease, 125,* 312–318.

Bennett, E. D., Jayson, M. I. V., Rubinstein, D., & Campbell, E. J. M. (1962). The ability of man to detect added non-elastic loads to breathing. *Clinical Science, 23,* 155–162.

Borg, G. A. V. (1982). Psychophysical basis of perceived exertion. *Medicine and Science in Sports and Exercise, 14,* 377–381.

Burki, N., Mitchell, L. K., Chaudhary, B. A., & Zechman, F. W. (1978). The ability of asthmatics to detect added resistive loads. *American Review of Respiratory Disease, 117,* 71–75.

Burki, N. (1979). Breathlessness and mouth occlusion pressure in patients with chronic obstruction of the airways. *Chest, 76,* 527–531.

Burns, B. H., & Howell, J. B. L. (1969). Disproportionately severe breathlessness in chronic bronchitis. *Quarterly Journal of Medicine, 23,* 277–294.

Campbell, E. J. M., Freedman, S., Smith, P. S., & Taylor, M. E. (1961). The ability of man to detect elastic loads to breathing. *Clinical Science, 20,* 223–231.

Campbell, E. J. M., & Howell, J. B. L. (1963). The sensation of dyspnea. *British Medical Journal, 2,* 868.

Campbell, E. J. M., Godfrey, S., Clark, T. J. M., Freedman, S., & Norman, J. (1969). The effect of muscular paralysis induced by tubocurare on the duration and sensation of breath-holding during hypercapnia. *Clinical Science, 36,* 323–328.

Campbell, E. J. M., Gandevia, S. C., Killian, K. J., Mahutte, C. K., & Riggs, J. R. A. (1980). Changes in the perception of inspiratory resistive loads during partial curarization. *Journal of Physiology (London), 309,* 93–100.

Chaudhary, B. A., & Burki, N. (1978). Effects of airway anesthesia on the ability to detect added inspiratory resistive loads. *Clinical Science and Molecular Medicine, 54,* 621–626.

Cherniack, R. M. (1959). The oxygen consumption and efficiency of the respiratory muscles in health and emphysema. *Journal of Clinical Investigations, 38,* 494–499.

Cohen, E. N. (1959). Blood brain barrier to d-tubocurarine. *Journal of Pharmacology and Experimental Therapy, 141,* 356–362.

Comroe, J. (1966). Some theories of the mechanism of dyspnoea. *Breathlessness,* In J. B. L. Howell & E. J. M. Campbell (Eds.), *Breathlessness* (pp. 1–7). Philadelphia: F. A. Davis.

Cournand, A., Richards, D. W., & Bader, R. A. (1954). The oxygen cost of breathing. *Transactions of the Association of American Physicians, 67,* 162–173.

Cross, B. A., Guz, A., Jain, J. K., Archer, S., Stevens, J., & Reynolds, F. (1976). The effect of anesthesia of the airway in dog and man: A study of respiratory reflexes, sensations and lung mechanic. *Clinical Science and Molecular Medicine, 50,* 439–454.

Derenne, J. P., Macklem, P. T., & Roussos, C. (1978). The respiratory muscles: mechanics, control and pathophysiology. Part III. *American Review of Respiratory Disease, 118,* 581–601.

Dudley, D. L., Martin, C. J., & Holmes, T. H. (1968). Dyspnea: psychologic and physiologic observations. *Journal of Psychosomatic Research, 11,* 325–339.

Eisele, J., Trenchard, D., Burki, N., & Guz, A. (1968). The effect of chest wall block on respiratory sensation and control in man. *Clinical Science, 35,* 23–33.

Eldridge, F. L. (1975). Relationship between respiratory nerve and muscle activity and muscle force output. *Journal of Applied Physiology, 39,* 567–574.

Epler, G. R., & Sabec, F. A., & Gaensler, E. A. (1980). Determination of severe disability in interstitial lung disease. *American Review of Respiratory Disease, 121,* 647–659.

Estenne, M., Yernault, J. C., & Detroyer, A. (1983). Mechanism of relief of dyspnea after thoracentesis in patients with large pleural effusions. *American Journal of Medicine, 74,* 819–831.

Fowler, W. S. (1954). Breaking point of breath-holding. *Journal of Applied Physiology, 6,* 539–545.

Gandevia, S. C., Killian, K. J., & Campbell, E. J. M. (1981). The effect of respiratory muscle fatigue on respiratory sensations. *Clinical Science, 60,* 463–466.

Guz, A., Noble, M. I. M., Widdicombe, J. G., Trenchard, D., Mucshin, W. W., & Mackey, A. R. (1966a). The role of vagal and glosso-pharyngeal afferent nerves in respiratory sensation, control of breathing and arterial pressure regulation in conscious man. *Clinical Science, 30,* 161–171.

Guz, A., Noble, M. I. M., Widdicombe, J. G., Trenchard, D., & Mucshin, W. W. (1966b). The effect of bilateral block of vagus and glossopharyngeal nerves on the ventilatory response to carbon dioxide in conscious man. *Respiration Physiology, 1,* 206–210.

Guz, A., Noble, M. I. M., & Eisele, J. H. (1970). Experimental results of vagal block in cardiopulmonary disease. In R. Porter, (Ed.), *Breathing: Hering-Breur Centenary Symposium* (pp. 315–329). London: Churchill.

Holle, R. H. O., Schoene, R. B., & Pavlin, E. J. (1984). Effect of respiratory muscle weakness on $P_{0.1}$ induced by partial curarization. *Journal of Applied Physiology, 57,* 1150–1157.

Killian, K. J., Bucens, D. D., & Campbell, E. J. M. (1982). Effect of breathing patterns on the perceived magnitude of added loads to breathing. *Journal of Applied Physiology, 52,* 578–584.

Killian, K. J., Gandevia, S. C., Summers, E., & Campbell, E. J. M. (1984). Effect of increased lung volume on perception of breathlessness, effort, and tension. *Journal of Applied Physiology, 57,* 686–691.

Killian, K. J., & Campbell, E. J. M. (1985a). Dyspnea. In C. Roussas & P. T. Macklem (Ed.) *The Thorax* (pp. 787–828). New York: Marcel Dekker.

Killian, K. J., Summers, E., Basalygo, M., & Campbell, E. J. M. (1985b). Effect of frequency on perceived magnitude of added loads to breathing. *Journal of Applied Physiology, 58,* 1616–1621.

Klassen, K. P., Morton, D. R., & Curtis, G. M. (1951). The effect of vagus section on the cough reflex, bronchial caliber and clearance of bronchial secretions. *Surgery, 29,* 483–490.

Knibestol, M., & Vallbo, A. B. (1980). Intensity of sensation related to activity of slowly adapting mechanoreceptor units in the human hand. *Journal of Physiology (London), 300,* 251–267.

Lederer, D. M., Altose, M. D., Kelsen, S. G., & Cherniack, N. S. (1977). Comparison of occlusion pressure and ventilatory responses. *Thorax, 32,* 212–220.

Light, R. W., Merrill, E. J., Despars, J. A., Gordon, G. H., & Mutilpassi, L. R. (1985). Prevalence of depression and anxiety in patients with COPD. *Chest, 87,* 35–38.

Marshall, R., Stone, R. W., & Christie, R. V. (1954). The relationship of dyspnea to respiratory effort in normal subjects, mitral stenosis and emphysema. *Clinical Science, 13,* 625–631.

Matthews, P. B. C. (1982). Where does Sherrington's 'muscular sense' originate? Muscles, joints, corollary discharges? *Annual Review of Neuroscience, 5,* 189–218.

McCloskey, D. I., Ebeling, P., & Goodwin, G. M. (1974). Estimation of weights and tensions and apparent involvement of a 'sense of effort'. *Experimental Neurology, 42,* 220–232.

McFadden, E. R., Kiser, R., & Degroot, W. J. (1973). Acute bronchial asthma: relations between clinical and physiologic manifestations. *New England Journal of Medicine, 288,* 221–225.

Mithoefer, J. C. (1959). Lung volume restrictions as a ventilatory stimulus during breath-holding. *Journal of Applied Physiology, 14,* 701–705.

Morgan, A. D., Peck, D. F., Buchanan, D. R., & McHardy, G. J. R. (1983). Effects of attitudes and beliefs on exercise tolerance in chronic bronchitis. *British Medical Journal, 286,* 171–173.

Morgan, W. K. C. (1979). Clinical significance of pulmonary function tests: disability or disinclination? *Chest, 75,* 712–715.

Morgan, W. K. C. (1982). Pulmonary disability and impairment. *Basics of Respiratory Disease, 10,* 1–6.

Morton, D. R., Klassen, K. P., & Curtis, G. M. (1951). The clinical physiology of the human bronchi II. The effect of vagus section upon pain of tracheobronchial origin. *Surgery, 30,* 800–809.

Noble, M. I. M., Eisele, J. H., Trenchard, D., & Guz, A. (1970). Effect of selective nerve blocks on respiratory sensation. In R. Porter (Ed.), *Breathing: Hering-Breur Centenary Symposium* (pp. 233–251). London: Churchill.

Noble, M. I. M., Eisele, J. H., Frankel, H. L., Else, W., & Guz, A. (1971). The role of the diaphragm in the sensation of holding the breath. *Clinical Science, 41,* 275–283.

Noble, M. I. M., Frankel, H. L., Else, W., & Guz, A. (1972). The sensation produced by threshold resistive loads to breathing. *European Journal of Clinical Investigation, 2,* 72–77.

Ogilvie, C. (1983). Dyspnoea. *British Medical Journal, 237,* 160–161.

Otis, A. B., Rahn, H., & Fenn, W. O. (1948). Alveolar gas changes during breath-holding. *American Journal of Physiology, 152,* 454–686.

Paintal, A. S. (1977). Thoracic receptors connected with sensation. *British Medical Bulletin, 33,* 169–174.

Patterson, J. L., Mullinax, P. F., Bain, T., Kreuger, J. J., & Richardson, D. W. (1962). Carbon dioxide-induced dyspnea in a patient with respiratory muscle paralysis. *American Journal of Medicine, 32,* 811–816.

Plum, F. & Leigh, R. J. (1981). Abnormalities of central mechanisms. In T. F. Hornbein (Ed.), *Regulation of Breathing, Part II.* New York: Marcel Dekker.

Roland, P. E., & Ladegaard-Pedersen, H. (1977). A quantitative analysis of sensations of tension and of kinesthesia in man. Evidence for a peripherally originating muscular sense and for a sense of effort. *Brain, 100,* 671–692.

Rosser, R., & Guz, A. (1981). Psychological approaches to breathlessness and its treatment. *Journal of Psychosomatic Research, 25,* 439–447.

Sharp, J. T. (1983). The respiratory muscles in emphysema. *Clinics in Chest Medicine, 4,* 421–432.

Smith, S. M., & Reese, R. E. (1951). The lack of cerebral effects of d-turbocurarine. *Anesthesiology, 8,* 1–13.

Smolley, L., Scheinman, S., Porcher, A., & Wanner, A. (1986a). Effects of inspiratory muscle training on dyspnea, central drive to breathe and length-tension inappropriateness in COPD. *American Review of Respiratory Disease, 133,* A102.

Smolley, L., Scheinman, S., Porcher, A., & Wanner, A. (1986b). Effects of thoracentesis on dyspnea, central drive to breathe and respiratory muscle strength in patients with large pleural effusions. *American Review of Respiratory Disease, 133,* A190.

Stark, R. D., O'Neill, P. A., Russell, N. J. W., Heapy, C. G., & Stretton, T. B., (1985). Effects of small-particle aerosols of local anesthetic on dyspnea in patients with respiratory disease. *Clinical Science, 69,* 29–36.

Stevens, S. S. (1957). On the psychophysical law. *Psychological Reviews, 64,* 153–181.

Stubbing, D. G., Ramsdale, E. H., Killian, K. J., & Campbell, E. J. M. (1983). Psychophysics of inspiratory muscle force. *Journal of Applied Physiology, 54,* 1216–1221.

West, D. V. M., Ellis, C. G., & Campbell, E. J. M. (1975). Ability of man to detect increases in his breathing. *Journal of Applied Physiology, 39,* 372–376.

Whitelaw, W. A., Derenne, J. P. H., & Milic-Emili, J. (1975). Occlusion pressure as a measure of respiratory center output in conscious man. *Respiration Physiology, 23,* 181–199.

Wiley, R. L., & Zechman, F. W. (1966). Perception of added airflow resistance in humans. *Respiration Physiology, 2,* 73–87.

Author Index

D

H

Y

Z

Subject Index

www.ingramcontent.com/pod-product-compliance
Ingram Content Group UK Ltd.
Pitfield, Milton Keynes, MK11 3LW, UK
UKHW021911150926
475560UK00003B/320